Drug  les for

D0379814

Cytochrome P450s
UGTs
P-Glycoproteins

Second Edition

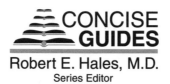

CONCISE
GUIDES

Robert E. Hales, M.D.
Series Editor

CONCISE GUIDE TO

Drug Interaction Principles for Medical Practice

Cytochrome P450s
UGTs
P-Glycoproteins

Second Edition

Kelly L. Cozza, M.D.

Scott C. Armstrong, M.D.

Jessica R. Oesterheld, M.D.

with chapter contributions by
David M. Benedek, M.D., Michael A. Cole, M.D.,
Elisabeth A. Pimentel, B.S., and Gary H. Wynn, M.D.

with section contribution by
Benjamin Smith, B.S.

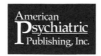

Washington, DC
London, England

Copyright © 2003 American Psychiatric Publishing, Inc.
ALL RIGHTS RESERVED

Manufactured in the United States of America on acid-free paper
07   06   05   04   03   5   4   3   2   1
Second Edition

Typeset in Adobe's Times and Helvetica

American Psychiatric Publishing, Inc.
1000 Wilson Boulevard
Arlington, VA 22209-3901
www.appi.org

Library of Congress Cataloging-in-Publication Data
Cozza, Kelly L.
    Concise guide to drug interaction principles for medical practice: cytochrome P450s, UGTs, P-glycoproteins / Kelly L. Cozza, Scott C. Armstrong, Jessica R. Oesterheld ; with chapter contributions by David M. Benedek, Michael A. Cole, Elisabeth A. Pimentel, Gary H. Wynn; with section contribution by Benjamin Smith.—2nd ed.
        p. ; cm. – (Concise guides)
    Previous edition published with title: Concise guide to the cytochrome P450 system.
    Includes bibliographical references and index.
    ISBN 1-58562-111-0 (alk. paper)
    1. Cytochrome P-450—Handbooks, manuals, etc. 2. Drugs—Metabolism—Handbooks, manuals, etc. 3. Psychopharmacology—Handbooks, manuals, etc. 4. Drug interactions—Handbooks, manuals, etc. I. Title: Cytochrome P450s, UGTs, P-glycoproteins. II. Armstrong, Scott C. III. Oesterheld, Jessica R. IV. Cozza, Kelly L. V. Title. VI. Concise guides (American Psychiatric Publishing)
    [DNLM: 1. Psychotropic Drugs—pharmacokinetics—Handbooks. 2. Cytochrome P-450 Enzyme System—metabolism—Handbooks. 3. Drug Interactions—Handbooks.]
QV 39 C882c 2003]
QP671.C83 C69 2003
615'.788—dc21

2002043890

British Library Cataloguing in Publication Data
A CIP record is available from the British Library.

Thanks again to my husband, Steve,
and my children, Vincent and Cecilia,
for their love and understanding during the preparation of this book.
A special thanks to all my mentors and patients at or affiliated with
Walter Reed Army Medical Center.
—*KLC*

Thanks to my wife, JoAnn, who was patient and understanding
of my time away while I researched and wrote this book;
to my three children, Joey, Katie, and Caleb;
and to my parents, Richard and Patricia.
—*SCA*

Thanks to my husband, Mark, who is always a trooper;
my children, Jennifer, Michael, Robert, Ben, and Amanda;
and my daughters-in-law, Jennifer and Kristen,
for their loving support.
—*JRO*

*We dedicate this book to our patients and to all clinicians
who may use this book in caring for them.
They are the reason we are doing this work.*

CONTENTS

PART I
Introduction and Basic Pharmacology of
Metabolic Drug Interactions

PART III
Drug Interactions by Medical Specialty

PART IV
Practical Matters

LIST OF TABLES

LIST OF FIGURES

CONTRIBUTORS

Scott C. Armstrong, M.D.
Co-Medical Director, Center for Geriatric Psychiatry, Tuality Forest
Grove Hospital, Forest Grove, Oregon; Clinical Associate Profes-
sor of Psychiatry, Oregon Health and Science University, Portland;
Fellow, American Psychiatric Association; Fellow, Academy of Psy-
chosomatic Medicine

David M. Benedek, M.D.
Chief, Forensic Psychiatry Service, Walter Reed Army Medical
Center, Washington, D.C.; Associate Professor of Psychiatry, Uni-
formed Services University of the Health Sciences, F. Edward
Hebert School of Medicine, Bethesda, Maryland

Michael A. Cole, M.D.
Staff Psychiatrist and Internist, Madigan Army Medical Center,
Tacoma, Washington

Kelly L. Cozza, M.D.
Psychiatrist, Infectious Disease Service, Department of Medicine,
Walter Reed Army Medical Center, Washington, D.C.; Assistant
Professor, Department of Psychiatry, Uniformed Services Univer-
sity of the Health Sciences, Bethesda, Maryland; Fellow, Academy
of Psychosomatic Medicine

Jessica R. Oesterheld, M.D.
Medical Director, The Spurwink School, Portland, Maine; Instructor in Family Medicine, University of New England School of Osteopathy, Biddle, Maine

Elisabeth A. Pimentel, B.S.
Medical student, Uniformed Services University of the Health Sciences, Bethesda, Maryland

Benjamin Smith, B.S.
Medical student, Uniformed Services University of the Health Sciences, Bethesda, Maryland

Gary H. Wynn, M.D.
Staff, Departments of Psychiatry and Medicine, Walter Reed Army Medical Center, Washington, D.C.; Clinical Instructor, Uniformed Services University of the Health Sciences, Bethesda, Maryland

INTRODUCTION

to the Concise Guides Series

The Concise Guides Series from American Psychiatric Publishing, Inc., provides, in an accessible format, practical information for psychiatrists, psychiatry residents, and medical students working in a variety of treatment settings, such as inpatient psychiatry units, outpatient clinics, consultation-liaison services, and private office settings. The Concise Guides are meant to complement the more detailed information to be found in lengthier psychiatry texts.

The Concise Guides address topics of special concern to psychiatrists in clinical practice. The books in this series contain a detailed table of contents, along with an index, tables, figures, and other charts for easy access. The books are designed to fit into a lab coat pocket or jacket pocket, which makes them a convenient source of information. References have been limited to those most relevant to the material presented.

Robert E. Hales, M.D., M.B.A.
Series Editor, Concise Guides

PREFACE TO THE SECOND EDITION

We are delighted to present a broader view of pharmacokinetic drug interactions, while maintaining a Concise Guide format. We have expanded the sections on metabolism (both phase I and phase II), updated all chapters and tables, and added illustrations. Web site addresses are found throughout the book. New in this edition are chapters on P-glycoproteins, minor P450 enzymes, narcotic and nonnarcotic analgesics, and legal matters.

To produce a well-balanced update, we invited more of our colleagues to participate. Dr. Oesterheld brought an enormous amount of enthusiasm and knowledge about her topics in this book, and her editing of the entire volume has been a fantastic new addition. She has made the complicated world of phase II metabolism and the emerging world of P-glycoproteins understandable and relevant. Dr. Benedek brought the need to know drug interactions into legal focus. Our young authors, Drs. Cole and Wynn, along with medical students Pimentel and Smith, continually reminded us why we work on this topic. Their energy and astute questioning kept us focused and forward-looking.

As in the first edition, references in each chapter support both the text and the tables. Most references are cited in the text; those not cited are included because they support data in the tables. The work contained in this guide was not funded or supported in any way by pharmaceutical companies or distributors.

We hope that this expanded coverage of pharmacokinetic drug interactions allows the reader to quickly and confidently predict, prevent, and use to the patient's advantage potential and actual drug interactions.

PREFACE TO THE FIRST EDITION

The development of this Concise Guide began as a necessity. As consecutive program directors for a busy military, tertiary-care, hospital-based consultation-liaison psychiatry service and fellowship program, we found ourselves being called on to evaluate drug interactions, as well as to teach about them to our students and colleagues. When we began to put this topic together, it was only to gain a better understanding of drug-drug interactions ourselves. It was frustrating to read articles and case reports that did not include full explanations of the topic. Some of the literature was contradictory, and the names of the enzymes seemed to change before our eyes. What began as a few tables, carried around in our pockets, became a formal lecture series. These P450 workshops grew from bedside and local grand rounds to pharmacy and therapeutics committee round tables.

Eventually, the topic followed us when we left the military. In time, we came to believe that our knowledge of the topic had evolved into something more than that of the average clinician. Our handout had grown from 8 pages to more than 50 pages by 1998. We find that software packages are typically designed for the pharmacist and do not have the depth necessary for a clinical psychiatrist to make quick yet well-informed decisions. We realized that a book was needed. However, there is one potential major limitation to a book: it may be somewhat outdated by the time of publication. The reader is cautioned that new drugs will have been introduced and older drugs will have new interactions described after the publication of this guide. During the preparation of this book, cisapride, mibefradil, and grepafloxacin were voluntarily removed from the United States market because of their P450-mediated interactions. This guide has been designed to enable psychiatrists to develop individualized tables and references for their own practices.

Because of length restrictions in the Concise Guides, references in each chapter of this book support both the text and the tables. Most references are cited within the text; those that are not cited are included because they support data in the tables.

The aforementioned limitations aside, we hope that readers will use this guide to quickly determine and even to anticipate drug interactions. It is designed to be used in the clinic and at the bedside as a tool for making rational and informed decisions when prescribing. We believe that this guide will provide clinicians with the information they need to prescribe appropriately in this age of polypharmacy.

Part I

**Introduction and Basic Pharmacology of
Metabolic Drug Interactions**

INTRODUCTION TO DRUG INTERACTIONS AND TO THIS CONCISE GUIDE

An understanding of drug interactions has become essential to the practice of medicine. The increasing pharmacopoeia, coupled with prolonged human life spans, makes polypharmacy commonplace. The better-studied metabolism phase, phase I, includes the P450 system (in this guide, we use the term *P450* rather than *cytochrome P450* or *CYP450*). The need for a thorough understanding of the P450 system became apparent in the 1980s, when the combination of terfenadine and antibiotics or of selective serotonin reuptake inhibitors and tricyclic antidepressants resulted in arrhythmias and sudden death. In recent years, research on glucuronidation and other phase II reactions and on efflux transporters such as P-glycoproteins has increased the understanding of drug-drug interactions. Despite burgeoning data and clear manufacturer warnings, patients are still at risk for these interactions.

■ WHY IS IT IMPORTANT TO UNDERSTAND PHARMACOKINETIC DRUG INTERACTIONS?

The following recent case demonstrates the importance of understanding drug-drug interactions:

> A 64-year-old woman with chronic schizophrenia required acute admission to a geriatric psychiatry unit from a group home setting

because of an iatrogenic drug interaction. The patient had responded well for several years to clozapine 125 mg twice a day. Two months before acute admission, clozapine therapy was stopped because she appeared to be having a toxic reaction; a clozapine level (1,043 ng/mL; usual range, 350–475 ng/mL) confirmed the clinical presentation. Her primary psychiatrist then initiated ziprasidone therapy, thinking the patient could not tolerate or metabolize clozapine because of her age. The patient's psychosis worsened, necessitating the acute hospitalization on the geriatric psychiatry unit. The inpatient psychiatrist (S.C.A.) asked for the list of medications that the patient had been taking at the time of the toxicity. It was discovered that the patient had been taking ciprofloxacin for a mild urinary tract infection. The inpatient psychiatrist determined that the ciprofloxacin increased the serum level of clozapine through inhibition of the P450 enzymes 1A2 and 3A4. This information permitted titration to the patient's original, therapeutic clozapine dose. She was discharged back to her group home. Subsequent outpatient clozapine levels ranged from 500 to 600 ng/mL.

If the patient's initial care providers had known about the ciprofloxacin-clozapine interaction, a different antibiotic could have been chosen or the clozapine dose could have been reduced or temporarily withheld, allowing the patient to maintain her usual level of functioning. Knowledge of this drug interaction would have led to better patient care and reduced health care costs.

Drug interactions have become an important preventable iatrogenic complication. In the United States, as many as 3% of hospitalizations per year are due to drug-drug interactions (Jankel and Fitterman 1993). The amount spent on these hospitalizations exceeds $1 billion (Johnson and Bootman 1995). In one large study involving Medicaid patients (n=315,084), the risk of hospitalization greatly increased when patients were prescribed azole antifungals (odds ratio, 3.43) or rifamycins (odds ratio, 8.07), two drug classes that have significant P450 drug-drug interaction profiles (Hamilton et al. 1998). In addition, a study by the Institute of Medicine in the United States indicates that adverse medication reactions—including drug-drug interactions—account for up to 7,000 deaths annually in the United States (Kohn et al. 2000). Clearly, drug-drug interactions are a problem that clinicians need to appreciate.

These data also seem to be an underrepresentation of the situation. Many interactions are not reported by patients to physicians or by physicians to monitoring agencies. Some bothersome side effects may in fact be effects of drug interactions (e.g., a patient's serum caffeine levels may be affected by newly administered medications, resulting in "jitters"). Adverse drug reactions such as tardive dyskinesia may be more pronounced in patients who are poor metabolizers at some P450 enzymes; some of these poor metabolizers are genetically predisposed, and others are made poor metabolizers via drug interactions. We suspect that most drug-drug interactions are less than lethal and go unrecognized, leading to ineffective or aborted drug therapy and/or increased care costs.

■ WHY DOES THE METABOLIC SYSTEM EXIST?

Metabolic enzymes may have originated from a common ancestral gene or protein in plants and animals billions of years ago. Initially, they may have helped maintain cell membrane integrity through their contribution to steroid metabolism. As animals evolved and ate plants to survive, the plants that developed toxins survived. Animals then needed to be able to detoxify these chemicals, and thus an elaborate detoxification system developed (Jefferson and Greist 1996).

P450 enzymes are oxidase systems (see Figure 1–1). These enzymes oxidize endogenous and exogenous compounds and usually render them less active (see Chapter 2 ["Definitions and Phase I Metabolism"]), preparing them for further transformation by phase II reactions such as glucuronidation or sulfation, and for elimination from the body. The P450 system's primary role is to metabolize endogenous compounds such as steroids and neuropeptides. A secondary role, especially for enzymes in the gastrointestinal or hepatic system, is to detoxify ingested chemicals. These exogenous,

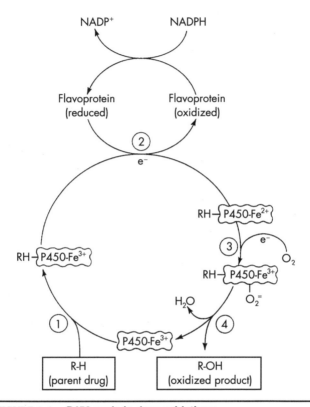

FIGURE 1–1.   **P450 cycle in drug oxidations.**

e^-=electron; $NADP^+$=oxidized form of nicotinamide adenine dinucleotide phosphate; NADPH=reduced form of NADP; R-H=parent drug. R-OH=oxidized metabolite.

Source.   Reprinted from Holford NHG: "Pharmacokinetics and Pharmacodynamics: Rational Dosing and the Time Course of Drug Action," in *Basic and Clinical Pharmacology,* 8th Edition. Edited by Katzung BG. New York, Lange Medical Books/McGraw-Hill, 2001, p. 53. Used with permission.

or xenobiotic, chemicals are compounds in foods, medicines, smoke, and anything else that is an ingested organic molecule. Medications are one group of "toxins" in the modern human environment (others include pesticides and organic solvents), and the role of the P450 system in metabolizing drugs is a relatively recent phenomenon in human history. P450 enzymes are indiscriminate in their activity; they will metabolize an ancient food chemical as readily as they will metabolize a modern drug. P450 enzymes are also multifunctional; each enzyme is capable of metabolizing many different compounds.

More than 40 individual P450 enzymes have been identified in humans. However, many of these enzymes play minor roles in drug metabolism. Six enzymes are responsible for more than 90% of human drug oxidation: 1A2, 3A4, 2C9, 2C19, 2D6, and 2E1 (Guengerich 1997). The enzymes 2A6, 2B6, 2C8, and 3A5 play clinically relevant but smaller roles in human metabolism. Each of these enzymes is discussed in this Concise Guide.

The six major P450 enzymes (and perhaps all human P450 enzymes) exhibit genetic variability via polymorphisms. Phase II enzymes may also exhibit genetic variability or polymorphisms. The clinical implications of this phase II variability are at times unclear and confusing. It is speculated that the variety of and differences in human genotypes are the result of isolated populations' evolving different abilities to survive local stressors—in this case, to metabolize indigenous organic compounds. As ethnic isolation has become replaced by diversity within the modern world, genotypic variability has become less predictable. The evolutionary advantage of genetic variability has disappeared for modern humans. Variability in drug response is now sometimes considered an obstacle rather than an advantage.

Gender may also play a role in the variability of metabolic enzyme systems. It is difficult to establish gender differences, however, because these differences can be obscured by the large interindividual variation in enzyme quantity and efficiency (e.g., 3A efficiency varies 3- to 13.9-fold [de Wildt et al. 1999] in the general population). Furthermore, to uncover metabolic enzyme-based gender distinctions in in vivo studies, one must factor out gender-based differences. It is difficult and costly to control factors related to weight and volume of distribution, ethnicity and polymorphism, smoking and alcohol consumption, obesity, age, cotherapy (including hormone replacement therapy and oral contraceptives), and gender differences in pharmacodynamics.

■ HOW TO USE THIS GUIDE

This Concise Guide is designed to be a practical pocket guide—a reference at the bedside, on rounds, or in the office. This text is divided into several sections.

Part I, "Introduction and Basic Pharmacology of Metabolic Drug Interactions," is a succinct review of pharmacology, written with clinicians in mind. We recommend reading this part first and then returning to particular chapters in the section as needed when consulting later chapters or reviewing other current literature. Phase I and phase II interactions are fully introduced in Part I, as are P-glycoproteins.

Part II, "P450 Enzymes," contains pertinent tables, short reviews, and carefully chosen clinical and research illustrations for individual P450 enzymes. This section will perhaps be frequently consulted once the reader is familiar with the nomenclature and the pertinent literature to date. We and many of our mentors carry lists such as these to refer to when we cannot remember where in the system a particular drug is metabolized or which drug inhibits or induces metabolism at which enzyme site. These chapters conclude with case vignettes, to provide an opportunity for study and to better illustrate P450-mediated drug interactions in clinical practice.

Part III, "Drug Interactions by Medical Specialty," is unique to this text. The drugs commonly used in medicine that have clinically significant pharmacokinetic phase I–, phase II–, or P-glycoprotein-related drug interactions are arranged by specialty (and listed in tables), with pertinent clinical and research data to support and clarify the issues. Some of the data in this section's tables are the same as in Parts I and II, so each part can stand alone.

Part IV, "Practical Matters," includes suggestions about prescribing multiple drugs and monitoring for drug interactions, a discussion of legal issues, and a chapter on how to review the literature. In that chapter, we share the approaches we developed in culling the enormous and sometimes confusing amount of information available in this area. We hope that this section will help clinicians to become more drug-interaction expert in their own fields, as they identify useful references and develop practice-specific drug lists of their own. Web site addresses and pertinent references are also listed in this chapter.

In the pocket guide, we reproduce the P450, UGT, P-glycoprotein, and medical subspecialty tables found throughout this text. A new Quick Guide table completes the pocket guide for even more convenience.

Finally, we remind the reader that drugs interact in many ways. An adverse drug reaction may occur without involvement of the P450 system, glucuronidation, or P-glycoproteins. Nevertheless, hepatic and gut wall P450-mediated interactions are in the majority. We do not review all types of interactions here (absorption, protein-binding, renal excretion and elimination, and pharmacodynamic interactions are excluded), and we refer the reader elsewhere for information on those specific interactions.

■ REFERENCES

de Wildt SN, Kearns GL, Leeder JS, et al: Glucuronidation in humans: pharmacogenetic and developmental aspects. Clin Pharmacokinet 36:439–452, 1999

Guengerich FP: Role of cytochrome P450 enzymes in drug-drug interactions. Adv Pharmacol 43:7–35, 1997

Hamilton RA, Briceland LL, Andritz MH: Frequency of hospitalization after exposure to known drug-drug interactions in a Medicaid population. Pharmacotherapy 18:1112–1120, 1998

Jankel CA, Fitterman LK: Epidemiology of drug-drug interactions as a cause of hospital admissions. Drug Saf 9:51–59, 1993

Jefferson JW, Greist JH: Brussels sprouts and psychopharmacology: understanding the cytochrome P450 enzyme system. The Psychiatric Clinics of North America. Annual of Drug Therapy 3:205–222, 1996

Johnson JA, Bootman JL: Drug-related morbidity and mortality: a cost-of-illness model. Arch Intern Med 155:1949–1956, 1995

Kohn L, Corrigan J, Donaldson M (eds): To Err Is Human: Building a Safer Health System. Washington, DC, National Academy Press, 2000

Tredger JM, Stoll S: Cytochrome P450: their impact on drug treatment. Hospital Pharmacist 9:167–173, 2002

2

DEFINITIONS AND PHASE I METABOLISM

Drug interactions reflect a shift in drug activity or effect in the body as a result of another drug's presence or activity. Drug interactions are usually considered either pharmacodynamic or pharmacokinetic. In this chapter, we outline pharmacodynamic and pharmacokinetic principles. Pharmacokinetics, specifically phase I P450 metabolism, is then fully described.

■ DRUG INTERACTIONS DEFINITIONS

Pharmacodynamic Interactions

Pharmacodynamic interactions are interactions due to one drug's influence on another drug's effect at the latter's intended receptor site or end organ. These interactions or alterations in drug function are not due to a change in absorption, distribution, metabolism, or elimination. When two drugs act at a receptor site in the brain, causing a combined, typically unwanted effect or negating a wanted effect, a pharmacodynamic interaction is said to have occurred. The potentially dangerous monoamine oxidase inhibitor–tricyclic antidepressant serotonin syndrome is an example of a pharmacodynamic interaction.

Pharmacokinetic Interactions

Pharmacokinetic interactions are interactions due to one drug's effect on the movement of another drug through the body. These interactions are alterations in the way the body would normally metabolize a drug in its effort to eliminate it. Pharmacokinetic interactions may result in delayed onset of effect, decreased or increased effect, toxicity, or altered excretion, and they directly affect the concentration of drug that reaches the target site. Pharmacokinetic interactions encompass alterations in absorption, distribution, metabolism, and excretion.

Absorption interaction: An alteration due to one drug's effect on another drug's route of entry into the body. Most absorption interactions occur in the gut; some examples of these interactions are those due to altered gastric pH, food coadministration, mechanical blockade or chelation, and loss of gut flora.

Distribution interaction: An alteration in how a drug travels throughout the body; typically a result of alterations in protein binding in plasma. Drug effect is directly related to the amount of free drug available to the target site. More or less drug is available if another drug displaces the protein-bound fraction of a drug. Warfarin is an example of a drug that is sensitive to protein-binding displacement by many other drugs.

Metabolism interaction: An alteration in the biotransformation of a compound into active drug or excretable inactive compounds; usually results in a change in drug concentration due to a blocking or "backing up" of or an increase in enzymatic metabolism. In this Concise Guide, metabolism is covered in great depth.

Excretion interaction: An alteration in the ability to eliminate an unaltered drug or metabolite from the body. An example of this type of interaction is the effect of sodium concentration or diuretics on lithium retention by the kidneys.

■ METABOLISM

The act of metabolism may have developed to assist humans in ridding their bodies of endogenous substances no longer needed (e.g., catecholamines, steroids, bilirubin). Over time, metabolism came to include biotransformation of exogenous substances, such as food, chemicals, environmental toxins, and drugs. Drugs are usually lipophilic, which allows them to enter their site of action at target organs or tissues via cell membranes and exert their effect. Lipophilic compounds are difficult to eliminate from the body. Metabolism—or biotransformation of these compounds into more polar, inactive metabolites—is necessary. These water-soluble metabolites then exit the body more readily via urine, bile, or stool. The workhorses of biotransformation are the metabolic enzymes.

Biotransformation occurs throughout the body, with the greatest concentration of activity in the liver and the gut wall. At the cellular level, biotransformation occurs in the endoplasmic reticulum. With many drugs, there is a *first-pass effect* as the drug crosses the gut wall and again as the drug passes through the liver, before reaching the systemic circulation and its target sites. Most drugs lose functional activity during the "first pass" as the body begins the process of preparing the drug for elimination. This first-pass effect can limit the oral availability of drugs and is a factor in determining whether a drug should be administered parenterally or orally. Several processes contribute to the first-pass effect: P450 metabolism in the gut wall (with 3A4 responsible for 70% of intestinal P450 activity) (DeVane 1998) and metabolism in the liver; phase II metabolic reactions in both gut and liver; and active transporters, especially intestinal P-glycoproteins (see Chapter 4 ["P-Glycoproteins"]). The brain, kidneys, lungs, and skin also have significant metabolic activity, and any cell with endoplasmic reticulum has the capacity for some metabolic reactions.

Drug biotransformation is generally accomplished in two phases: phase I and phase II. Some drugs undergo these processes in order, some undergo them simultaneously, and some undergo only phase I or phase II. In the remainder of this chapter, we review phase I. The reader is referred to Chapter 3 ("Metabolism in Depth: Phase II") for a full discussion of phase II. At the time of publication, a slide show on biotransformation could be found at www.sci.tamucc.edu/pals/moslen/dominski/sld001.htm.

Phase I Metabolism

Phase I reactions typically add small, polar groups to a parent drug by adding or exposing a functional group on a compound or drug through oxidative reactions such as *N*-dealkylation, *O*-dealkylation, hydroxylation, *N*-oxidation, *S*-oxidation, or deamination (Table 2–1). The resulting compounds may then lose all pharmacological activity, and they are ready for reactions to form highly water-soluble conjugates and for elimination by means of phase II metabolism. As mentioned in the previous paragraph, many drugs are not metabolized in this linear fashion, and some may undergo conjugation reactions of phase II before phase I, or these reactions may occur simultaneously. Some drugs do not lose pharmacological activity at all; instead, their activity is enhanced. Some drugs (e.g., terfenadine) are pro-drugs and must be metabolized to their active metabolite. The cytochrome P450 monooxygenase system is a phase I system.

P450 System or Cytochrome P450 Monooxidase System

More than 200 P450 enzymes exist in nature, and a collection of at least 40 enzymes is found in humans (Figure 2–1). Six enzymes are responsible for about 90% of all the metabolic activity of P450 enzymes—1A2, 3A4, 2C9, 2C19, 2D6, and 2E1—and all play an important role in xenobiotic oxidative metabolism. Minor but clinically relevant enzymes include 2A6, 2B6, and 2C8. All of these enzymes are on the smooth endoplasmic reticulum of hepatocytes and the luminal epithelium of the small intestine. These proteins are closely associated with nicotinamide adenine dinucleotide phosphate (reduced form) (NADPH) cytochrome P450 reductase, which donates or is the source of the electrons needed for oxidation (Wilkinson 2001). (For details on the enzymatic reactions, see Table 2–1 and the references at the end of this chapter.)

The P450 enzymes contain red-pigmented heme, and when bound to carbon monoxide they absorb light at a wavelength of 450 nm. In the term *cytochrome P450, cyto* stands for *microsomal vesicles, chrome* for *colored, P* for *pigmented,* and *450* for *450 nanometers.* Each enzyme is encoded by one particular gene—one gene, one

TABLE 2–1. Major reactions involved in phase I drug metabolism

Reaction	Phase I	Examples
Oxidative reactions		
N-Dealkylation	$RNHCH_3 \longrightarrow RNH_2 + CH_2O$	Imipramine, diazepam, codeine, erythromycin, morphine, tamoxifen, theophylline, caffeine
O-Dealkylation	$ROCH_3 \longrightarrow ROH + CH_2O$	Codeine, indomethacin, dextromethorphan
Aliphatic hydroxylation	$RCH_2CH_3 \longrightarrow RCHCH_3$ with OH	Tolbutamide, ibuprofen, pentobarbital, meprobamate, cyclosporine, midazolam
Aromatic hydroxylation		Phenytoin, phenobarbital, propranolol, phenylbutazone, ethinyl estradiol, amphetamine, warfarin

TABLE 2–1. Major reactions involved in phase I drug metabolism *(continued)*

Reaction		Examples
Phase I		
Oxidative reactions		
N-Oxidation	$RNH_2 \longrightarrow RNHOH$	Chlorpheniramine, dapsone, meperidine
	$\begin{matrix} R_1 \\ R_2 \end{matrix} NH \longrightarrow \begin{matrix} R_1 \\ R_2 \end{matrix} N{-}OH$	Quinidine, acetaminophen
S-Oxidation	$\begin{matrix} R_1 \\ R_2 \end{matrix} S \longrightarrow \begin{matrix} R_1 \\ R_2 \end{matrix} S{=}O$	Cimetidine, chlorpromazine, thioridazine, omeprazole
Deamination	$RCHCH_3 \rightarrow R{-}\overset{OH}{\underset{NH_2}{C}}{-}CH_3 \rightarrow R{-}\overset{O}{C}{-}CH_3 + NH_2$	Diazepam, amphetamine

TABLE 2–1. Major reactions involved in phase I drug metabolism *(continued)*

Reaction	Examples
Hydrolysis reactions	
Phase I	
$\underset{R_1COR_2}{\overset{O}{\parallel}} \longrightarrow R_1COOH + R_2OH$	Procaine, aspirin, clofibrate, meperidine, enalapril, cocaine
$\underset{R_1CNR_2}{\overset{O}{\parallel}} \longrightarrow R_1COOH + R_2NH_2$	Lidocaine, procainamide, indomethacin

Source. Adapted from Wilkinson GR: "Pharmacokinetics: The Dynamics of Drug Absorption, Distribution, and Elimination," in *Goodman and Gilman's The Pharmacological Basis of Therapeutics,* 10th Edition. Edited by Hardman JG, Limbird LE, Gilman AG. New York, McGraw-Hill, 2001, p. 14. With permission of the McGraw-Hill Companies.

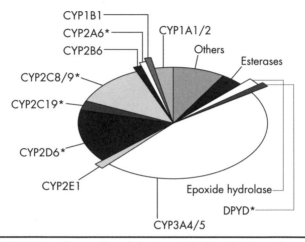

FIGURE 2–1. **Proportion of drugs metabolized by the major phase I enzymes.**

The relative size of each pie section indicates the estimated percentage of phase I metabolism that each enzyme contributes to the metabolism of drugs based on literature reports. Enzymes that have functional allelic variants are indicated by an asterisk (*). In many cases, more than one enzyme is involved in a particular drug's metabolism. CYP=cytochrome P450; DPYD=dihydropyrimidine dehydrogenase.

Source. Adapted from Wilkinson GR: "Pharmacokinetics: The Dynamics of Drug Absorption, Distribution, and Elimination," in *Goodman & Gilman's The Pharmacological Basis of Therapeutics,* 10th Edition. Edited by Hardman JG, Limbird LE, Gilman AG. New York, McGraw-Hill, 2001, p. 15. With permission of the McGraw-Hill Companies.

enzyme. The enzymes are grouped into families and subfamilies according to the similarity of their amino acid sequences. Enzymes in the same family are homologous for 40%–55% of amino acid sequences, and enzymes within the same subfamily are homologous for more than 55%. (See Table 2–2 for more on P450 nomenclature.)

Until the early 1990s, it was standard to label a family using a Roman numeral; an enzyme might be labeled *CYPIID6*. Today, Arabic numerals are used; the same enzyme is now labeled *CYP2D6*.

TABLE 2–2.   **P450 nomenclature**

Category	Addition(s) to *P450*	Examples
Family	Arabic numeral	P450 1, P450 2
Subfamily	Arabic numeral + uppercase letter	P450 1A, P450 2D
Single gene or protein	Arabic numeral + uppercase letter + Arabic numeral	P450 1A2, P450 2D6

The P450 system is also referred to as the *cytochrome P450 system, CYP450 system,* and *P450 system.* For brevity, we use *P450 system* throughout this book. Individual enzymes are designated several ways in the literature; a particular enzyme might be labeled *cytochrome P450 2D6, CYP2D6,* or *2D6.* In this book, we use the shortest forms, labeling individual P450 enzymes *2D6* or *3A4,* for example. Finally, the P450 enzymes are often called *isoenzymes* or *isozymes* in the literature, but these terms are misnomers because they refer to enzymes that catalyze one reaction. To avoid confusion, the term *enzymes* is used throughout this text.

Other Phase I Systems

Other phase I metabolism systems include the alcohol dehydrogenase, flavin monooxygenase, esterase, and amidase systems. The monoamine oxidase system is also considered a part of phase I, but it is not the P450 system. This group includes monoamine oxidases, which have been studied in relation to depression and Parkinson's disease. Strolin and Tipton (1998) wrote a thorough review of non-P450 phase I metabolism.

■ METABOLIC VARIABILITY: INHIBITION, INDUCTION, AND PHARMACOGENETICS

Drug response varies greatly across groups and individuals. This variability is due to many pharmacological factors. In phase I and phase II metabolism, this variability may be a reflection of enzyme inhibition, enzyme induction, and/or genetic differences.

Inhibition

Drugs metabolized at a common human enzyme will at times be competing or sharing metabolic sites within the endoplasmic reticulum in the liver and gut. A drug's affinity for an enzyme is called its *inhibitory potential,* or *Ki.* These values are routinely determined in vitro via human liver microsome studies (see Chapter 23 ["How to Retrieve and Review the Literature"] for a discussion of in vitro studies). Drugs with little affinity for an enzyme have a high Ki and probably will not bind. Drugs with a low Ki, or great affinity for enzyme binding, are very likely to bind and may compete with drugs for the same site. Drugs with a Ki less than 2.0 μM are typically considered potent inhibitors. When drugs are coadministered, the drug with the greater affinity (lower Ki) will competitively inhibit the binding of the drug with lower affinity (high Ki) (Owen and Nemeroff 1998). (See Figure 2–2.) Some drugs bind to an enzyme and inhibit its activity without needing the enzyme for their own metabolism. Some drugs may be both substrates of an enzyme (may require that enzyme for metabolism) and inhibitors of the same enzyme. Drugs that inhibit an enzyme may slow down the enzyme's activity or block the activity needed for metabolism of other drugs there, which will result in increased levels of any drug dependent on that enzyme for biotransformation. This inhibition leads to prolonged pharmacological effect and may result in drug toxicity. Inhibition is immediate in its effect, and when treatment with the offending drug is discontinued, the enzyme quickly returns to normal function. Symptoms caused by drug-drug inhibition have a rapid onset and disappear quickly.

The P450 system is greatly affected by competitive inhibition. Ketoconazole has a low Ki for 3A4, or a high affinity for enzyme binding at 3A4. When coadministered with terfenadine, this drug prevents the metabolism of the parent compound of terfenadine, leading to an increased serum level of toxic terfenadine, which

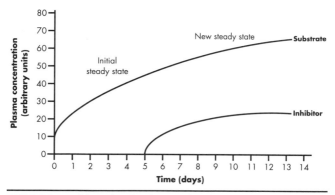

FIGURE 2–2.   **Alteration in plasma kinetics in the presence of a potent *inhibitor* for that P450 enzyme and substrate.**

causes arrhythmias (Monahan 1990). Without coadministration of a potent inhibitor, terfenadine is rapidly metabolized at 3A4 to its nontoxic but pharmacodynamically active compound fexofenadine. Each human P450 enzyme is fully discussed in the chapters that follow, with tables of inhibitors provided. The drug interaction program at http://www.mhc.com provides many of the Ki values of commonly prescribed drugs.

Induction

Some xenobiotics (drugs and environmental substances such as cigarette smoke) increase the synthesis of P450 proteins, actually increasing the number of sites available for biotransformation. When more sites are available, more compound is metabolized at a time. This induction process may lead to decreases in the amount of parent drug administered and increases in the amount of metabolites produced. An inducer may cause the level of a coadministered drug to decrease to below the level needed for therapeutic effect, resulting in loss of clinical efficacy (see Figure 2–3). For example, coadministration of the potent inducer rifampin and methadone has

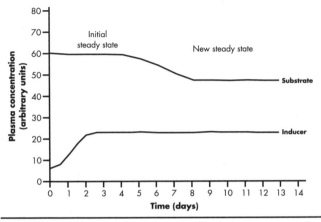

FIGURE 2–3.   **Alteration in plasma kinetics in the presence of a potent *inducer* for that P450 enzyme and substrate.**

led to opiate withdrawal (see Chapter 18 ["Pain Management II: Narcotic Analgesics"]). Drugs that require P450 metabolism for activation may become toxic if active metabolites are produced more quickly than expected. Such a phenomenon is hypothesized to occur with the induction of valproic acid: the production of toxic metabolites is increased, leading to hepatotoxicity (see Chapter 15 ["Neurology"]). 3A4, 2D6, 1A2, 2C9, 2C19, and 2E1 may all be induced.

Pharmacogenetics: Polymorphisms

Clinicians have noted for decades that drug metabolism greatly varies across racial groups. The genetic variability (polymorphisms) of P450 enzymes is arguably the most important clinical pharmacogenetic consideration (Eichelbaum and Evert 1996). The concept of racially polymorphic enzymes makes intuitive sense. Enzymes exist in part to metabolize exogenous substances in human environments, and therefore different populations developed different enzyme capabilities, based on exposure to particular environmental stressors.

Each person has two copies (or *alleles*) of each gene. The most common pair of alleles is usually referred to as the "wild type." Some individuals will have variations to the wild-type alleles. These variations are called *genetic polymorphisms.* Genetic polymorphisms can arise from a variety of alterations of the alleles, to include minor base pair changes, missense mutations, entire allelic deletions, or extra alleles. Those with nonworking or missing alleles are considered *poor metabolizers* (PMs): their metabolism is slower or they are less able to biotransform a compound at a specific enzyme site compared with the rest of a population. *Ultraextensive metabolizers,* also called ultrarapid metabolizers in older literature, require more drug than expected to achieve therapeutic effect, because of the rapidity and extensiveness with which their enzymes metabolize a compound. They typically have extra allelic copies of the wild-type genome. Average metabolizers, called *extensive metabolizers* or rapid metabolizers in older literature, may be "converted" to PMs by P450 inhibitors. Although these "converted" individuals are not genetically determined to metabolize poorly, they mimic genetic PMs and are thus "phenotypic" PMs. Most P450 and some phase II enzymes are polymorphic. See the sections on polymorphisms in Chapter 3 ("Metabolism in Depth: Phase II") and throughout Part II ("P450 Enzymes") for examples.

Genetic Polymorphisms in Depth

The polymorphic variability of drug metabolism was empirically recognized before the P450 system was well understood. Slow and rapid acetylators of isoniazid were recognized in the 1950s. Glucose-6-phosphate dehydrogenase deficiency leading to hemolytic anemia was appreciated as a genetically based variation in drug metabolism. In the 1970s, Ziegler and Biggs (1977) noted that black patients had significantly higher nortriptyline levels than did other patients, and the investigators assumed there were genetic differences. These differences in nortriptyline metabolism are now believed to result from genetic polymorphisms related to 2D6 and 3A4.

Genotypic or phenotypic testing of P450 enzymes is being incorporated into some practice protocols (Crespi and Miller 1999; Tanaka and Breimer 1997). For example, activity of 2D6, which has a polymorphism that renders some people PMs for drugs that use 2D6, may be premeasured through administration of a probe drug, such as dextromethorphan. Probes are drugs that are metabolized, often exclusively, by an enzyme, resulting in a measurable and reliable metabolite. Dextromethorphan is exclusively metabolized by 2D6 to dextrorphan. A patient who has no dextrorphan after ingesting dextromethorphan likely lacks 2D6 activity. Predetermining 2D6 phenotypes would help one to adequately treat patients who require tramadol, which is essentially a pro-drug metabolized by 2D6 to the more active analgesic compound M1 (Dayer et al. 1997) (see Chapter 18 ["Pain Management II: Narcotic Analgesics"]). Knowing before initiation of pharmacotherapy that a patient is a PM would allow one to alter treatment for better analgesia. See Chapter 5 ("2D6") for further discussion.

Another illustration of "probing" for genetic variability to guide treatment is found in cancer chemotherapy. A person who lacks thiopurine methyltransferase, a phase II conjugation enzyme (these individuals make up 0.3% of the population), may have a fatal response to normal doses of thiopurines (Keuzenkamp-Jansen et al. 1996) (see Chapter 16 ["Oncology"]). Most clinicians do not routinely genotype patients. It is expected that in the future, as physicians continue to prescribe multiple drugs, increasing reliance will be placed on the use of probes or similar methods to genetically fingerprint patients (Tanaka and Breimer 1997). Such methods will become most useful in situations in which drugs either are activated by enzymes (pro-drugs; e.g., tramadol [2D6] and cyclophosphamide [2C19]) or are dangerous at high levels (e.g., some antiarrhythmics [metabolized by 2D6] and S-warfarin [2C9]) (Linder and Valdes 1999). A well-written lecture on pharmacogenetics can be found at http://www.aphanet.org/govt/pohcycomm2000/pharmacobackground.html.

■ SUMMARY

Drug interactions occur for many reasons. Pharmacokinetic interactions are due to an alteration in drug absorption, distribution, metabolism, or elimination. Most drug interactions are due to alterations in enzymatic processes of phase I and phase II metabolism. An understanding of phase I metabolism alone does not explain why there is so much variability in patient response to drugs. Much of this variability is due to alterations in the P450 system through the environmental and genetic influences of inhibition, induction, and genetic variability.

■ REFERENCES

Crespi CL, Miller VP: The use of heterologously expressed drug metabolizing enzymes—state of the art and prospects for the future. Pharmacol Ther 84:121–131, 1999

Dayer P, Desmeules J, Collart L: Pharmacology of tramadol. Drugs 53 (suppl 2):18–24, 1997

DeVane CL: Principles of pharmacokinetics and pharmacodynamics, in The American Psychiatric Press Textbook of Psychopharmacology, 2nd Edition. Edited by Schatzberg AF, Nemeroff CB. Washington, DC, American Psychiatric Press, 1998, pp 155–169

Eichelbaum M, Evert B: Influence of pharmacogenetics on drug disposition and response. Clin Exp Pharmacol Physiol 23:983–985, 1996

Keuzenkamp-Jansen CW, Leegwater PA, De Abreu RA, et al: Thiopurine methyltransferase: a review and a clinical pilot study. J Chromatogr B Biomed Appl 678:15–22, 1996

Linder MW, Valdes R Jr: Pharmacogenetics in the practice of laboratory medicine. Mol Diagn 4:365–379, 1999

Monahan BP, Ferguson CL, Killeavy ES, et al: Torsades de pointes occurring in association with terfenadine use. JAMA 264:2788–2790, 1990

Owen JR, Nemeroff CB: New antidepressants and the cytochrome P450 system: focus on venlafaxine, nefazodone and mirtazapine. Depress Anxiety 7 (suppl 1):24–32, 1998

Strolin BM, Tipton KF: Monoamine oxidases and related amine oxidases as phase I enzymes in the metabolism of xenobiotics. J Neural Transm Suppl 52:149–171, 1998

Tanaka E, Breimer DD: In vivo function tests of hepatic drug-oxidizing capacity in patients with liver disease. J Clin Pharm Ther 22:237–249, 1997

Wilkinson GR: Pharmacokinetics: the dynamics of drug absorption, distribution, and elimination, in Goodman and Gilman's The Pharmacological Basis of Therapeutics, 10th Edition. Edited by Hardman JG, Limbird LE, Gilman AG. New York, McGraw-Hill, 2001, pp 3–29

Ziegler VE, Biggs JT: Tricyclic plasma levels: effect of age, race, sex, and smoking. JAMA 238:2167–2169, 1977

3

METABOLISM IN DEPTH: PHASE II

In phase II or conjugation reactions, water-soluble molecules are added to a drug, usually making an inactive, easily excretable compound. Covalent linkages are made between the drug and glucuronic acid, sulfate, acetate, amino acids, and/or glutathione (Wilkinson 2001) (Table 3–1).

Phase II enzymes have not been as well studied because recent research focus has been on the P450 or phase I enzymes. Phase I enzymes were the first to come to researchers' attention because these enzymes are more apt to produce active or toxic metabolites when they oxidize, by "taking away" methyl, alkyl, or hydroxyl groups. The vast majority of clinically important drug interactions involve P450. Nevertheless, the attention paid to phase II enzymes has increased, and it has become clear that this system has a great effect on metabolic drug interactions as well. What follows is an overview of three of the best-studied phase II enzymatic processes: glucuronidation, sulfation, and methylation (see Table 3–1).

■ GLUCURONIDATION

The most abundant phase II enzymes belong to the family of uridine 5′-diphosphate glucuronosyltransferases (UGTs). This family is a major detoxification system, and the liver is the main site of glucuronidation (McGurk et al. 1998). UGTs are also found throughout the gastrointestinal tract, where they are an integral part of prehepatic first-pass metabolism (Tukey and Strassburg 2000). In ad-

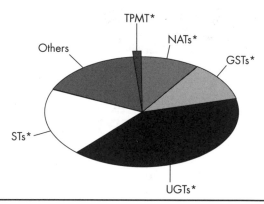

FIGURE 3–1. **Proportion of drugs metabolized by the major phase II enzymes.**

The relative size of each pie section indicates the estimated percentage of phase II metabolism that each enzyme contributes to the metabolism of drugs based on literature reports. Enzymes that have functional allelic variants are indicated by an asterisk (*). In many cases, more than one enzyme is involved in a particular drug's metabolism. GST=glutathione S-transferase; NAT=N-acetyltransferase; ST=sulfotransferase; TPMT=thiopurine methyltransferase; UGT=uridine 5'-diphosphate glucuronosyltransferase.

Source. Adapted from Wilkinson GR: "Pharmacokinetics: The Dynamics of Drug Absorption, Distribution, and Elimination," in *Goodman & Gilman's The Pharmacological Basis of Therapeutics,* 10th Edition. Edited by Hardman JG, Limbird LE, Gilman AG. New York, McGraw-Hill, 2001, p. 15. With permission of the McGraw-Hill Companies.

dition, UGTs work in the kidneys, brain, placenta, and elsewhere in the body. UGTs are found in the endoplasmic reticulum (next to the P450 enzymes) and in the nucleus and nuclear membrane (Radominska-Pandya et al. 2002). In terms of both quantity of substrates and variety of substrates conjugated, UGTs are the most important phase II enzymes. Many endogenous products, including bilirubin, bile acids, thyroxine, and steroids, are substrates of UGTs. It is postulated that nuclear and nuclear membrane UGTs regulate these important endogenous compounds.

TABLE 3–1. Major reactions involved in phase II drug metabolism

Reaction		Examples
Conjugation reactions	**Phase II**	
Glucuronidation	UDP-glucuronic acid	Acetaminophen, morphine, oxazepam, lorazepam
Sulfation		Acetaminophen, steroids, methyldopa

TABLE 3–1. **Major reactions involved in phase II drug metabolism** *(continued)*

Reaction	Examples
Acetylation	Sulfonamides, isoniazid, dapsone, clonazepam

acetyl-coenzyme A

Source. Adapted from Wilkinson GR: "Pharmacokinetics: The Dynamics of Drug Absorption, Distribution, and Elimination," in *Goodman and Gilman's The Pharmacological Basis of Therapeutics*, 10th Edition. Edited by Hardman JG, Limbird LE, Gilman AG. New York, McGraw-Hill, 2001, p. 14. With permission of the McGraw-Hill Companies.

After glucuronidation, intestinal bacterial β-glucuronidases break down glucuronidation products and release unconjugated drug via enterohepatic recirculation. This "recycling" system slowly clears conjugated compounds and releases glucuronides for reuse. Some forms of glucuronidated drugs (acyl forms) are "immune" to these bacterial actions and can bind to plasma proteins and produce hypersensitivity reactions. In 1993, zomepirac was removed from the United States market because of the high incidence of hypersensitivity reactions caused by its acyl glucuronide (Spielberg 1994).

Many drugs are metabolized through both phase I metabolism and glucuronidation, but some drugs are directly conjugated by UGTs. Most benzodiazepines are first metabolized by the P450 system and then glucuronidated (see Chapter 19 ["Psychiatry"]). Lorazepam, oxazepam, and temazepam are directly glucuronidated. Because UGTs are less affected than P450 enzymes by chronic hepatic disease, these three drugs are the preferred benzodiazepines for use in patients with chronic hepatic disease. More than 1,000 exogenous compounds—including chemicals, carcinogens, flavonoids, and drugs—are substrates of UGTs (Tukey and Strassburg 2000). Drugs primarily handled by UGTs include lamotrigine, valproate, nonsteroidal anti-inflammatory drugs, zidovudine, and most opioids (e.g., morphine and codeine). Like the P450 enzymes, UGTs have both unique and overlapping drug substrates, and they are vulnerable to drug inhibition and induction. Competitive inhibition between substrates of the same UGT may occur, and UGT inhibitors and inducers may be metabolized on other UGTs or through other metabolic systems.

UGT amino acids have been sequenced, and, as in the case of the P450 enzymes, a nomenclature based on amino acid similarity has been developed: the root symbol (UGT) is followed by the family (Arabic numeral), subfamily (uppercase letter), and gene (Arabic numeral)—for example, UGT1A1. The Web site address for the committee responsible for UGT nomenclature is http://www.unisa.edu.au/pharm_medsci/Gluc_trans/default.htm.

This nomenclature was developed in 1997. Few specific probe substrates (drugs metabolized—often exclusively—by the UGT, resulting in a measurable and reliable metabolite) are known for each UGT, and there is little agreement among researchers on specific UGT inducers and inhibitors. Further, most current information about UGT-based drug interactions was obtained through in vitro experiments and may not be relevant to living individuals. For example, there is in vitro evidence that diclofenac significantly inhibits codeine glucuronidation (Ammon et al. 2000), but in vivo testing has failed to support this interaction (Ammon et al. 2002). In some cases, a UGT-based drug interaction is known to occur (e.g., valproate interacts with naproxen [Addison et al. 2000]) but the particular UGT has not been definitively identified. Some drugs currently known to be substrates of the seven best-characterized hepatic UGTs are listed in Tables 3–2 and 3–3.

UGT subfamily 1A1 and UGT family 2B are important in endogenous and drug metabolism. Hepatic subfamily UGT1A includes UGT1A1, UGT1A3, UGT1A4, UGT1A6, and UGT1A9. They are all products of a single complex gene located on chromosome 2. They have in common exons 2–5, but exon 1 is unique to each enzyme. Bilirubin is a substrate of only UGT1A1, and genetic alterations are responsible for congenital hyperbilirubinemias: Crigler-Najjar syndrome type I (inactive protein) and Gilbert syndrome and Crigler-Najjar syndrome type II (partially active protein). Individuals with Gilbert syndrome (representing about 8%–12% of Caucasian populations) have a fluctuating mild hyperbilirubinemia.

Like slow metabolizers of the P450 enzyme 2D6, individuals with congenital hyperbilirubinemias have increased blood concentrations of substrates of UGT1A1. Because UGT1A1 is inducible by phenobarbital, this drug has been used to reduce levels of bilirubin in patients with partially inactive UGT1A1 (Jansen 1999; Sugatani et al. 2001). Individuals with Gilbert syndrome who are given the anticancer drug irinotecan have been shown to have an increased risk of toxicity, because UGT1A1 is the major metabolic pathway for its active metabolite, SN-38 (Ando et al. 2002; Iyer et al. 1999, 2002). The importance of genotyping individuals before treatment with irinotecan has been advocated (Rauchschwalbe et al. 2002). Both ethinyl estradiol (common in oral contraceptives) and buprenorphine are substrates of UGT1A1, and individuals with Gilbert syndrome may also have higher blood levels of these compounds and may be more likely to have increased side effects. Although telmisartan, an angiotensin II antagonist, is also conjugated by UGT1A1, only a small percentage of the drug is handled by this route. Drug interactions involving UGT1A1 are not yet well documented.

Because UGT1A4 catalyzes amines, many psychotropic agents (e.g., amitriptyline, chlorpromazine, imipramine, lamotrigine, olanzapine, clozapine, promethazine) are substrates. Probenecid, a broadly potent UGT inhibitor, affects the clearance of olanzapine but not risperidone, the latter primarily being handled by P450 enzymes (Markowitz et al. 2002).

Unlike UGT1A, UGT2B enzymes are produced from separate genes. Located on chromosome 4, the best characterized include *UGT2B4, UGT2B7, UGT2B10, UGT2B11, UGT2B15,* and *UGT2B17.* Genetic polymorphisms are known to exist for *UGT2B4, UGT2B7,* and *UGT2B15,* but their clinical significance has not been demonstrated.

UGT2B7 exists in two forms, which differ only by a single amino acid. Whether each has unique substrates has not been clarified. UGT2B7 has a wide substrate spectrum; drugs catalyzed include carboxylic acid nonsteroidal anti-inflammatory drugs (e.g., ibuprofen, ketoprofen), zidovudine, benzodiazepines, (e.g., lorazepam, *R*-oxazepam, and temazepam), epirubicin, and chloramphenicol (Barbier et al. 2000; Radominska-Pandya et al. 2001). UGT2B7 exclusively catalyzes morphine and codeine and many of their derivatives (see Table 3–2). Most glucuronidated drugs have decreased plasma protein binding and increased hydrophilicity and are inactive, but morphine-6-glucuronate is more than 20 times more potent than morphine at the receptor site. Whereas UGT1A3 glucuronidates morphine in the 3-hydroxy position, only UGT2B7 catalyzes morphine in the 6-hydroxy position. Morphine-3-glucuronate antagonizes the effects of both morphine and its 6-glucuronidate and may be responsible for the development of tolerance to morphine (Liston et al. 2001).

TABLE 3–2. Some UGT1A substrates

	1A1	1A3	1A4	1A6	1A9
Chromosome	2	2	2	2	2
Polymorphism	CN-I, CN-II, GS			Yes	
Some endogenous substrates	Bilirubin Estriol	Estrones	Androsterone Progestins	Serotonin	2-Hydroxyestradiols Thyroxine

Some substrate drugs	Acetaminophen
	Atorvastatin
	Buprenorphine
	Cerivastatin
	Ciprofibrate
	Clofibrate
	Ethinyl estradiol
	Flutamide
	  metabolite
	Gemfibrozil
	Nalorphine
	Naltrexone
	Simvastatin
	SN-38
	Telmisartan
	Troglitazone
		Amitriptyline
		Atorvastatin
		Buprenorphine
		Cerivastatin
		Chlorpromazine
		Clozapine
		Cyproheptadine
		Diclofenac
		Diflunisal
		Diphenhydramine
		Doxepin
		Fenoprofen
		Gemfibrozil
		4-Hydroxytamoxifen
		Ibuprofen
		Imipramine
			Amitriptyline
			Chlorpromazine
			Clozapine/Desmethyl
			  metabolites
			Cyproheptadine
			Diphenhydramine
			Doxepin
			4-Hydroxytamoxifen
			Imipramine
			Lamotrigine
			Loxapine
			Meperidine
			Olanzapine
			Promethazine
			Retigabine
				Acetaminophen
				Entacapone
				Flutamide
				  metabolite
				Ketoprofen
				Naftazone
				SN-38
					Acetaminophen
					Clofibric acid
					Dapsone
					Diclofenac
					Diflunisal
					Ethinyl estradiol
					Estrone
					Flavonoids
					Furosemide
					Ibuprofen
					Ketoprofen
					Labetalol
					Mefenamic acid
					Naproxen
					R-Oxazepam
					Propofol

TABLE 3–2. Some UGT1A substrates *(continued)*

1A1	1A3	1A4	1A6	1A9
	Losartan			Propranolol
	Loxapine			Retinoic acid
	Morphine			*SN-38*
	Nalorphine			Tolcapone
	Naloxone			*Valproate*
	Naltrexone			
	Naproxen			
	Naringenin			
	Norbuprenorphine			
	Promethazine			
	Simvastatin			
	SN-38			
	Tripelennamine			
	Valproate			

Note. *Italics* indicate that the UGT is a minor pathway for the substrate.
CN-I=Crigler-Najjar syndrome type I; CN-II=Crigler-Najjar syndrome type II; GS=Gilbert syndrome; UGT=uridine 5'-diphosphate glucuronosyltransferase.

TABLE 3–3.   **Some UGT2B substrates**

	2B7	2B15
Chromosome	4	4
Polymorphism	Yes	Yes
Some endogenous substrates	Androsterone Bile acid	Catechol estrogens 2-Hydroxyestrone Testosterone
Some substrate drugs	Chloramphenicol Clofibric acid Codeine Cyclosporine Diclofenac *Entacapone* Epirubicin *Fenoprofen* Hydromorphone *Ibuprofen* Ketoprofen Lorazepam Losartan Morphine Nalorphine Naloxone Naltrexone Naproxen Norcodeine *R*-Oxazepam Oxycodone Tacrolimus Temazepam *Tolcapone* Valproate Zidovudine Zomepirac	Dienestrol *Entacapone* *S*-Oxazepam Phenytoin metabolites *Tolcapone*

Note.   *Italics* indicate that the UGT is a minor pathway for the substrate.
CN-I=Crigler-Najjar syndrome type I; CN-II=Crigler-Najjar syndrome type II;
UGT=uridine 5′-diphosphate glucuronosyltransferase.

Some UGT levels are diminished in neonates (Burchell et al. 1989; de Wildt et al. 1999), and some decrease in the elderly (Sonne 1993). Some of the UGTs are more efficient in men than in women, which may account for differences in concentrations of acetaminophen and other drugs (Meibohm et al. 2002; Morissette et al. 2001). Like P450 enzymes, glucuronidation is affected by many environmental factors—smoking (Benowitz and Jacob 2000; Yue et al. 1994), foods (e.g., watercress [Hecht et al. 1999]), and disease states (e.g., hypothyroidism [Sonne 1993])—but specifics about individual UGTs are lacking.

■ SULFATION

Sulfation, or sulfonation (an older term), is another important phase II conjugation. The process involves the transfer of a sulfuryl group from a donor substrate, 3′-phosphoadenosine 5′-phosphosulfate (PAPS), to an acceptor compound via sulfotransferase (SULT). Sulfation is PAPS dependent in that PAPS can easily by "used up" in human liver in 2 minutes (Klaassen and Boles 1997), although more can be made quickly. This "turnover" of PAPS, along with sulfation and desulfation, creates an active recycling process.

There exists a cytosolic superfamily of 10 SULTs that are tissue- and substrate-specific. A nomenclature similar to the nomenclatures used for P450 enzymes and UGTs is just emerging and is generally accepted (http://www.fccc.edu/research/labs/raftogianis/sult/accessions.html). There are two families of important drug-conjugating human SULTs: SULT1 and SULT2. Subfamilies SULT1A, SULT1B, SULT1C, SULT1E, SULT2A, and SULT2B handle small endogenous compounds (e.g., steroids, thyroid hormones, catechol estrones, neurotransmitters) and exogenous compounds (e.g., ethinyl estradiol, acetaminophen, budesonide [SULT2A1 {Meloche et al. 2002}]). A major step in troglitazone's metabolism is sulfation (SULT1A1 [Honma et al. 2002]). Although sulfation of many drugs produces water-soluble, less-toxic metabolites, other conjugates are active (e.g., minoxidil), and some are reactive and can "attach" to DNA or RNA. Sulfation often produces promutagens (Glatt 2000).

Less information is available about specific SULT inhibitors, inducers, and substrates than about UGT inhibitors, inducers, and substrates. Environmental influences are known to occur. One of the more interesting of these influences is the apparent inhibition of SULTs by components such as vanillin, wine, tartrazine (a synthetic coloring agent), tea, and coffee (Burchell and Coughtrie 1997; Coughtrie et al. 1998). Several SULTs are known to be polymorphic (e.g., SULT1A1), but the clinical significance is unknown (Raftogianis et al. 2000).

■ METHYLATION

Enzyme subfamilies that conjugate through methylation are almost too numerous to count. The effects of S-adenosylmethionine (SAMe, or "sammy") (which is used to treat many illnesses, including depression) may be related to methylation enzymes, because SAMe is a methyl donor compound (Bottiglieri and Hyland 1994). Three of the better-studied and more interesting methyltransferases are catechol O-methyltransferase (COMT), histamine N-methyltransferase (HNMT), and thiopurine methyltransferase (TPMT).

Catechol O-Methyltransferase

The best appreciated of the methyltransferases, COMT has been known for more than 70 years (Kopin 1994). COMT is one of two means by which catecholamines are metabolized, the other being monoamine oxidases (a non-P450 phase I system). COMTs also metabolize steroid catechols. COMTs are located in virtually all regions, the two most important of which may be the brain and the liver. There are two main forms of COMT: membrane-bound COMT and soluble COMT (Ellingson et al. 1999), and genetic polymorphisms have been noted (Kuchel 1994). Three COMT genes have been identified that differ in activity level (Lee et al. 2002). Many studies have examined the genetic diversity of COMT as a factor in illness, including breast cancer, hypertension, obsessive-compulsive disorder, bipolar disorder, and schizophrenia.

Selective and reversible inhibition of COMT was developed as a strategy for enhancing dopamine availability in patients with Parkinson's disease (Goldstein and Lieberman 1992). Tolcapone and entacapone are COMT-inhibiting drugs, but how they inhibit COMT is unclear.

Histamine *N*-Methyltransferase

HNMT metabolizes histamine by adding a methyl group to histamine; then monoamine oxidase further catabolizes the methylhistamine. HNMT is located in many regions, particularly the liver and the kidney (De Santi et al. 1998). Its gene is located on chromosome 2, and HNMT has genetic polymorphic variability, but the clinical significance of the polymorphisms are currently unclear (Preuss et al. 1998). A common group of inhibitors, the 4-aminoquinolones (e.g., chloroquine and hydroxychloroquine), are believed to be inhibitors of HNMT, and this inhibition may account for their usefulness in treating rheumatoid arthritis, systemic lupus erythematosus (Cumming et al. 1990), and other inflammatory disorders. Another group of inhibitors of HNMTs is the steroidal neuromuscular relaxants, such as pancuronium and vecuronium. Inhibition of HNMT may explain instances of flushing and hypotension with the use of these drugs (Futo et al. 1990).

Thiopurine Methyltransferase

TPMT is best known for its rare polymorphic character, with a complete absence of enzyme occurring in about 10% of Caucasian populations (McLeod and Siva 2002). In fact, TPMT's routine phenotyping in patients with leukemia who require drugs such as 6-mercaptopurine is perhaps the first use of phenotype testing to enter general practice (Weinshilboum et al. 1999). Other drugs known to be conjugated by TPMT are thioguanine and azathioprine (Nishida et al. 2002). In women, TPMT has a slightly lower activity (Meibohm et al. 2002). For further details, see Chapter 2 ("Definitions and Phase I Metabolism") and Chapter 16 ("Oncology").

40

■ REFERENCES

Addison RS, Parker-Scott SL, Hooper WD, et al: Effect of naproxen coadministration on valproate disposition. Biopharm Drug Dispos 21: 235–242, 2000

Ammon S, von Richter O, Hofmann U, et al: In vitro interaction of codeine and diclofenac. Drug Metab Dispos 28:1149–1152, 2000

Ammon S, Marx C, Behrens C, et al: Diclofenac does not interact with codeine metabolism in vivo: a study in healthy volunteers. BMC Clin Pharmacol 2:2, 2002

Ando Y, Ueoka H, Sugiyama T, et al: Polymorphisms of UDP-glucuronosyltransferase and pharmacokinetics of irinotecan. Ther Drug Monit 24: 111–116, 2002

Barbier O, Turgeon D, Gerare C, et al: 3′-Azido-3′-deoxythimidine (AZT) is glucuronidated by human UDP-glucuronosyltransferase 2B7 (UGT2B7). Drug Metab Dispos 28:497–502, 2000

Benowitz NL, Jacob P 3rd: Effects of cigarette smoking and carbon monoxide on nicotine and cotinine metabolism. Clin Pharmacol Ther 67:653–659, 2000

Bottiglieri T, Hyland K: S-Adenosylmethionine levels in psychiatric and neurological disorders: a review. Acta Neurol Scand Suppl 154:19–26, 1994

Burchell B, Coughtrie MW: Genetic and environmental factors associated with variation of human xenobiotic glucuronidation and sulfation. Environ Health Perspect 105 (suppl 4):739–747, 1997

Burchell B, Coughtrie M, Jackson M, et al: Development of human liver UDP-glucuronosyltransferases. Dev Pharmacol Ther 13:70–77, 1989

Coughtrie MW, Sharp S, Maxwell K, et al: Biology and function of the reversible sulfation pathway catalysed by human sulfotransferases and sulfatases. Chem Biol Interact 109:3–27, 1998

Court MH, Duan SX, Guillemette C, et al: Stereoselective conjugation of oxazepam by human UDP-glucuronosyltransferases (UGTs): S-oxazepam is glucuronidated by UGT2B15, while R-oxazepam is glucuronidated by UGT2B7 and UGT1A9. Drug Metab Dispos 30:1257–1265, 2002

Cumming P, Reiner PB, Vincent SR: Inhibition of rat brain histamine-N-methyltransferase by 9-amino-1,2,3,4-tetrahydroacridine (THA). Biochem Pharmacol 40:1345–1350, 1990

De Santi C, Donatelli P, Giulianotti PC, et al: Interindividual variability of histamine N-methyltransferase in the human liver and kidney. Xenobiotica 28:571–577, 1998 de Wildt SN, Kearns GL, Leeder JS, et al: Glucuronidation in humans: pharmacogenetic and developmental aspects. Clin Pharmacokinet 36:439–452, 1999

Ellingson T, Duppempudi S, Greenberg BD, et al: Determination of differential activities of soluble and membrane-bound catechol-*O*-methyltransferase in tissues and erythrocytes. J Chromatogr B Biomed Sci Appl 729:347–353, 1999

Futo J, Kupferberg JP, Moss J: Inhibition of histamine *N*-methyltransferase (HNMT) in vitro by neuromuscular relaxants. Biochem Pharmacol 39:415–420, 1990

Glatt H: Sulfotransferases in the bioactivation of xenobiotics. Chem Biol Interact 129:141–170, 2000

Goldstein M, Lieberman A: The role of the regulatory enzymes of catecholamine synthesis in Parkinson's disease. Neurology 42:8–14, 41–48, 1992

Hawes EM: N+-Glucuronidation, a common pathway in human metabolism of drugs with a tertiary amine group. Drug Metab Dispos 26:830–837, 1998

Hecht SS, Carmella SG, Murphy SE: Effects of watercress consumption on urinary metabolites of nicotine in smokers. Cancer Epidemiol Biomarkers Prev 8:907–913, 1999

Honma W, Shimada M, Sasano H, et al: Phenol sulfotransferase, ST1A3, as the main enzyme catalyzing sulfation of troglitazone in human liver. Drug Metab Dispos 30:944–952, 2002

Iyer L, Hall D, Das S, et al: Phenotype-genotype correlation of in vitro SN-38 (active metabolite of irinotecan) and bilirubin glucuronidation in human liver tissue with UGT1A1 promoter polymorphism. Clin Pharmacol Ther 65:576–582, 1999

Iyer L, Das S, Janisch L, et al: UGT1A1*28 polymorphism as a determinant of irinotecan disposition and toxicity. Pharmacogenomics J 2:43–47, 2002

Jansen PL: Diagnosis and management of Crigler-Najjar syndrome. Eur J Pediatr 158 (suppl 2):S89–S94, 1999

Klaassen CD, Boles JW: Sulfation and sulfotransferases 5: the importance of 3′-phosphoadenosine 5′-phosphosulfate (PAPS) in the regulation of sulfation. FASEB J 11:404–418, 1997

Kopin IJ: Monoamine oxidase and catecholamine metabolism. J Neural Transm Suppl 41:57–67, 1994

Kuchel O: Clinical implications of genetic and acquired defects in catecholamine synthesis and metabolism. Clin Invest Med 17:354–373, 1994

Lee MS, Kim HS, Cho EK, et al: COMT genotype and effectiveness of entacapone in patients with fluctuating Parkinson's disease. Neurology 58:564–567, 2002

Lin JH: Complexities of glucuronidation affecting in vitro in vivo extrapolation. Curr Drug Metab 3:623–646, 2002

Liston HL, Markowitz JS, DeVane CL: Drug glucuronidation in clinical psychopharmacology. J Clin Psychopharmacol 21:500–505, 2001

Markowitz JS, DeVane CL, Liston HL, et al: The effects of probenecid on the disposition of risperidone and olanzapine in healthy volunteers. Clin Pharmacol Ther 71:30–38, 2002

McGurk KA, Brierley CH, Burchell B: Drug glucuronidation by human renal UDP-glucuronosyltransferases. Biochem Pharmacol 55:1005–1012, 1998

McLeod HL, Siva C: The thiopurine *S*-methyltransferase gene locus—implications for clinical pharmacogenomics. Pharmacogenomics 3:89–98, 2002

Meibohm B, Beierle I, Derendorf H: How important are gender differences in pharmacokinetics? Clin Pharmacokinet 41:329–342, 2002

Meloche CA, Sharma V, Swedmark S, et al: Sulfation of budesonide by human cytosolic sulfotransferase, dehydroepiandrosterone-sulfotransferase (DHEA-ST). Drug Metab Dispos 30:582–585, 2002

Morissette P, Albert C, Busque S, et al: In vivo higher glucuronidation of mycophenolic acid in male than in female recipients of a cadaveric kidney allograft and under immunosuppressive therapy with mycophenolate mofetil. Ther Drug Monit 23:520–525, 2001

Nishida A, Kubota T, Yamada Y, et al: Thiopurine *S*-methyltransferase activity in Japanese subjects: metabolic activity of 6-mercaptopurine 6-methylation in different TPMT genotypes. Clin Chim Acta 323:147–150, 2002

Preuss CV, Wood TC, Szumlanski CL, et al: Human histamine *N*-methyltransferase pharmacogenetics: common genetic polymorphisms that alter activity. Mol Pharmacol 53:708–717, 1998

Radominska-Pandya A, Little JM, Czernik PJ: Human UDP-glucuronosyltransferase 2B7. Curr Drug Metab 2:283–298, 2001

Radominska-Pandya A, Pokrovskaya ID, Xu J, et al: Nuclear UDP-glucuronosyltransferases: identification of UGT2B7 and UGT1A6 in human liver nuclear membranes. Arch Biochem Biophys 399:37–48, 2002

Raftogianis R, Creveling C, Weinshilboum R, et al: Estrogen metabolism by conjugation. J Natl Cancer Inst Monogr 27:113–124, 2000

Rauchschwalbe SK, Zuhlsdorf MT, Schuhly U, et al: Predicting the risk of sporadic elevated bilirubin levels and diagnosing Gilbert's syndrome by genotyping UGT1A1*28 promoter polymorphism. Int J Clin Pharmacol Ther 40:233–240, 2002

Sonne J: Factors and conditions affecting the glucuronidation of oxazepam. Pharmacol Toxicol 73 (suppl 1):1–23, 1993

Spielberg TE: Examining product risk in context: the case of zomepirac (letter). JAMA 272:1252, 1994

Sugatani J, Kojima H, Ueda A, et al: The phenobarbital response enhancer module in the human bilirubin UDP-glucuronosyltransferase UGT1A1 gene and regulation by the nuclear receptor CAR. Hepatology 33:1232–1238, 2001

Tukey RH, Strassburg CP: Human UDP-glucuronosyltransferases: metabolism, expression, and disease. Annu Rev Pharmacol Toxicol 40:581–616, 2000

Weinshilboum RM, Otterness DM, Szumlanski CL: Methylation pharmacogenetics: catechol *O*-methyltransferase, thiopurine methyltransferase, and histamine *N*-methyltransferase. Annu Rev Pharmacol Toxicol 39:19–52, 1999

Wilkinson GR: Pharmacokinetics: the dynamics of drug absorption, distribution, and elimination, in Goodman & Gilman's The Pharmacological Basis of Therapeutics, 10th Edition. Edited by Hardman JG, Limbird LE, Gilman AG. New York, McGraw-Hill, 2001, pp 3–29

Yue QY, Tomson T, Sawe J: Carbamazepine and cigarette smoking induce differentially the metabolism of codeine in man. Pharmacogenetics 4:193–198, 1994

4

P-GLYCOPROTEINS

Forty years ago, it was known that certain cancers (e.g., leukemias, breast cancer) could acquire resistance to previously effective oncology drugs. This process was named multidrug resistance (MDR), and the question of why many drugs become ineffective at the same time has been gradually answered. The *MDR1* gene on chromosome 7 of cancer cells was found to overexpress a protein that can actively transport some cancer drugs (e.g., vinca alkaloids and paclitaxel) across membranes in association with an energy source, adenosine triphosphate (ATP). The membrane-based glycoprotein was named P-glycoprotein (*P* designates *permeability*). MDR develops when the *MDR1* gene directs P-glycoproteins to multiply and to extrude all their substrates from or "bounce" all substrates out of the cell. (MDR develops because all P-glycoprotein substrates have been affected at the same time.)

A family of transporters with a distinctive sequence was soon identified and was named the ATP-binding cassette family. A Web site of ATP-binding cassette transporter nomenclature has been established at http://nutrigene.4t.com/humanabc.htm. Human P-glycoproteins were later divided into Pgp1 and Pgp3 (and they were renamed PGY1 and PGY3 in this nomenclature); researchers and clinicians continue to use the older terminology. PGY3 functions in phospholipid transport, while PGY1 is an efflux transporter. In this chapter, the term *P-glycoprotein(s)* will be used to stand for PGY1 only.

P-glycoproteins transport endogenous substances such as steroids, cytokines, and glucuronate and sulfate conjugates (Conrad et al. 2001). Only in recent years has a pharmacokinetic role in drug interactions been characterized for these transporters. P-glycoproteins are present on the villus tips of enterocytes in the jejunum (the primary site of absorption of oral drugs); in the colon, gonads, renal proximal tubules, placenta, and biliary system; and in the capillary endothelial cells of the blood-brain barrier. P-glycoproteins can transport certain hydrophobic substances across cells into the gut, into bile, into urine, and out of the gonads and the brain. The gonads and the brain can be considered "drug-free zones," and P-glycoproteins are postulated to play a protective role in the body by excluding drugs from these areas (Wilkinson 2001).

The gastrointestinal tract is not a passive barrier for medications. As part of first-pass drug elimination, 3A4 and conjugation enzymes in luminal jejunal cells have been shown to metabolize drugs before they are absorbed. P-glycoproteins also control the absorption of xenobiotics by "pumping" drugs out of the luminal cells and back into the gut for excretion (Doherty and Charman 2002). A similar action occurs at the renal tubules.

Drugs can be P-glycoprotein substrates, inhibitors, and/or inducers (see Table 4–1). They may also be none of these.

If P-glycoprotein function is inhibited or induced, absorption of drug substrates is altered. For example, quinidine has been known to increase digoxin levels. For many years, the mechanism of this interaction was undetermined, but it was known that P450 enzymes were not involved. Recently, it was shown that quinidine inhibits P-glycoprotein activity in the intestine and the kidney, and digoxin is a substrate of (or relies on) P-glycoprotein. During coadministration, digoxin is absorbed back into the body rather than bounced out (Fromm et al. 1999; Su and Huang 1996). Other drugs that are P-glycoprotein inhibitors can also increase digoxin concentrations; these drugs are nifedipine, nitrendipine, felodipine (Klotz 2002), atorvastatin (Boyd et al. 2000), verapamil, clarithromycin (Verschraagen et al. 1999; Wakasugi et al. 1998), propafenone (Woodland et al. 1997), cyclosporine, amiodarone, and itraconazole. Although intestinal P-glycoproteins may play a part in most of these drug interactions, digoxin toxicity occurs primarily as a result of P-glycoprotein inhibition in the renal tubules.

TABLE 4–1.   Some P-glycoprotein nonsubstrates, substrates, inhibitors, and inducers

Nonsubstrates	Substrates	Inhibitors	Inducers
Alfentanil	Aldosterone	Amiodarone	Dexamethasone
Amantadine	Amitriptyline	Amitriptyline	Doxorubicin
Chlorpheniramine	Amoxicillin	Atorvastatin	?Nefazodone (chronic)
Citalopram	Amprenavir	Bromocriptine	Phenobarbital
Clozapine	Carbamazepine	Chloroquine	Prazosin
Fentanyl	Chloroquine	Chlorpromazine	Rifampin
Fluconazole	Cimetidine	Clarithromycin	Ritonavir (chronic)
Flunitrazepam	Ciprofloxacin	Cyclosporine	St. John's wort
Fluoxetine	Colchicine	Cyproheptadine	Trazodone
Haloperidol	Corticosteroids	Desipramine	?Venlafaxine
Itraconazole	Cyclosporine	Diltiazem	
Ketoconazole	Digitoxin	Erythromycin	
Lidocaine	Digoxin	Felodipine	
Methotrexate	Diltiazem	Fentanyl	
Midazolam	Docetaxel	Fluphenazine	
Sumatriptan	L-Dopa	Garlic	
Yohimbine	Doxorubicin	Grapefruit juice	
	Enoxacin	Green tea (catechins)	
	Erythromycin	Haloperidol	
	Estradiol	Hydrocortisone	

TABLE 4–1. Some P-glycoprotein nonsubstrates, substrates, inhibitors, and inducers *(continued)*

Nonsubstrates	Substrates	Inhibitors	Inducers
	Fexofenadine	Hydroxyzine	
	Grepafloxacin	Imipramine	
	Indinavir	Itraconazole	
	Irinotecan	Ketoconazole	
	Lansoprazole	Lansoprazole	
	Loperamide	Lidocaine	
	Losartan	Lovastatin	
	Lovastatin	Maprotiline	
	Mibefradil	Methadone	
	Morphine	Mibefradil	
	Nelfinavir	Midazolam	
	Nortriptyline	Nefazodone (acute)	
	Ondansetron	Nelfinavir	
	Phenytoin	Ofloxacin	
	Quetiapine	Omeprazole	
	Quinidine	Orange juice (Seville)	
	Ranitidine	Pantoprazole	
	Rifampin	Phenothiazines	
	Ritonavir	Pimozide	
	Saquinavir	Piperine	

TABLE 4–1. Some P-glycoprotein nonsubstrates, substrates, inhibitors, and inducers *(continued)*

Nonsubstrates	Substrates	Inhibitors	Inducers
	Tacrolimus	Probenecid	
	Talinolol	Progesterone	
	Teniposide	Propafenone	
	Terfenadine	Propranolol	
	Vinblastine	Quinidine	
	Vincristine	Ritonavir (initial)	
		Saquinavir	
		Simvastatin	
		Spironolactone	
		Tamoxifen	
		Terfenadine	
		Testosterone	
		Trifluoperazine	
		Valspodar	
		Verapamil	
		Vinblastine	
		Vitamin E	

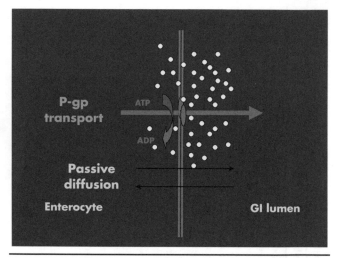

FIGURE 4–1. **Digoxin transport across the gastrointestinal (GI) lumen.**
ADP=adenosine diphosphate; ATP=adenosine triphosphate; P-gp=P-glycoprotein.
Source. Available at: http://www.cc.nih.gov/ccc/principles/pdf/00-01/pharma-cogenetics.pdf. Accessed December 18, 2002. Used with permission.

In contrast, rifampin has been shown to decrease digoxin concentrations by inducing P-glycoprotein in the intestinal tract (Greiner et al. 1999); digoxin is pumped back into the gastrointestinal tract. Another P-glycoprotein inducer, St. John's wort, can increase intestinal P-glycoprotein 1.5-fold (Durr et al. 2000). When St. John's wort is administered with digoxin, the concentration of the latter drug is reduced. St. John's wort is also known to induce 3A4 (Hennessy et al. 2002) (see Chapter 6 ["3A4"]). Drugs that are both 3A4 and P-glycoprotein substrates (e.g., cyclosporine [Ernst 2002]) are doubly affected. It has been shown that both 3A4 induction and P-glycoprotein induction are due mainly to the pregnane X receptor, although other mechanisms and receptors may also be involved (Lin 2003).

Not only are some drugs double inducers—some are double inhibitors. Two authors coined the term *drug efflux-metabolism alliance* to describe this association (Benet and Cummins 2001). Although there is no definite evidence that the activity of P-glycoprotein inhibitors and that of 3A4 inhibitors are coregulated, a considerable number of drugs are both P-glycoprotein and 3A4 inhibitors (e.g., ketoconazole, erythromycin [Wacher 1995]). These double inhibitors are very likely to produce clinically significant drug-drug interactions.

P-glycoproteins protect the brain by pumping out drugs that might enter by crossing the blood-brain barrier. Most psychotropic drugs are not substrates of P-glycoprotein and therefore achieve adequate central nervous system (CNS) concentrations. This finding makes intuitive sense given that psychotropics need to be at appropriate concentrations to be effective within the CNS. All first-generation antihistamines cause sedation, whereas second-generation antihistamines do not. The reason for this difference is that the former are not P-glycoprotein substrates and the latter are (Chishty et al. 2001). Second-generation antihistamines are kept out of the brain. Loperamide (Imodium A-D), an over-the-counter opiate antidiarrheal, is a P-glycoprotein substrate. It is normally transported out of the brain by P-glycoprotein and therefore has no central opiate effects. When this drug is given with quinidine (a P-glycoprotein inhibitor), loperamide concentrations in the brain increase, and signs of respiratory depression can ensue (Sadeque et al. 2000). Because drug clearance is not altered, there is no increase in systemic blood concentrations of the offending drug. The only clues to the existence of an interaction are CNS-related symptoms.

Because all human immunodeficiency virus (HIV) protease inhibitors are P-glycoprotein substrates, they may be kept out of the CNS (and the gonads and the fetus). It has been speculated that the ability of these drugs to achieve therapeutic CNS concentrations may therefore be limited by the P-glycoprotein system and that a potential sanctuary for viral replication may exist in the brain. HIV protease inhibitors are also P-glycoprotein substrates in the gut. Ritonavir (when taken initially) is a potent 3A4 and P-glycoprotein inhibitor. Combinations of protease inhibitors (e.g., lopinavir and low-dose ritonavir) have been formulated to produce an iatrogenic, therapeutic drug interaction (van Heeswijk et al. 2001). Another example is the experimental use of valspodar (SC 833), a P-glycoprotein inhibitor, with vincristine to reverse MDR (Bates et al. 2001). Whether P-glycoprotein inhibitors can reverse MDR but will inevitably cause systemic drug toxicity by also inhibiting the P-glycoprotein protection of normal cells is yet to be shown (Lin 2003).

Clearly, more study is needed to fully elucidate the role of P-glycoproteins in drug interactions. Since intestinal P-glycoprotein kinetics are "saturable," P-glycoproteins may play a part in drug interactions only when the concentration of the substrate drug is low (Lin 2003). Will drug interactions that occur in the intestine be found to be less significant than those that occur at the blood-brain barrier?

Many factors can alter P-glycoprotein function and influence P-glycoprotein-based interactions. Genetic differences of P-glycoproteins are known to exist, and more than 15 polymorphisms have been identified (Lin 2003). A polymorphism at exon 26 has been shown to influence the level of intestinal P-glycoprotein and concentration of digoxin (Lin 2003). This genotype has also been shown to be a risk factor for the side effect of orthostatic hypotension of the P-glycoprotein substrate nortriptyline (Roberts et al. 2002). There are racial differences of this polymorphism: 61% of African Americans and 26% of whites show this genotype (Kim et al. 2001; Schaeffeler et al. 2001). Women have about one-third fewer hepatic P-glycoproteins than men, which may account for more efficient metabolism of certain drugs by women (Cummins et al. 2000; Meibohm et al. 2002). Herbal supplements (e.g., St. John's wort) and even vitamins (certain formulations of vitamin E are P-glycoprotein inhibitors) can influence P-glycoproteins. Even foods can alter P-glycoprotein function; for example, black pepper (Bhardwaj et al. 2002), grapefruit juice, and Seville orange juice (Di Marco et al. 2002) are P-glycoprotein inhibitors. Hormones (e.g., levothyroxine [Siegmund et al. 2002]) can affect of P-glycoproteins as well.

Because P-glycoprotein-based drug interactions are a relatively new concept, well-substantiated reports of clinical interactions are relatively few, but they are beginning to accumulate. Although P-glycoproteins are the only transporters considered in this short review, many transporters exist in the intestine, the liver, and elsewhere (e.g., the organic anion transporting polypeptide). A list of intestinal transporters and their substrates, inducers, and inhibitors may be found at http://bigfoot.med.unc.edu/watkinsLab/intesinfo.htm.

■ REFERENCES

Bates S, Kang M, Meadows B, et al: A phase I study of infusional vinblastine in combination with the P-glycoprotein antagonist PSC 833 (valspodar). Cancer 92:1577–1590, 2001

Benet LZ, Cummins CL: The drug efflux-metabolism alliance: biochemical aspects. Adv Drug Deliv Rev 50 (suppl 1):S3–S11, 2001

Bhardwaj RK, Glaeser H, Becquemont L, et al: Piperine, a major constituent of black pepper, inhibits human P-glycoprotein and CYP3A4. J Pharmacol Exp Ther 302:64–50, 2002

Boyd RA, Stern RH, Stewart BH, et al: Atorvastatin coadmistration may increase digoxin concentrations by inhibition of intestinal P-glycoprotein-mediated secretion. J Clin Pharmacol 40:91–98, 2000

Chishty M, Reichel A, Siva J, et al: Affinity for the P-glycoprotein efflux pump at the blood-brain barrier may explain the lack of CNS side-effects of modern antihistamines. J Drug Target 9:223–228, 2001

Conrad S, Kauffmann HM, Ito K, et al: Identification of human multidrug resistance protein 1 (MRP1) mutations and characterization of a G671V substitution. J Hum Genet 46:656–663, 2001

Cummins CL, Wu CY, Benet LZ: Sex-related differences in the clearance of cytochrome P450 3A4 substrates may be caused by P-glycoprotein. Clin Pharmacol Ther 72:474–489, 2002

Di Marco MP, Edwards DJ, Wainer IW, et al: The effect of grapefruit juice and seville orange juice on the pharmacokinetics of dextromethorphan: the rule of gut CYP3A and P-glycoprotein. Life Sci 71:1149–1160, 2002

Doherty MM, Charman WN: The mucosa of the small intestine: how clinically relevant as an organ of drug metabolism? Clin Pharmacokinet 41:235–253, 2002

Durr D, Stieger B, Kullak-Ublick GA, et al: St John's wort induces intestinal P-glycoprotein/*MDR1* and intestinal and hepatic CYP3A4. Clin Pharmacol Ther 68:598–604, 2000

Ernst E: St John's wort supplements endanger the success of organ transplantation. Arch Surg 137:316–319, 2002

Fromm MF, Kim RB, Stein CM, et al: Inhibition of P-glycoprotein-mediated drug transport: a unifying mechanism to explain the interaction between digoxin and quinidine. Circulation 99:552–557, 1999

Greiner B, Eichelbaum M, Fritz P, et al: The role of intestinal P-glycoprotein in the interaction of digoxin and rifampin. J Clin Invest 104:147–153, 1999

Hennessy M, Kelleher D, Spiers JP, et al: St Johns wort increases expression of P-glycoprotein: implications for drug interactions. Br J Clin Pharmacol 53:75–82, 2002

Kim RB, Leake BF, Choo EF, et al: Identification of functionally variant *MDR1* alleles among European Americans and African Americans. Clin Pharmacol Ther 70:189–199, 2001

Klotz U: Interaction potential of lercanidipine, a new vasoselective dihydropyridine calcium antagonist. Arzneimittelforschung 52:155–161, 2002

Lin JH: Drug-drug interaction mediated by inhibition and induction of P-glycoprotein. Adv Drug Deliv Rev 55:53–81, 2003

Lin JH, Yamazaki M: Role of p-glycoprotein in pharmacokinetics: clinical implications. Clin Pharmacokinet 42:59–98, 2003

Meibohm B, Bererle I, Derendorf H: How important are gender differences in pharmacokinetics? Clin Pharmacokinet 41:329–342, 2002

Roberts RL, Joyce PR, Mulder RT, et al: A common P-glycoprotein polymorphism is associated with nortriptyline-induced postural hypotension in patients treated for major depression. Pharmacogenomics 2:191–196, 2002

Sadeque AJ, Wandel C, He H, et al: Increased drug delivery to the brain by P-glycoprotein inhibition. Clin Pharmacol Ther 68:231–237, 2000

Schaeffeler E, Eichelbaum M, Brinkmann U, et al: Frequency of C3435T polymorphism of *MDR1* gene in African people (letter). Lancet 358: 383–384, 2001

Siegmund W, Altmannsberger S, Paneitz A, et al: Effect of levothyroxine administration on intestinal P-glycoprotein expression: consequences for drug disposition. Clin Pharmacol Ther 72:256–264, 2002

Su SF, Huang JD: Inhibition of the intestinal digoxin absorption and exsorption by quinidine. Drug Metab Dispos 24:142–147, 1996 van Heeswijk RP, Veldkamp A, Mulder JW, et al: Combination of protease inhibitors for the treatment of HIV-1-infected patients: a review of pharmacokinetics and clinical experience. Antivir Ther 6:201–229, 2001

Verschraagen M, Koks CH, Schellens JH, et al: P-glycoprotein system as a determinant of drug interactions: the case of digoxin-verapamil. Pharmacol Res 40:301–306, 1999

Wacher VJ, Wu CY, Benet LZ: Overlapping substrate specificities and tissue distribution of cytochrome P450 3A and P-glycoprotein: implications for drug delivery and activity in cancer chemotherapy. Mol Carcinog 13:129–134, 1995

Wakasugi H, Yano I, Ito T, et al: Effect of clarithromycin on renal excretion of digoxin: interaction with P-glycoprotein. Clin Pharmacol Ther 64: 123–128, 1998

Wilkinson GR: Pharmacokinetics: the dynamics of drug absorption, distribution, and elimination, in Goodman & Gilman's The Pharmacological Basis of Therapeutics, 10th Edition. Edited by Hardman JG, Limbird LE, Gilman AG. New York, McGraw-Hill, 2001, pp 3–29

Woodland C, Verjee Z, Giesbrecht E, et al: The digoxin-propafenone interaction: characterization of a mechanism using renal tubular cell monolayers. J Pharmacol Exp Ther 283:39–45, 1997

Part II

P450 Enzymes

5

2D6

2D6 is discussed first in reviews of the P450 enzymes because of its historical role in the development of an understanding of drug interactions. In 1988, Vaughan noted very high serum levels of desipramine and nortriptyline when fluoxetine was concomitantly administered. More reports followed Vaughan's report on two cases, and by 1990 the P450 system was recognized as being responsible for this potentially dangerous interaction (von Ammon Cavanaugh 1990). In 1991, Muller et al. identified 2D6 as the enzyme that fluoxetine inhibits, and Skjelbo and Brosen (1992) confirmed this finding the following year. In the early 1990s, 2D6 was the most studied of the hepatic enzymes. However, the other P450 enzymes and phase II enzymes have since caught up with 2D6 in terms of amount of research. Nevertheless, 2D6 is an important metabolic enzyme for many drugs.

■ WHAT DOES 2D6 DO?

Located in the endoplasmic reticulum, 2D6 is involved in phase I metabolism of endogenous and exogenous compounds. Through oxidative metabolism, it hydroxylates, demethylates, or dealkylates these compounds; the actual oxidative reaction depends on the compound. Examples of 2D6's diverse oxidative reactions include hydroxylation of tricyclic antidepressants (Sawada and Ohtani 2001), fluoxetine's N-demethylation to norfluoxetine (Fjordside et al. 1999), and N-dealkylation of metoclopramide (Desta et al. 2002). 2D6 is involved in metabolism of endogenous chemicals as well, such as central nervous system hydroxylation of progesterone (Hiroi et al. 2001).

2D6 activity does not appear to change with age (Shulman and Ozdemir 1997); however, 2D6 activity may appear to be altered because of age-associated changes in hepatic blood flow or a decrease in renal elimination of metabolites. Premenopausal women may have a slight increase in 2D6 activity compared with men (Hagg et al. 2001).

For many medications, particularly psychotropic medications, 2D6 is considered a low-capacity, high-affinity enzyme. It accounts for only a small percentage of liver P450 content but appears to clear oxidatively more than its share of exogenous compounds. As a low-capacity, high-affinity enzyme, 2D6 will preferentially metabolize drugs at lower concentrations. As the concentration of a drug increases, the metabolism spills over to 3A4 or 1A2, which are high-capacity, low-affinity enzymes (Olesen and Linnet 1997). Thus, if a drug that has several metabolic pathways but relies on 2D6 as its major pathway is given to a patient with poor 2D6 activity (see "Does 2D6 Have Any Polymorphisms"), the other P450 enzymes that are high capacity, low affinity will clear the drug, but the drug's clearance will likely be slower and less efficient, and levels will increase.

■ WHERE DOES 2D6 DO ITS WORK?

2D6 is found in many tissues, including the brain (Hiroi et al. 2001), the prostate (Finnstrom et al. 2001), bone marrow (Hodges et al. 2000), and the heart (Thum and Borlak 2000). Although metabolism of drugs may occur at these sites, 2D6 plays its role in drug metabolism primarily in the liver. 2D6 actually makes up only 1.5% of the total P450 content in the liver, the smallest percentage with regard to the major drug-metabolizing P450 enzymes in humans. Nevertheless, 2D6 is a very active primary or secondary participant in the metabolism of many drugs.

■ DOES 2D6 HAVE ANY POLYMORPHISMS?

The fact that 2D6 is polymorphic has been known for years (Vesell et al. 1971). In the 1980s, 2D6 was named in relation to its probes (drugs metabolized—often exclusively—by the enzyme, resulting in a measurable and reliable metabolite); it was called the debrisoquin/sparteine enzyme (Eichelbaum 1986). By 1990, its polymorphic character was well recognized, and 2D6 was given its current name (Lennard 1990).

Clinically, the polymorphic expressions of the 2D6 alleles are important to remember about this enzyme. The 2D6 gene is located on chromosome 22 (see the *PubMed LocusLink* review at http://www.ncbi.nlm.nih.gov/LocusLink/LocRpt.cgi?l=1565). Numerous polymorphisms of 2D6 exist; Alam and Sharma (2001) reported more than 30 human alleles. The alterations of alleles in the wild type fall into six categories: one amino acid change or deletion, frameshift, splicing defect, stop codon, insertion, and entire gene deletion. From these polymorphic alleles, the following genotypes can be distinguished: homozygous or heterozygous extensive ("normal") metabolizers (EMs); homozygous poor metabolizers (PMs); and ultraextensive metabolizers (UEMs), who have duplicate or multiple copies of the *2D6* gene (DeVane and Nemeroff 2002). There are ethnic differences in the distribution of EMs, PMs, and UEMs. PMs are reported to make up 5%–14% of Caucasian populations (Daly et al. 1996; de Leon et al. 1998). A recent review indicated that Asians, Pacific Islanders, Africans, and African Americans have a higher percentage of reduced-function or nonfunctional 2D6 alleles (between 40% and 50%) than do Caucasians (26%) (Bradford 2002); therefore, the percentages of PMs in the former groups are most likely higher. Previous reports indicated a lower incidence of PMs in these groups (Belpaire and Bogaert 1996). UEMs are generally rare, representing 1%–3% of the population (Eichelbaum and Evert 1996).

Any drug that is primarily metabolized by 2D6 and ingested by a PM will have a delayed metabolism. The PM will accumulate the parent drug and incur the risk of enhanced side effects. The drug may be secondarily metabolized by another P450 enzyme that is higher in capacity but that has a lower affinity for the drug or substrate. Often, the alternative enzyme is 3A4. This shifting to a less efficient enzyme leads PMs to have higher drug levels of the parent compound.

PMs usually require lower doses to achieve desired effects. In most clinical situations, patients are not identified as PMs at 2D6. When a drug dependent on 2D6 is given to a PM, the untoward effects are likely assumed to be due to an unknown drug interaction or some other idiosyncratic reaction. Treatment with the poorly tolerated (and metabolized) drug may be abandoned. However, many drugs can be given to a 2D6 PM; the clinician need only decrease the dose. Not anticipating that patients may be PMs is potentially dangerous. For example, the action of some antiarrhythmics depends on 2D6 metabolism. If a patient lacks 2D6 activity, severe toxicity may occur if an antiarrhythmic such as encainide is prescribed (Funck-Brentano et al. 1992).

A drug may be less effective for a PM at 2D6 as well, particularly if the drug needs to be activated at 2D6. For example, tramadol is O-demethylated by 2D6 to an active analgesic, racemic M1. Higher levels of M1 were associated with better ongoing pain control in patients with polyneuropathy (Sindrup et al. 1999). In a pain model study, Poulsen et al. (1996) demonstrated that PMs at 2D6 had poorer analgesia and lower levels of (+)-M1 (see "Codeine" in Chapter 18 ["Pain Management II: Narcotic Analgesics"] for more details). Although tramadol's analgesia is thought to be due to other mechanisms as well as to the (+)-M1's μ receptor activity, a clinician might repeatedly increase the dose of tramadol in an attempt to achieve the desired effect in a PM, with possibly poor results—leaving the patient and the clinician frustrated.

Risperidone is metabolized by 2D6 to its active 9-hydroxy metabolite. In PMs at 2D6, the drug is primarily metabolized by 3A4. Evidence suggests that PMs at 2D6 have a poorer tolerance of side effects and higher drug levels, even though the 3A4 route is available (Bork et al. 1999).

In an effort to reduce the number of ineffective therapies and dangerous outcomes due to 2D6 interactions, detection of PMs at 2D6 may soon become a routine part of medical practice. Chou et al. (2000) studied 100 psychiatric inpatients in relation to their 2D6 genotypes and clinical outcomes. They found that PMs (12% of the study group) had more adverse medication effects and longer, more expensive hospital stays. Andreassen et al. (1997) found that PMs were more likely to develop tardive dyskinesia over 11 years while exposed to antipsychotics. Similarly, Ellingrod et al. (2000) showed that heterozygotes for 2D6 (with wild type/mutation) were at higher risk of developing movement disorders when exposed to antipsychotics compared with homozygotes for 2D6 (wild type/wild type). Finally, Schillevoort et al. (2002) demonstrated that when being treated with 2D6-dependent antipsychotic drugs (see the table entitled "Drugs Metabolized by 2D6," at the end of this chapter), PMs were four times more likely to use antiparkinsonian medications than were EMs—and this was not the case among patients using non-2D6-dependent antipsychotics.

Given these study findings, it would seem prudent for clinicians to consider genotype testing of 2D6 before instituting drug therapy. However, this approach is rarely taken, despite the fact that testing is relatively inexpensive. A simpler method is to first administer a drug (probe) primarily metabolized by 2D6 and then look for specific 2D6 metabolites. Dextromethorphan, the over-the-counter cough remedy, is one such drug; debrisoquin and sparteine are two others. Once a patient is given a fixed single dose of dextromethorphan, the clinician can determine whether 2D6 activity is present by measuring dextrorphan, the active metabolite specific to 2D6 (created by 2D6's O-demethylation of dextromethorphan), in the blood or urine (Schadel et al. 1995). The cost of this test is approximately $100. An even simpler method is to ask a patient if he or she has ever had a bad reaction to dextromethorphan! In the near future, a more likely way to determine a patient's 2D6 genotype will be through the use of microarray chip technology (de Longueville et al. 2002). With this technology, it may be possible to check not only 2D6 alleles but also perhaps all known P450 and other metabolic enzyme alleles, using just a drop of blood or saliva.

■ WHAT DRUGS SIGNIFICANTLY INHIBIT 2D6 ACTIVITY?

Selective Serotonin Reuptake Inhibitors

Fluoxetine

Fluoxetine is the best-known inhibitor of 2D6, and it was the first drug discovered to have clinically relevant P450 inhibition (Vaughan 1988). Fluoxetine is a 50/50 racemic mix. Both the *R* and *S* forms are substrates of 2D6 and are metabolized to the active and racemic-mix metabolites *R/S*-norfluoxetine. Other P450 enzymes are involved in fluoxetine's metabolism as well—particularly 2C9, which de-methylates fluoxetine and which fluoxetine also potently inhibits (von Moltke et al. 1997).

In PMs at 2D6, fluoxetine and norfluoxetine have roughly the same clinical effectiveness because of alternative metabolism at 2C9. In addition, the *S*-isomer of norfluoxetine is a potent selective serotonin reuptake inhibitor (SSRI) itself, whereas *R*-norfluoxetine is not. Therefore, PMs will have less active metabolite (*S*-norfluoxetine) but more active parent compound—with the result that the process is essentially equaled out (Prozac 2001).

Fluoxetine and norfluoxetine have extremely long half-lives. The advantage to this is that daily dosing is not necessary: indeed, weekly dosing is available for fluoxetine, since the half-life of chronically administered fluoxetine is 4–6 days and the half-life of norfluoxetine is 4–16 days. The disadvantage, of course, is that if fluoxetine is added to a regimen with another drug that is dependent on 2D6 activity for clearance, inhibition of the second drug's metabolism will continue to be impaired for 4–8 weeks after fluoxetine therapy is discontinued.

Fluoxetine and its metabolite, norfluoxetine, are very potent inhibitors of 2D6, with Ki values between 0.22 and 1.48 μM (Stevens and Wrighton 1993). In vivo studies have shown fluoxetine to significantly inhibit the metabolism of clozapine, desipramine, imipramine, and thioridazine—primarily through inhibition of 2D6 and possibly also through moderate inhibition of 3A4 and other enzymes. Multiple case studies have demonstrated that numerous other drugs (benztropine, clomipramine, dextromethorphan, fluphenazine, haloperidol, nortriptyline, perphenazine, propranolol, risperidone, and trazodone) have increased levels or side effects due to fluoxetine's 2D6 inhibition. Many of these drugs have narrow therapeutic indexes and/or margins of safety. For example, because fluoxetine inhibits the metabolism of thioridazine and mesoridazine, there is the risk of lengthening the QTc interval and causing torsades de pointes. Therefore, both thioridazine and mesoridazine are contraindicated during fluoxetine therapy—and a lengthy wash-out period for fluoxetine is indicated before administration of these antipsychotics can be started (Armstrong and Cozza 2001).

Monoamine oxidase inhibitors are also contraindicated during treatment with fluoxetine (and other SSRIs) because of the risk of a pharmacodynamic drug-drug interaction (serotonin syndrome) that is potentially lethal.

Paroxetine

Paroxetine is as potent an inhibitor of 2D6 as fluoxetine, having a Ki of 2.0 μM (von Moltke et al. 1995). Unlike fluoxetine, paroxetine does not have a long half-life (21 hours), does not have active metabolites, and does not significantly inhibit other P450 enzymes other than 2C9 (Paxil 2001) and possibly 2B6. Its oxidative metabolism is accomplished mainly by 2D6, with subsequent phase II glucuronidation and sulfation. Because of paroxetine's potent inhibition of 2D6, the manufacturer recommends caution when it is used with drugs metabolized by 2D6—certain antidepressants (e.g., nortriptyline, amitriptyline, imipramine, and desipramine), phenothiazines, and Type IC antiarrhythmics (e.g., propafenone, flecainide, and encainide). Like fluoxetine, it is contraindicated with thioridazine and mesoridazine therapy.

Sertraline

In vitro studies (Hemeryck et al. 2000) indicate that sertraline's inhibition of 2D6 is less potent than that of fluoxetine, norfluoxetine, and paroxetine. However, clinically significant inhibition of 2D6 by sertraline may be dose related (Sproule et al. 1997). For example, 50 mg of sertraline (a low dose) increased nortriptyline (dependent on 2D6 for clearance) levels only 2% in 14 elderly depressed patients (Solai et al. 1997). Interestingly, in 7 patients given sertraline at a dosage of 100–150 mg/day, nortriptyline levels increased an average of 40%—with a range of 12% to 239%. We believe that the higher dose ranges of sertraline (>150 mg/day) lead to clinically significant 2D6 inhibition.

Other Antidepressants

Bupropion

Bupropion is metabolized predominantly at 2B6, a minor metabolic P450 enzyme (see Chapter 11 ["Other Relevant P450 Enzymes"]). In addition, bupropion has many alternative sites of metabolism, including 1A2, 2A6, 2C9, 2E1, and 3A4 (Wellbutrin 2001). This plethora of metabolic sites makes inhibition of bupropion metabolism nearly impossible, and we are unaware of any clinical data supporting the concern that potent inhibitors of 3A4 or other P450 enzymes could increase bupropion levels to the point of causing seizures.

The manufacturer provided data from a study of 15 healthy volunteers with normal 2D6 activity in whom 150 mg of Wellbutrin SR twice a day significantly increased the maximum drug concentration, area under the curve, and half-life of a single dose of desipramine (50 mg) (Wellbutrin 2001). The manufacturer recommends that treatment with drugs that are predominantly metabolized by 2D6 and that have narrow therapeutic windows (nortriptyline, desipramine, imipramine, β-blockers, type IC antiarrhythmics, and the potentially arrhythmogenic antipsychotics haloperidol, risperidone, and thioridazine) be initiated at lower doses in patients receiving bupropion.

Other Medications

Cimetidine

Cimetidine appears to be a potent and indiscriminate inhibitor of several enzymes, including 2D6, 3A4, and 1A2 (Martinez et al.

1999) Other histamine, subtype 2 (H_2), receptor blockers, such as ranitidine, are not as problematic (see Chapter 13 ["Internal Medicine"]). Multiple case reports indicate that cimetidine increases tricyclic levels; in one study, it increased imipramine's half-life from 10.8 to 22.7 hours (Wells et al. 1986). Cimetidine has been found to increase serum paroxetine levels by 50% (Greb et al. 1989).

Quinidine

Quinidine is a commonly used antimalarial drug and class IA antiarrhythmic agent. It is the *d*-isomer of quinine and a very potent inhibitor of 2D6, with a reported Ki of 0.053 μM (von Moltke et al. 1994). It is metabolized by 3A4 preferentially, and PMs at 2D6 will clear the drug adequately (Quinaglute 1999). Quinine is also an inhibitor of 2D6 (Hiroi et al. 1995). The manufacturer does advise caution during administration with drugs dependent on 2D6 for clearance.

Ritonavir

Ritonavir is a human immunodeficiency virus (HIV) protease inhibitor. It is a P450 inhibitor of 2D6, with a Ki of 0.16 μM (von Moltke et al. 1998a). It also seems to be a "pan-inhibitor," significantly inhibiting 3A4, 2C9, and 2C19, but not 1A2 or 2E1 (von Moltke et al. 1998b). The manufacturer of Norvir (ritonavir) indicates that a single 100-mg dose of desipramine used with ritonavir increases the desipramine's area under the curve by 145% (Norvir 2000). Because of ritonavir's 2D6 inhibition, the manufacturer contraindicates its use with most antiarrhythmics. Caution is also suggested with concomitant administration of tricyclics or antipsychotics with ritonavir (see section on antiretrovirals in Chapter 14: "Infectious Diseases").

Terbinafine

Terbinafine, an antifungal agent available in topical and oral forms, is an inhibitor of 2D6, with a Ki ranging from 22 to 44 μM (Abdel-

Rahman et al. 1999). The findings of Abdel-Rahman et al. (1999) suggest that terbinafine is not a potent 2D6 inhibitor, but recent cases of severe toxicity due to excessive levels of tricyclics have been reported with terbinafine given in conjunction with imipramine (Teitelbaum and Pearson 2001) and nortriptyline (van der Kuy and Hooymans 1998) (see section on antifungals in Chapter 14: "Infectious Diseases").

Other Possible Potent Inhibitors

Ticlopidine is an antiplatelet agent known to be a potent 2C19 inhibitor (see Chapter 9 ["2C19"]). Ko et al. (2000) demonstrated that ticlopidine is also a fairly strong inhibitor of 2D6, having a Ki of 3.4 μM during in vitro tests with human liver microsomes. Pimozide is metabolized primarily by 3A4 and to a lesser extent by 1A2. In vitro tests with human liver microsomes revealed that pimozide may inhibit 2D6 potently, with a Ki of approximately 1.0 μM (Desta et al. 1998). Fluvoxamine is generally thought to be a potent inhibitor of 1A2, 2C9, 2C19, and possibly 2B6. However, an in vitro study by Olesen and Linnet (2000) showed fluvoxamine's Ki for 2D6 to be fairly low (4.9 μM). This may be significant, given that serum fluvoxamine levels normally range from 4 to 7 μM in therapeutic conditions.

■ ARE THERE DRUGS THAT INDUCE 2D6 ACTIVITY?

It is unclear whether 2D6 is inducible. Using 10-hydroxylation of nortriptyline as a probe for 2D6 activity, von Bahr et al. (1998) found that pentobarbital appears to induce other P450 enzymes but not 2D6. However, there is some evidence that phenobarbital and smoking may decrease serum concentrations of 2D6 substrates. It is unclear whether this decrease is due to induction or to other mechanisms.

■ REFERENCES

Abdel-Rahman SM, Marcucci K, Boge T, et al: Potent inhibition of cytochrome P-450 2D6-mediated dextromethorphan O-demethylation by terbinafine. Drug Metab Dispos 27:770–775, 1999

Alam DA, Sharma RP: Cytochrome enzyme genotype and the prediction of therapeutic response to psychotropics. Psychiatric Annals 31:715–722, 2001

Andreassen OA, MacEwan T, Gulbrandsen AK et al: Non-functional CYP2D6 alleles and risk for neuroleptic-induced movement disorders in schizophrenic patients. Psychopharmacology (Berl) 131:174–179, 1997

Armstrong SC, Cozza KL: Consultation-liaison psychiatry drug-drug interactions update. Psychosomatics 42:157–159, 2001

Belpaire FM, Bogaert MG: Cytochrome P450: genetic polymorphism and drug interactions. Acta Clin Belg 51:254–260, 1996

Bork JA, Rogers T, Wedlund PJ, et al: A pilot study on risperidone metabolism: the roles of cytochromes P450 2D6 and 3A. J Clin Psychiatry 60:469–476, 1999

Bradford LD: CYP2D6 allele frequency in European Caucasians, Asians, Africans and their descendants. Pharmacogenomics 3:229–243, 2002

Caccia S: Metabolism of the new antidepressants: an overview of the pharmacological and pharmacokinetic implications. Clin Pharmacokinet 34:281–302, 1998

Chou WH, Yan FX, de Leon J, et al: Extension of a pilot study: impact from the cytochrome P450 2D6 polymorphism on outcome and costs associated with severe mental illness. J Clin Psychopharmacol 20:246–251, 2000

Daly AK, Brockmoller J, Broly F, et al: Nomenclature for human CYP2D6 alleles. Pharmacogenetics 6:193–201, 1996

de Leon J, Barnhill J, Rogers T, et al: Pilot study of cytochrome P450-2D6 genotype in a psychiatric hospital. Am J Psychiatry 155:1278–1280, 1998

de Longueville F, Surray D, Meneses-Lorente G, et al: Gene expression profiling of drug metabolism and toxicology markers using a low-density DNA microarray. Biochem Pharmacol 64:137–149, 2002

Desta Z, Kerbusch T, Soukhova N, et al: Identification and characterization of human cytochrome P450 isoforms interacting with pimozide. J Pharmacol Exp Ther 285:428–437, 1998

Desta Z, Wu GM, Morocho AM, et al: The gastroprokinetic and antiemetic drug metoclopramide is a substrate and inhibitor for cytochrome P450 2D6. Drug Metab Dispos 30:336–343, 2002

DeVane CL, Nemeroff CB: 2002 guide to psychotropic drug interactions. Primary Psychiatry 9:28–57, 2002

Eichelbaum M: Polymorphic oxidation of debrisoquine and sparteine. Prog Clin Biol Res 214:157–167, 1986

Eichelbaum M, Evert B: Influence of pharmacogenetics on drug disposition and response. Clin Exp Pharmacol Physiol 23:983–985, 1996

Ellingrod VL, Schultz SK, Arndt S: Association between cytochrome P4502D6 (CYP2D6) genotype, antipsychotic exposure, and abnormal involuntary movement scale (AIMS) score. Psychiatr Genet 10:9–11, 2000

Ereshefsky L: Pharmacokinetics and drug interactions: update for newer antipsychotics. J Clin Psychiatry 57 (suppl 11):12–25, 1997

Finnstrom N, Bjelfman C, Soderstrom TG, et al: Detection of cytochrome P450 mRNA transcripts in prostate samples by RT-PCR. Eur J Invest 31:880–886, 2001

Fjordside L, Jeppesen U, Eap CB, et al: The stereoselective metabolism of fluoxetine in poor and extensive metabolizers of sparteine. Pharmacogenetics 9:55–60, 1999

Funck-Brentano C, Thomas G, Jacqz-Aigrain E, et al: Polymorphism of dextromethorphan metabolism: relationships between phenotype, genotype and response to the administration of encainide in humans. J Pharmacol Exp Ther 263:780–786, 1992

Gillen C, Haurand M, Kobelt DJ, et al: Affinity, potency, and efficacy of tramadol and its metabolites at the cloned human mu-opioid receptor. Naunyn Schmiedebergs Arch Pharmacol 362:116–121, 2000

Greb WH, Buscher G, Dierdorf HD, et al: The effect of liver enzyme inhibition by cimetidine and enzyme induction by phenobarbitone on the pharmacokinetics of paroxetine. Acta Psychiatr Scand Suppl 350:95–98, 1989

Greenblatt DJ, von Moltke LL, Harmatz JS, et al: Drug interactions with newer antidepressants: role of human cytochromes P450. J Clin Psychiatry 59 (suppl 15):19–27, 1998

Hagg S, Spigset O, Dahlqvist R: Influence of gender and oral contraceptives on CYP2D6 and CYP2C19 activity in healthy volunteers. Br J Pharmacol 51:169–173, 2001

Hemeryck A, De Vriendt C, Belpaire FM: Effect of selective serotonin re-uptake inhibitors on the oxidative metabolism of propafenone in in vitro studies using human liver microsomes. J Clin Psychopharmacol 20: 428–434, 2000

Hiroi T, Ohishi N, Imaoka S, et al: Mepyramine, a histamine H_1 receptor antagonist, inhibits the metabolic activity of rat and human P450 2D forms. J Pharmacol Exp Ther 272:939–944, 1995

Hiroi T, Kishimoto W, Chow T, et al: Progesterone oxidation by cytochrome P450 2D isoforms in the brain. Endocrinology 142:3901–3908, 2001

Hodges VM, Molloy GY, Wickramasinghe SN: Demonstration of mRNA for five species of cytochrome P450 in human bone marrow, bone marrow-derived macrophages and human haemopoietic cell lines. Br J Haematol 108:151–156, 2000

Ko JW, Desta Z, Soukhova NV, et al: In vitro inhibition of the cytochrome P450 (CYP) system by the antiplatelet drug ticlopidine: potent effect on CYP2C19 and CYP2D6. Br J Clin Pharmacol 49:343–351, 2000

Lennard MS: Genetic polymorphism of sparteine/debrisoquine oxidation: a reappraisal. Pharmacol Toxicol 67:273–283, 1990

Martinez C, Albet C, Agundez JA, et al: Comparative in vitro and in vivo inhibition of cytochrome P450 CYP1A2, CYP2D6, and CYP3A by H_2-receptor antagonists. Clin Pharmacol Ther 65:369–376, 1999

Muller N, Brockmoller J, Roots I: Extremely long plasma half-life of ami-triptyline in a woman with the cytochrome P450IID6 29/29-kilobase wild-type allele—a slowly reversible interaction with fluoxetine. Ther Drug Monit 13:533–536, 1991

Norvir (package insert). North Chicago, IL, Abbott Laboratories, 2000

Olesen OV, Linnet K: Hydroxylation and demethylation of the tricyclic antidepressant nortriptyline by cDNA-expressed human cytochrome P-450 isozymes. Drug Metab Dispos 25:740–744, 1997

Olesen OV, Linnet K: Fluvoxamine-clozapine drug interaction: inhibition in vitro of five cytochrome P450 isoforms involved in clozapine metabolism. J Clin Psychopharmacol 20:35–42, 2000

Paxil (package insert). Research Triangle, NC, GlaxoSmithKline, 2001

Poulsen L, Arendt-Nielsen L, Brosen K: The hypoalgesic effect of tramadol in relation to CYP2D6. Clin Pharmacol Ther 60:636–644, 1996

Prozac (package insert). Indianapolis, IN, Eli Lilly & Co, 2001

Quinaglute (package insert). Wayne, NJ, Berlex Laboratories, 1999

Sawada Y, Ohtani H: Pharmacokinetics and drug interactions of antidepressant agents (in Japanese). Nippon Rinsho 59:1539–1545, 2001

Schadel M, Wu D, Otton SV, et al: Pharmacokinetics of dextromethorphan and metabolites in humans: influence of the CYP2D6 phenotype and quinidine inhibition. J Clin Psychopharmacol 15:263–269, 1995

Schillevoort I, de Boer A, van der Weide J, et al: Antipsychotic-induced extrapyramidal syndromes and cytochrome P450 2D6 genotype: a case controlled study. Pharmacogenetics 12:235–240, 2002

Shulman RW, Ozdemir V: Psychotropic medications and cytochrome P450 2D6: pharmacologic considerations in the elderly. Can J Psychiatry 42 (suppl 1):4S–9S, 1997

Sindrup SH, Madsen C, Brosen K, et al: The effect of tramadol in painful polyneuropathy in relation to serum drug and metabolite levels. Clin Pharmacol Ther 66:636–641, 1999

Skjelbo E, Brosen K: Inhibitors of imipramine metabolism by human liver microsomes. Br J Clin Pharmacol 34:256–261, 1992

Solai LK, Mulsant BH, Pollock BG, et al: Effect of sertraline on plasma nortriptyline levels in depressed elderly. J Clin Psychiatry 58:440–443, 1997

Sroule BA, Otton SV, Cheung SW, et al: CYP2D6 inhibition in patients treated with sertraline. J Clin Psychopharmacol 17:102–106, 1997

Stevens JC, Wrighton SA: Interaction of the enantiomers of fluoxetine and norfluoxetine with the human liver cytochromes P450. J Pharmacol Exp Ther 266:964–971, 1993

Teitelbaum ML, Pearson VE: Imipramine toxicity and terbinafine (letter). Am J Psychiatry 158:2086, 2001

Thum T, Borlak J: Gene expression in distinct regions of the heart. Lancet 355:979–983, 2000

van der Kuy PH, Hooymans PM: Nortriptyline intoxication induced by terfenadine. BMJ 316:441, 1998

Vaughan DA: Interaction of fluoxetine with tricyclic antidepressants (letter). Am J Psychiatry 145:1478, 1988

Vesell ES, Passananti GT, Greene FE, et al: Genetic control of drug levels and of the induction of drug-metabolizing enzymes in man: individual variability in the extent of allopurinol and nortriptyline inhibition of drug metabolism. Ann N Y Acad Sci 179:752–773, 1971

von Ammon Cavanaugh S: Drug-drug interactions of fluoxetine with tricyclics. Psychosomatics 31:273–276, 1990

von Bahr C, Steiner E, Koike Y, et al: Time course of enzyme induction in humans: effect of pentobarbital on nortriptyline metabolism. Clin Pharmacol Ther 64:18–26, 1998 von Moltke LL, Greenblatt DJ, Cotreau-Bibbo MM, et al: Inhibition of desipramine hydroxylation in vitro by serotonin-reuptake-inhibitor antidepressants, and by quinidine and ketoconazole: a model system to predict drug interactions in vivo. J Pharmacol Exp Ther 268:1278–1283, 1994

von Moltke LL, Greenblatt DJ, Court MH: Inhibition of alprazolam and desipramine hydroxylation in vitro by paroxetine and fluvoxamine: comparison with other selective serotonin reuptake inhibitor antidepressants. J Clin Psychopharmacol 15:125–131, 1995

von Moltke LL, Greenblatt DJ, Duan SX, et al: Human cytochromes mediating N-demethylation of fluoxetine in vitro. Psychopharmacology (Berl) 132:402–407, 1997

von Moltke LL, Greenblatt DJ, Duan SX, et al: Inhibition of desipramine hydroxylation (cytochrome P450-2D6) in vitro by quinidine and by viral protease inhibitors: relation to drug interactions in vivo. J Pharm Sci 87: 1184–1189, 1998a

von Moltke LL, Greenblatt DJ, Grassi JM, et al: Protease inhibitors as inhibitors of human cytochromes P450: high risk associated with ritonavir. J Clin Pharmacol 38:106–111, 1998b

Wellbutrin (package insert). Research Triangle, NC, GlaxoSmithKline, 2001

Wells BG, Pieper JA, Self TH: The effect of ranitidine and cimetidine on imipramine disposition. Eur J Pharmacol 31:285–290, 1986

■ STUDY CASES

Case 1

A 37-year-old Caucasian man who had tested positive for HIV was severely depressed and began nortriptyline therapy. He improved clinically at a dosage of 75 mg/day, and the serum tricyclic level was 87 ng/mL (therapeutic range, 50–150 ng/mL). His infectious disease physician prescribed ritonavir and saquinavir. The psychiatrist was notified about the new medication and told the patient to obtain a tricyclic level measurement 5–7 days after initiation of treatment with ritonavir and saquinavir. The patient did so and returned complaining of increasing depressive symptoms. His serum tricyclic level was 203 ng/mL.

Comment

2D6 (and 3A4) inhibition: The psychiatrist and infectious disease physician correctly anticipated that ritonavir and saquinavir might increase tricyclic levels. Indeed, the tricyclic level increased beyond the therapeutic range, which may have reduced nortriptyline's effectiveness. The presumed mechanism for this interaction is ritonavir's potent inhibition of several P450 enzymes, including 2D6, 3A4, 2C9, and 2C19. Nortriptyline is metabolized primarily by 2D6, with 3A4 as a secondary route.

References

Tseng AL, Foisy MM: Management of drug interactions in patients with HIV. Ann Pharmacother 31:1040–1058, 1997
Venkatakrishnan K, von Moltke LL, Greenblatt DJ: Nortriptyline E-10-hydroxylation in vitro is mediated by human CYP2D6 (high affinity) and CYP3A4 (low affinity): implications for interactions with enzyme-inducing drugs. J Clin Pharmacol 39:567–577, 1999

Case 2

A 17-year-old Caucasian boy with bipolar disorder, a seizure disorder, and mild mental retardation was taking haloperidol (5 mg/day), valproic acid (1,750 mg/day), benztropine (4 mg/day), gabapentin (300 mg/day), and buspirone (10 mg/day). Paroxetine therapy (20 mg/day) was started because of depressive symptoms. On the eighth day of paroxetine therapy, the patient reported that he had a dry mouth and nausea; was disoriented to time, disorganized, forgetful, and lethargic; and had slurred speech. Vital signs were unremarkable, and he exhibited no extrapyramidal symptoms. Pupils were dilated and sluggish to respond. Treatment with paroxetine, haloperidol, benztropine, and valproic acid was discontinued. Serum levels were as follows: valproic acid, 119 µg/mL (previous levels, 103–105 µg/mL); haloperidol, 2.9 ng/mL (therapeutic range, 5–12 ng/mL); and gabapentin, 4.1 µg/mL (therapeutic range, 4–16 µg/mL). His serum benztropine level was 35.9 ng/mL; levels greater than 25 ng/mL are considered toxic. Two days after discontinuation of the medications, the patient reported feeling better. He resumed treatment with haloperidol and valproic acid without incident.

Comment

2D6 inhibition: Benztropine is an older drug whose metabolism has not been well characterized. Seven cases in the literature indicate that SSRIs may interact with benztropine because of inhibition of benztropine metabolism. Because fluoxetine, paroxetine, and sertraline inhibit 2D6, it is hypothesized that benztropine is at least in part metabolized by 2D6. We suggest that in this case, paroxetine's inhibition increased serum benztropine levels, causing a mild anticholinergic delirium.

References

Armstrong SC, Schweitzer SM: Delirium associated with paroxetine and benztropine combination. Am J Psychiatry 154:581–582, 1997

Byerly MJ, Christensen RC, Evans OL: Delirium associated with a combination of sertraline, haloperidol and benztropine. Am J Psychiatry 153:965–966, 1996

Roth A, Akyol S, Nelson JC: Delirium associated with a combination of a neuroleptic, an SSRI and benztropine. J Clin Psychiatry 55:492–495, 1994

Case 3

A 29-year-old man with major depression was treated with paroxetine 40 mg/day. Because of partial efficacy, desipramine 100 mg/day was added. The patient developed signs of delirium. The trough blood level of desipramine was greater than 400 ng/mL.

Comment

2D6 inhibition: Paroxetine inhibits 2D6, which desipramine uses for its clearance. Tricyclics do have alternative pathways, but this reaction is common. Similarly, in a PM at 2D6, one would expect lower doses of desipramine to achieve therapeutic levels.

References

Alderman J, Preskorn SH, Greenblatt DJ, et al: Desipramine pharmacokinetics when coadministered with paroxetine or sertraline in extensive metabolizers. J Clin Psychopharmacol 17:284–291, 1997

Brosen K, Hansen JG, Nielsen KK, et al: Inhibition by paroxetine of desipramine metabolism in extensive but not in poor metabolizers of sparteine. Eur J Clin Pharmacol 44:349–355, 1993

Case 4

A 17-year-old boy with schizophrenia experienced severe extrapyramidal side effects when administered risperidone 4 mg/day. Genotyping indicated he was a PM at 2D6, raising his serum levels of risperidone and 9-hydroxyrisperidone.

Comment

PM at 2D6: Often clinicians are more concerned about severe adverse drug reactions in a PM at 2D6, but in this case, determining the patient's genotype helped explain his sensitivity to risperidone. The clinician then chose an antipsychotic not predominantly cleared by 2D6. Olanzapine, quetiapine, and ziprasidone are three atypical antipsychotics that are not dependent on 2D6 for metabolism.

References

Bork JA, Rogers T, Wedlund PJ, et al: A pilot study on risperidone metabolism: the roles of cytochromes P450 2D6 and 3A. J Clin Psychiatry 60: 469–476, 1999

Kohnke MD, Griese EU, Stosser D, et al: Cytochrome P450 2D6 deficiency and its clinical relevance in a patient treated with risperidone. Pharmacopsychiatry 35:116–118, 2002

■ DRUGS METABOLIZED BY 2D6

Antidepressants

Tricyclic antidepressants[1]
Amitriptyline
Clomipramine
Desipramine
Doxepin
Imipramine
Nortriptyline[2]
Trimipramine

Other antidepressants
Fluoxetine[3]
Fluvoxamine[3]
Maprotiline[3]
Mirtazapine[3]
Nefazodone
Paroxetine
Sertraline
Trazodone[3]
Venlafaxine[3]

Antipsychotics

Chlorpromazine
Clozapine[4]
Fluphenazine[3]
Haloperidol[3]
Perphenazine[3]
Quetiapine[3]
Risperidone[3]
Thioridazine[3]

Other psychotropics

Aripiprazole
Atomoxetine

Other drugs

Analgesics
Codeine[5]
Hydrocodone
Lidocaine[2]
Methadone[2]
Oxycodone
Tramadol[6]

Cardiovascular drugs[3]
Alprenolol
Bufuralol
Carvedilol
Diltiazem
Encainide
Flecainide
Metoprolol
Mexiletine
Nifedipine
Nisoldipine
Propafenone
Propranolol[7]
Timolol

Miscellaneous drugs
Amphetamine
Benztropine[2]
Cevimeline
Chlorpheniramine
Delavirdine[2]
Dexfenfluramine
Dextromethorphan[8]
Donepezil[2]
Indoramin
Loratadine[3]

78

DRUGS METABOLIZED BY 2D6 (continued)

		Miscellaneous drugs (continued)	
		Metoclopramide	Phenformin
		Minaprine	Tacrine[2]
		Ondansetron[2]	Tamoxifen[2]

[1]Tricyclic antidepressants (TCAs) use several enzymes for metabolism. The secondary tricyclics are preferentially metabolized by 2D6, the tertiary tricyclics by 3A4. TCAs are also oxidatively metabolized by 1A2 and 2C19.
[2]Oxidatively metabolized primarily by 2D6.
[3]Metabolized by other P450 enzymes.
[4]2D6 is a minor pathway; 3A4 and 1A2 are more prominent.
[5]O-Demethylated to morphine by 2D6, a minor pathway.
[6]Metabolized to a more active pain-relieving compound, M1.
[7]β-Blockers are partly or primarily metabolized by 2D6.
[8]Used as a probe for 2D6 activity.

■ INHIBITORS OF 2D6

Antidepressants	*Antipsychotics*	*Other inhibitors* (continued)
Amitriptyline	Chlorpromazine	Lansoprazole
Bupropion	Clozapine	Lopinavir/Ritonavir
Desipramine	Fluphenazine	Loratadine
Fluoxetine	Haloperidol	Methadone
Fluvoxamine[1]	Perphenazine	Methylphenidate
Imipramine	Risperidone	**Metoclopramide**
Norfluoxetine	Thioridazine	Mibefradil
Paroxetine	*Other inhibitors*	Pimozide[1]
Sertraline[2]	Amiodarone	**Quinidine**
Venlafaxine	Chlorpheniramine	**Ritonavir**
	Celecoxib	Terbinafine
	Cimetidine	Ticlopidine[1]
	Clomipramine	Valproic acid
	Diphenhydramine	Yohimbine
	Doxorubicin	

Note. Names of potent inhibitors are in **bold** type.

[1] In vitro evidence exists only for the *potential* for potent inhibition of 2D6.

[2] Sertraline's inhibition seems to be dose specific, with higher doses resulting in more potent inhibition than lower doses.

6

3A4

3A4 is the workhorse of the P450 system. It accounts for 30% of P450 activity in the liver and 70% of P450 activity in the small intestine (DeVane and Nemeroff 2002; Zhang et al. 1999). Because so much of human P450 activity is due to 3A4, it comes as no surprise that 3A4 performs the bulk of oxidative drug metabolism in humans. This makes 3A4 arguably the most important human P450 enzyme to understand. Indeed, the list of medications metabolized by 3A4 is constantly growing, and 3A4 may account for more than half of all drug oxidation in human liver (Guengerich 1999). Until the mid-1990s, the literature included references to 3A3 or 3A3/4. It is now understood, however, that 3A3 is not a separate P450 enzyme but a transcript variant of 3A4.

■ WHAT DOES 3A4 DO?

3A4 is involved in phase I metabolism of endogenous and exogenous compounds. This activity includes hydroxylation, demethylation, and dealkylation of substrates. 3A4's ability to affect so many compounds through multiple enzymatic steps is probably due to the multiple enzymatic sites on the 3A4 molecule. 3A4 is an important enzyme in the metabolism of endogenous steroids, cholesterol, and lipids through hydroxylation. Children and young adults seem to have more 3A4 function than do adults, and this enzyme may be more active in women than in men, but studies of age and gender differences with regard to 3A4 have yielded conflicting results (see Tanaka 1999).

■ WHERE DOES 3A4 DO ITS WORK?

Small intestine enterocytes have both 3A4 and P-glycoprotein (Doherty and Charman 2002). Gut lumen 3A4 inactivates an ingested drug, and P-glycoprotein "bounces" the drug back into the intestinal lumen, preventing absorption. In this way, 3A4 and P-glycoprotein in the mucosal cells serve to keep the body safe from ingested noxious exogenous compounds. Teleologically, there may be a close relationship between 3A4 and P-glycoprotein because they are located near each other on chromosome 7 (see Chapter 4 ["P-Glycoproteins"]).

3A4 has a vast amount of metabolic activity, and it is often thought of as a high-capacity/low-affinity enzyme as compared with other P450 enzymes—particularly 2D6, 2C9, and 2C19, which are low-capacity/high-affinity enzymes. 3A4 may function as a "sink," where many drugs go to be metabolized at relatively high levels. At low levels, the low-capacity/high-affinity enzymes perform more of the enzymatic activity. If 3A4 is inhibited, the drugs may spill over to the other enzymes, but because these enzymes are low capacity, serum levels of the drugs may increase significantly and lead to toxicity (see Olesen and Linnet 1997).

■ DOES 3A4 HAVE ANY POLYMORPHISMS?

Variations and polymorphisms of 3A4 have been described, but their clinical implications in drug metabolism have not been determined (Westlind et al. 1999). 3A4 represents one variation of the 3A subfamily in humans. The two other major human 3A enzymes are 3A5 and 3A7. All three are coded on chromosome 7 (see the *PubMed LocusLink* review at http://www.ncbi.nlm.nih.gov/Locus-Link/LocRpt.cgi?l=1574). These three enzymes are not technically polymorphisms; they are genetic variations in a P450 subfamily. The 3A region on chromosome 7 (7q21.1–22.1) codes for a superfamily of genes (perhaps up to 850 genes) that are all related to the

3A subfamily. It is not clear what all the genes code for. Some variability exists in these other 3A region genes. For example, some are actually pseudogenes that code for promoter regions. Variations in these promoter regions may alter the rate of transcription to messenger RNA. 3A7 is expressed in utero, quickly dissipates after birth, and is replaced by 3A4. It is not clear what differences 3A7 brings to chemical metabolism.

Despite the apparent genetic complexity of the 3A subfamily, all humans have considerable 3A activity. No one is a clear genotypic poor metabolizer at 3A, unlike polymorphisms that exist with 2D6, 2C9, 2C19, or 2A6. In fact, because 3A is the workhorse of the P450 enzymes, teleologically it would not make sense for populations to essentially lack 3A activity. Such a polymorphism might not be compatible with life.

Recently, it was determined that 33% of Caucasians and up to 60% of African Americans preferentially express 3A5 as their liver 3A enzyme (Kuehl et al. 2001). 3A5 is 83% homologous in amino acid sequence to 3A4. It is unclear how these differences in gene expression change drug metabolism; however, there is some speculation that 3A5 is less inducible than 3A4, and in vitro evidence suggests that 3A4 is 10 times more sensitive than 3A5 to inhibition by fluconazole.

MacPhee et al. (2002) noted that black transplant patients required higher dosing of tacrolimus, and hypothesized that this may be due to 3A5 activity differences. Their genotyping determined that the higher dosing requirements were associated with the *3AP1* G allele. Whether this allele was found in black and other ethnic patients, it was associated with greater dose requirements. The *3AP1* G_{44} allele is linked to hepatic 3A5 expression.

Taken together, the variations, polymorphisms, and complexity of the 3A subfamily gene region point to a wide variation in 3A/3A4 enzymatic activity. Clinical observations indicate that expression of 3A and 3A4 varies widely from individual to individual, being 10- to 30-fold greater in some persons (Ketter et al. 1995).

■ ARE THERE DRUGS THAT INHIBIT 3A4 ACTIVITY?

Yes. Many drugs and drug classes moderately or potently inhibit 3A4. Clinically, this is the most important fact to remember about this system. Drugs with evidence of potent competitive or noncompetitive 3A4 inhibition (Ki values<2.0 μM in in vitro human liver microsome studies and/or demonstrated strong inhibition in substantial in vivo or clinical studies) include the azole antifungals itraconazole (von Moltke et al. 1996a) and ketoconazole (Boxenbaum 1999); diltiazem (Sutton et al. 1997); the macrolide antibiotics clarithromycin, erythromycin (Pai et al. 2000), and troleandomycin (Venkatakrishnan et al. 1998); norfluoxetine; nefazodone (von Moltke et al. 1996a); the quinolone antibiotics ciprofloxacin and norfloxacin (McLellan et al. 1996); quinupristin/dalfopristin (Rubinstein et al. 1999); and the protease inhibitors indinavir and ritonavir (Iribarne et al. 1998). Ketoconazole and ritonavir seem to be the most potent of all the 3A4 inhibitors; in some in vitro human liver microsome studies, Ki was measured in nanomolars rather than micromolars.

Many drugs that inhibit 3A4 less potently may have the potential for increasing levels of other drugs. Despite their notoriety for inhibiting P450 enzymes, the selective serotonin reuptake inhibitors (SSRIs) are not the strongest inhibitors of 3A4. SSRIs, except for citalopram (which is a mild inhibitor), are only moderate inhibitors of 3A4. The only psychotropic drug known to be a potent inhibitor of 3A4 is nefazodone, a non-SSRI antidepressant (Owen and Nemeroff 1998).

Another moderate 3A4 inhibitor is a chemical (or chemicals) in grapefruit and grapefruit juice (Fuhr 1998; He et al. 1998). The action of this chemical (or these chemicals) is probably through inhibition of gut wall 3A4, although there is some evidence that the effect may due to P-glycoprotein inhibition (Wang et al. 2001). Regardless of the mechanism, when a second drug is ingested after grapefruit juice has been drunk, serum levels of the second drug increase if it is a substrate of 3A4 or P-glycoprotein.

With so many drugs metabolized by 3A4, one would expect many serious consequences of inhibition of 3A4 activity, particularly in the case of drugs that are highly dependent on 3A4 activity and that have narrow therapeutic windows or margins of safety. Many psychotropic drugs are partly to fully metabolized by 3A4 (DeVane and Nemeroff 2002), and when these drugs are combined with any of the potent 3A4 inhibitors, the inhibitors may wreak havoc on drug levels and cause significant toxicity and adverse side effects. For example, two deaths in 1997 were associated with concomitant use of clarithromycin and pimozide (Desta et al. 1999; Food and Drug Administration 1996). Clarithromycin, a commonly used macrolide that potently inhibits 3A4, had been added to pimozide, which is metabolized by 3A4. High serum levels of pimozide can cause significant and life-threatening prolongation of the QTc interval. Orap's (pimozide's) package insert now contraindicates use with *any* azole antifungal, macrolide antibiotic, or protease inhibitor (Orap 1999).

Some of these 3A4 inhibitors, such as azole antifungal agents, macrolide antibiotics, and quinolone antibiotics, are medications commonly prescribed by physicians who may be unfamiliar with the patients (i.e., in urgent or emergency care settings). We recommend that primary care physicians and psychiatrists ask their patients to contact them after any new medication is prescribed. In this way, the regular physician can determine whether extra caution or monitoring is necessary if a 3A4 inhibitor has been prescribed. For example, the levels of clozapine or any tertiary tricyclic may be increased to toxic ranges when widely used antibiotics such as clarithromycin are administered for respiratory tract infections or itraconazole is administered for fungal infections.

Inhibition of 3A4: Historical Issues

In the late 1990s, several 3A4-related casualties occurred, and the drugs were removed from the United States market by manufacturers. These cases are reminders of the potentially serious nature of 3A4 inhibition.

Nonsedating Antihistamines

In 1997, terfenadine was voluntarily withdrawn from the United States market by its manufacturer. Astemizole was withdrawn in 1999. These histamine, subtype 1 (H_1), receptor antagonists were pro-drugs that required 3A4 for metabolism to their active ingredients. However, the parent compounds were toxic to the cardiac conduction system. At high levels, they increased the QTc interval, leading to the potential for supraventricular tachycardia and/or torsades de pointes. Significant interactions occurred when inhibitors of 3A4 were prescribed with these drugs. Terfenadine is no longer available, but its nontoxic active metabolite, fexofenadine, is. Fexofenadine is excreted by the kidneys unchanged and, even at high serum levels, is not associated with cardiac toxicity (see "Allergy Drugs" in Chapter 13 ["Internal Medicine"]).

Mibefradil

Mibefradil, a calcium-channel blocker, was voluntarily removed from the United States market in 1998 because of its toxicity as a potent inhibitor of 3A4 and 2D6. The drug also inhibited 1A2. Although warnings were updated as interactions and potential interactions became apparent, physicians continued to prescribe it. Just before the manufacturer's withdrawal, the Food and Drug Administration (1998) published a Talk Paper that included a long list of drugs that could have dangerous effects when administered with mibefradil. Deaths and cardiac shock occurred in numerous cases when the drug was used along with other cardiotropic drugs fully or partly metabolized by 3A4, such as calcium-channel blockers and β-blockers (Krum and McNeil 1998; Mullins et al. 1998). Because many other calcium-channel blockers are available without such strong 3A4 inhibition, the manufacturer removed it from distribution.

Cisapride

Cisapride was removed from the United States market in 2000. This agent is metabolized by 3A4 and can have serious cardiac effects similar to those of nonsedating antihistamines. A total of 341 cases of cardiac arrhythmia have been reported, including 80 fatalities (Propulsid [drug warning] 2000). Eighty-five percent of these interactions involved 3A4 inhibitors or drugs that could cause arrhythmia (Food and Drug Administration 2000). Before this interaction was well known, a study of the use of low-dose cisapride to reduce SSRI-induced nausea did not reveal any adverse cardiac events (Bergeron and Plier 1994).

Inhibition of 3A4: Current Issues

Dresser et al. (2000) wrote a thorough review of the consequences of 3A4 inhibition. They cautioned against coadministering potent 3A4 inhibitors and drugs with narrow safety margins, such as drugs that can increase the QTc interval (pimozide) or cause excessive sedation (triazolobenzodiazepines), hypotension (calcium-channel blockers), or rhabdomyolysis (hydroxymethylglutaryl–coenyzme A [HMG-CoA] reductase inhibitors). In this section, we describe some issues regarding 3A4 inhibition that a primary care physician or a psychiatrist is likely to encounter.

Triazolobenzodiazepines

Triazolobenzodiazepines (alprazolam, midazolam, estazolam, and triazolam) are substrates of 3A4 and in this way differ from other benzodiazepines, which are metabolized through multiple other routes, particularly phase II enzymes. Caution is warranted when these drugs are used with most SSRIs, nefazodone, and other inhibitors of 3A4. The manufacturer of nefazodone has recommended a 50% reduction in the dose of alprazolam and a 75% reduction in the dose of triazolam when they are coadministered with nefazodone (Serzone 2001). Case reports and reports of small controlled studies have indicated enhanced effects (including severe sedation and delirium) when triazolobenzodiazepines are used with inhibitors of 3A4, such as ritonavir (von Moltke et al. 1998), erythromycin (Tokinaga et al. 1996), and diltiazem (Kosuge et al. 1997).

Nonbenzodiazepine Hypnotics

The nonbenzodiazepine hypnotics zolpidem and zaleplon are metabolized by 3A4. Enhanced effects are expected when these drugs are used with 3A4 inhibitors. Greenblatt et al. (1998) reported that in five healthy volunteers, use of zolpidem and ketoconazole increased the half-life and levels of zolpidem, which led to impairment in motor or cognitive skills. Norvir's (ritonavir's) package insert recommends against concomitant use of ritonavir and zolpidem because of the potential for enhanced central nervous system (CNS) effects (Norvir 2000). No case reports or reports of studies have indicated that other 3A4 inhibitors enhance the CNS effects of these drugs. This lack may be due to the excellent safety margin of these drugs and to the fact that few patients or physicians probably recognize oversedation as a drug-drug interaction. Most patients and physicians probably consider such reactions common and expected side effects or adverse drug reactions.

Selective Serotonin Reuptake Inhibitors

Although they are only moderate inhibitors of 3A4, SSRIs may be problematic. Fluoxetine's active metabolite, norfluoxetine, is considered a more potent inhibitor of 3A4 than fluoxetine. Therefore, reports of fluoxetine's role in enhancing 3A4 substrates may be inconsistent. Nevertheless, there are case reports of fluoxetine increasing the 3A4 substrates alprazolam (Lasher et al. 1991), cyclosporine (Horton and Bonser 1995), midazolam (von Moltke et al. 1996b), nifedipine (Azaz-Livshits and Danenberg 1997), and tertiary tricyclics (multiple cases and series).

Buspirone

Buspirone is mainly metabolized by 3A4. Enhanced effects of the drug (chiefly sedation) have been reported with coadministration of buspirone and either erythromycin or itraconazole, the latter two drugs increasing buspirone levels 5–13 times (Kivisto et al. 1997). One would expect the same result with coadministration of buspirone and other 3A4 inhibitors.

Grapefruit Juice

There is ample evidence that a chemical or chemicals in grapefruit juice inhibit 3A4. This interaction occurs with administration of drugs that are dependent on 3A4 (or substrates for P-glycoprotein) and have narrow therapeutic or safety ranges; the list includes cisapride (Kivisto et al. 1997), cyclosporine, some HMG-CoA reductase inhibitors (Kane and Lipsky 2000), and triazolam (Hukkinsen 1995). Although earlier reports indicated that grapefruit juice increases clozapine levels, the best study to date indicated that the effect, if present at all, is modest and not clinically relevant (Lane et al. 2001). This study was conducted in Taiwan, and therefore it is possible that the 3A4 (or P-glycoprotein) is of a different polymorphism. Grapefruit juice may also worsen side effects of oral contraceptives, because the juice can increase peak levels of ethinyl estradiol by 137% (Weber et al. 1996).

Drug Sparing and Augmentation

Some authors have advocated using inexpensive 3A4 inhibitors, such as grapefruit juice or ketoconazole, as sparing agents (to reduce the amount spent on expensive drugs such as cyclosporine or some protease inhibitors). We advise against this strategy. For example, the concentration of grapefruit juice is not constant, even within the same brand. Timing grapefruit juice ingestion (i.e., planning juice ingestion a few hours before or after 3A4-dependent medications are taken) could be disastrous, leading to wildly fluctuating serum levels of the drug being spared.

Keogh et al. (1995) reported that concomitant use of ketoconazole and cyclosporine reduced the dose of the latter drug by 80% and reduced the amount spent on that drug per patient by an average of $5,200. A subsequent report indicated that long-term use of ketoconazole may have risks, such as reduction of bone mineralization (L.W. Moore et al. 1996).

Psychiatrists have engaged in enhancement of drug effects for some time. Cimetidine was used for years to augment the effects of clozapine, until potential toxicity was recognized (Szymanski et al.

1991). Cimetidine is an inhibitor of 2D6, 3A4, and 1A2 (Rendic 1999) and can increase clozapine levels. Some clinicians have used SSRIs to augment clozapine's effects, and some physicians have proposed using an SSRI to decrease the amount spent on clozapine. Maintaining safe serum levels of clozapine with these drug combinations is difficult, and at times the risk of very high levels of clozapine may outweigh any gains. One series indicated a 43% increase in serum clozapine or norclozapine levels when administered with fluoxetine, paroxetine, or sertraline (Centorrino et al. 1996), none of which are considered extremely potent inhibitors of 3A4. Fluvoxamine (which inhibits both 3A4 and, more potently, 1A2, the two main enzymes needed for metabolism of clozapine) is the worst offender. Wetzel et al. (1998) demonstrated a threefold increase in the serum level and half-life of clozapine or norclozapine with the addition of just 50 mg of fluvoxamine per day. Coadministration of fluvoxamine and clozapine has been found, in a well-monitored setting, to be both safe and economically beneficial in schizophrenic patients requiring clozapine (Lu et al. 2000). However, we believe that this strategy has a potential for disaster if the fluvoxamine is stopped inadvertently or if the dose of fluvoxamine is increased by a clinician to a "therapeutic" level to help with depression or compulsions. Extremely close and probably impractical monitoring would be needed to ensure safety with this regimen.

■ ARE THERE DRUGS THAT INDUCE 3A4 ACTIVITY?

Yes. The best-known inducer of 3A4 is carbamazepine. For years it was known that carbamazepine induces its own metabolism. Neurologists and psychiatrists recognized that after initiation of carbamazepine therapy, an upward dose adjustment would be necessary within 4–8 weeks to maintain stable carbamazepine levels. The mechanism is now known: carbamazepine induces 3A4, and the drug is also metabolized by 3A4 (Levy 1995). Carbamazepine induces not only 3A4 but also phase II conjugation enzymes (Ketter et al. 1999).

Oxcarbazepine, a drug developed to have fewer drug interactions and adverse side effects than carbamazepine, does induce 3A4 and can induce the metabolism of oral contraceptives, rendering them less effective (Fattore et al. 1999). Other antiepileptics are inducers as well, including phenytoin, phenobarbital, and primidone (Anderson 1998).

There is evidence that the antitubercular drugs rifampin and rifabutin (Strayhorn et al. 1997), the nonnucleoside reverse transcriptase inhibitors nevirapine and efavirenz (Barry et al. 1997; Tseng and Foisy 1997), troglitazone (Caspi 1997), and dexamethasone and prednisone (Pichard et al. 1992) all induce 3A4. Modafinil, a CNS stimulant, has been shown to induce its own metabolism at high doses, and 3A4 is the enzyme induced (Provigil 1999). Provigil's manufacturer did report the case of a 41-year-old woman taking cyclosporine whose cyclosporine levels were reduced by 50% when modafinil 200 mg/day was administered (see Provigil 1999).

There is growing evidence that the herbal supplement St. John's wort may induce 3A4 (L.B. Moore et al. 2000; Roby et al. 2000) and/or P-glycoprotein (Hennessy et al. 2002). Use of the supplement has led to decreased cyclosporine levels, ultimately causing transplant rejection (Barone et al. 2000; Karliova et al. 2000; Ruschitzka et al. 2000). St. John's wort has also been shown to decrease digoxin levels (Johne et al. 1999). Given these reports, St. John's wort may affect numerous other drugs and make them less effective.

Though a potent inhibitor of 3A4, ritonavir *induces* 3A4 metabolism after a few weeks. The mechanism is unclear but may involve a feedback loop response to a cell's chronic exposure to ritonavir, which has a low K_i (high affinity) for 3A4. Ritonavir has been found to increase the metabolism of meperidine, resulting in increased levels of the neurotoxic metabolite normeperidine, and to reduce the area under the curve and maximal drug concentration of ethinyl estradiol (Piscitelli et al. 2000; Ouellet et al. 1998).

What Is Stimulation of 3A4?

Unlike other P450 enzymes, 3A4 is capable of being stimulated. Stimulation is similar to induction in that enhanced 3A4 activity occurs. It differs in that it is immediate; induction is delayed by 1–3 weeks. Stimulation is termed *homotropic* if performed by a substrate of 3A4 and *heterotropic* if performed by other effectors or drugs (Tang and Stearns 2001). To date, only a few in vitro human studies have shown this effect. Stimulation may be yet another factor in the wide variability seen in 3A4 activity and capacity.

■ REFERENCES

Anderson GD: A mechanistic approach to antiepileptic drug interactions. Ann Pharmacother 32:554–563, 1998

Azaz-Livshits TL, Danenberg HD: Tachycardia, orthostatic hypotension and profound weakness due to concomitant use of fluoxetine and nifedipine. Pharmacopsychiatry 30:274–275, 1997

Barone GW, Gurley BJ, Ketel BL, et al: Drug interaction between St John's wort and cyclosporine. Ann Pharmacother 34:1013–1016, 2000

Barry M, Gibbons S, Mulchay F: Protease inhibitors in patients with HIV disease: clinically important pharmacokinetic considerations. Clin Pharmacokinet 32:194–209, 1997

Bergeron R, Plier P: Cisapride for the treatment of nausea produced by selective serotonin inhibitors. Am J Psychiatry 151:1084–1086, 1994

Boxenbaum H: Cytochrome P450 3A4 in vivo ketoconazole competitive inhibition: determination of Ki and dangers associated with high clearance drugs in general. J Pharm Sci 2:47–52, 1999

Caspi A: Troglitazone. Pharmacy and Therapeutics 22:198–205, 1997

Centorrino F, Baldessarini RJ, Frankenburg FR, et al: Serum levels of clozapine and norclozapine in patients treated with selective serotonin reuptake inhibitors. Am J Psychiatry 153:820–822, 1996

Desta Z, Kerbusch T, Flockhart DA: Effect of clarithromycin on the pharmacokinetics and pharmacodynamics of pimozide in healthy poor and extensive metabolizers of cytochrome P450 2D6 (CYP2D6). Clin Pharmacol Ther 65:10–20, 1999

DeVane CL, Nemeroff CB: 2002 guide to psychotropic drug interactions. Primary Psychiatry 9:28–57, 2002

De Wildt SN, Kearns GL, Leeder JS, et al: Cytochrome P450 3A: ontogeny and drug disposition. Clin Pharmacokinet 37:485–505, 1999

Doherty MM, Charman WN: The mucosa of the small intestine: how clinically relevant as an organ of drug metabolism? Clin Pharmacokinet 41:235–253, 2002

Dresser GK, Spence JD, Bailey DG: Pharmacokinetic-pharmacodynamic consequences and clinical relevance of cytochrome P450 3A4 inhibition. Clin Pharmacokinet 38:41–57, 2000

Edwards DJ, Bellevue FH 3rd, Woster PM: Identification of 6′,7′-dihydroxybergamottin, a cytochrome P450 inhibitor, in grapefruit juice. Drug Metab Dispos 24:1287–1290, 1996

Fattore C, Cipolla G, Gatti G, et al: Induction of ethinylestradiol and levonorgestrel metabolism by oxcarbazepine in healthy women. Epilepsia 40:783–787, 1999

Food and Drug Administration: Report of pimozide and macrolide antibiotic interaction. FDA Medical Bulletin 26:3, 1996

Food and Drug Administration: Roche Laboratories announces withdrawal of Posicor from the market (FDA Talk Paper T98–33). Rockville, MD, National Press Office, June 8, 1998

Food and Drug Administration: Janssen Pharmaceutica stops marketing cisapride in the US (FDA Talk Paper T00–14). Rockville, MD, National Press Office, March 23, 2000

Fuhr U: Drug interactions with grapefruit juice: extent, probable mechanism and clinical relevance. Drug Saf 18:251–272, 1998

Greenblatt DJ, von Moltke LL, Harmatz JS, et al: Kinetic and dynamic interaction study of zolpidem with ketoconazole, itraconazole, and fluconazole. Clin Pharmacol Ther 64:661–671, 1998

Guengerich FP: Cytochrome P-450 3A4: regulation and the role in drug metabolism. Annu Rev Pharmacol Toxicol 39:1–17, 1999

He K, Iyer KR, Hayes RN, et al: Inactivation of cytochrome P450 3A4 by bergamottin, a component of grapefruit juice. Chem Res Toxicol 11:252–259, 1998

Hennessy M, Kelleher D, Spiers JP, et al: St John's wort increases expression of P-glycoprotein: implications for drug interactions. Br J Clin Pharmacol 53:75–82, 2002

Horton RC, Bonser RS: Interaction between cyclosporin and fluoxetine. BMJ 311:422, 1995

Hukkinsen SK: Plasma concentrations of triazolam are increased by concomitant ingestion of grapefruit juice. Clin Pharmacol Ther 58:127–131, 1995

Iribarne C, Berthou F, Carlhant D, et al: Inhibition of methadone and buprenorphine N-dealkylations by three HIV-1 protease inhibitors. Drug Metab Dispos 26:257–260, 1998

Ishizaki T, Horai Y: Cytochrome P450 and the metabolism of proton pump inhibitors—emphasis on rabeprazole (review article). Aliment Pharmacol Ther 13 (suppl 3):27–36, 1999

Johne A, Brockmoller J, Bauer S, et al: Pharmacokinetic interaction of digoxin with an herbal extract from St John's wort *(Hypericum perforatum)*. Clin Pharmacol Ther 66:338–345, 1999

Kane GC, Lipsky JJ: Drug-grapefruit juice interactions. Mayo Clin Proc 75:933–942, 2000

Karliova M, Treichel U, Malago M, et al: Interaction of *Hypericum perforatum* (St John's wort) with cyclosporin A metabolism in a patient after liver transplantation. J Hepatol 33:853–855, 2000

Keogh A, Spratt P, McCosker C, et al: Ketoconazole to reduce the need for cyclosporine after cardiac transplantation. N Engl J Med 333:628–633, 1995

Ketter TA, Flockhart DA, Post RM, et al: The emerging role of cytochrome P450 3A in psychopharmacology. J Clin Psychopharmacol 15:387–398, 1995

Ketter TA, Frye MA, Cora-Locatelli G, et al: Metabolism and excretion of mood stabilizers and new anticonvulsants. Cell Mol Neurobiol 19:511–532, 1999

Kivisto KT, Lamberg TS, Kantola T, et al: Plasma buspirone concentrations are greatly increased by erythromycin and itraconazole. Clin Pharmacol Ther 62:348–354, 1997

Kosuge K, Nishimoto M, Kimura M, et al: Enhanced effect of triazolam with diltiazem. Br J Clin Pharmacol 43:367–372, 1997

Krum H, McNeil JJ: The short life and rapid death of a novel antihypertensive and antianginal agent. Med J Aust 169:408–409, 1998

Kuehl P, Zhang J, Lin Y, et al: Sequence diversity in CYP3A promoters and characterization of the genetic basis of polymorphic CYP3A5 expression. Nat Genet 27:383–391, 2001

Lane H-Y, Jann MW, Chang Y-C, et al: Repeated ingestion of grapefruit juice does not alter clozapine's steady-state plasma levels, effectiveness, and tolerability. J Clin Psychiatry 62:812–817, 2001

Lasher TA, Fleishaker JC, Steenwyk RC, et al: Pharmacokinetic pharmacodynamic evaluation of the combined administration of alprazolam and fluoxetine. Psychopharmacology (Berl) 104:323–327, 1991

Levy RH: Cytochrome P450 isoenzymes and antiepileptic drugs. Epilepsia 36 (suppl 5):S8–S13, 1995

Lu ML, Lane HY, Chen KP, et al: Fluvoxamine reduces the clozapine dosage needed in refractory schizophrenic patients. J Clin Psychiatry 61: 594–599, 2000

MacPhee IA, Fredericks S, Tai T, et al: Tacrolimus pharmacogenetics: polymorphisms associated with expression of cytochrome P4503A5 and P-glycoprotein correlate with dose requirement. Transplantation 74:1486–1489, 2002

McLellan RA, Drobitch RK, Monshouwer M, et al: Fluoroquinolone antibiotics inhibit cytochrome P450-mediated microsomal drug metabolism in rat and human. Drug Metab Dispos 24:1134–1138, 1996

Monsarrat B, Chatelut E, Alvinerie P, et al: Modification of paclitaxel metabolism by drug induction of cytochrome P450A4 in a cancer patient (abstract). Proceedings of the Annual Meeting of the American Association for Cancer Research 38:A31, 1997

Moore LB, Goodwin B, Jones SA, et al: St John's wort induces hepatic drug metabolism through activation of the pregnane X receptor. Proc Natl Acad Sci U S A 97:7500–7502, 2000

Moore LW, Alloway RR, Acchiardo SR, et al: Clinical observations of metabolic changes occurring in renal transplant recipients receiving ketoconazole. Transplantation 61:537–541, 1996

Mullins ME, Horowitz BZ, Linden DH, et al: Life-threatening interaction of mibefradil and beta-blockers with dihydropyridine calcium channel blockers. JAMA 280:157–158, 1998

Norvir (package insert). Chicago, IL, Abbott Laboratories, 2000

Olesen OV, Linnet K: Metabolism of the tricyclic antidepressant amitriptyline by cDNA-expressed human cytochrome P450 enzymes. Pharmacology 55:235–243, 1997

Orap (package insert). Sellersville, PA, Gate Pharmaceuticals, 1999

Ouellet D, Hsu A, Qian J, et al: Effect of ritonavir on the pharmacokinetics of ethinyl oestradiol in healthy female volunteers. Br J Clin Pharmacol 46: 111–116, 1998

Owen JR, Nemeroff CB: New antidepressants and the cytochrome P450 system: focus on venlafaxine, nefazodone, and mirtazapine. Depress Anxiety 7 (suppl 1):24–32, 1998

Pai MP, Graci DM, Amsden GW: Macrolide drug interactions: an update. Ann Pharmacother 34:495–513, 2000

Pichard L, Fabre I, Daujat M, et al: Effect of corticosteroids on the expression of cytochromes P450 and on cyclosporin A oxidase activity in primary cultures of human hepatocytes. Mol Pharmacol 41:1047–1055, 1992

Piscitelli SC, Kress DR, Bertz RJ, et al: The effect of ritonavir on the pharmacokinetics of meperidine and normeperidine. Pharmacotherapy 20: 549–553, 2000

Propulsid (drug warning). Titusville, NJ, Janssen Pharmaceutica, April 12, 2000

Provigil (package insert). West Chester, PA, Cephalon, Inc., 1999

Rendic S: Drug interactions of H_2-receptor antagonists involving cytochrome P450 (CYPs) enzymes: from the laboratory to the clinic. Croat Med J 40:357–367, 1999

Roby CA, Anderson GD, Kantor E, et al: St John's wort: effect on CYP3A4 activity. Clin Pharmacol Ther 67:451–457, 2000

Rubinstein E, Prokocimer P, Talbot GH: Safety and tolerability of quinupristin/dalfopristin: administration guidelines. J Antimicrob Chemother 44 (suppl A):37–46, 1999

Ruschitzka F, Meier PJ, Turina M, et al: Acute heart transplant rejection due to Saint John's wort (letter). Lancet 355:548–549, 2000

Serzone (package insert). Princeton, NJ, Bristol-Myers Squibb, 2001

Strayhorn VA, Baciewicz AM, Self TH: Update on rifampin drug interactions, III. Arch Intern Med 157:2453–2458, 1997

Sutton D, Butler AM, Nadin L, et al: Role of CYP3A4 in human diltiazem N-demethylation: inhibition of CYP3A4 activity by oxidated diltiazem metabolites. J Pharmacol Exp Ther 282:294–300, 1997

Szymanski S, Lieberman JA, Picou D, et al: A case report of cimetidine-induced clozapine toxicity. J Clin Psychiatry 52:21–22, 1991

Tanaka E: Gender-related differences in pharmacokinetics and their clinical significance. J Clin Pharm Ther 24:339–346, 1999

Tang W, Stearns RA: Heterotropic cooperativity of cytochrome P450 3A4 and potential drug-drug interactions. Curr Drug Metab 2:185–198, 2001

Tokinaga N, Kondo T, Kaneko S, et al: Hallucinations after a therapeutic dose of benzodiazepine hypnotics with co-administration of erythromycin. Psychiatry Clin Neurosci 50:337–339, 1996

Tseng AL, Foisy MM: Management of drug interactions in patients with HIV. Ann Pharmacother 31:1040–1058, 1997

Venkatakrishnan K, von Moltke LL, Duan SX, et al: Kinetic characterization and identification of the enzymes responsible for the hepatic biotransformation of adinazolam and N-desmethyladinazolam in man. J Pharm Pharmacol 50:265–274, 1998 von Moltke LL, Greenblatt DJ, Duan SX, et al: Inhibition of terfenadine metabolism in vitro by azole antifungal agents and by selective serotonin reuptake inhibitor antidepressants: relation to pharmacokinetic interactions in vivo. J Clin Psychopharmacol 16:104–112, 1996a

von Moltke LL, Greenblatt DJ, Schmider J, et al: Midazolam hydroxylation by human liver microsomes in vitro: inhibition by fluoxetine, norfluoxetine, and by the azole antifungal agents. J Clin Pharmacol 36:783–791, 1996b

von Moltke LL, Greenblatt DJ, Grassi JM, et al: Protease inhibitors as inhibitors of human cytochrome P450: high risk associated with ritonavir. J Clin Pharmacol 38:106–111, 1998

Wang EJ, Casciano CN, Clement RP, et al: Inhibition of P-glycoprotein transport function by grapefruit juice psoralen. Pharm Res 18:432–438, 2001

Weber A, Jager R, Borner A, et al: Can grapefruit juice influence ethinyl-estradiol bioavailability? Contraception 53:41–47, 1996

Westlind A, Lofberg L, Tindberg N, et al: Interindividual differences in hepatic expression of CYP3A4: relationship to genetic polymorphism in the 5'-upstream regulatory region. Biochem Biophys Res Commun 259: 201–205, 1999

Wetzel H, Anghelescu I, Szegedi A, et al: Pharmacokinetic interactions of clozapine with selective serotonin reuptake inhibitors: differential effects of fluvoxamine and paroxetine in a prospective study. J Clin Psychopharmacol 18:2–9, 1998

Zhang QY, Dunbar D, Ostrooska A, et al: Characterization of human small intestinal cytochromes P-450. Drug Metab Dispos 27:804–809, 1999

■ STUDY CASES

Case 1

A 38-year-old Caucasian man who had tested positive for the human immunodeficiency virus (HIV) and who had several chronic problems, including allergic rhinitis, degenerative joint disease, and gastroesophageal reflux, began nelfinavir and nevirapine therapy. He became increasingly depressed, and treatment with doxepin was begun. Over time, the doxepin dose was titrated to 300 mg/day, with few side effects and questionable efficacy, despite good compliance. Serum tricyclic levels were low, ranging from 35 to 50 ng/mL. Viral load suppression was never achieved, and the patient's CD4 count continued to decrease.

Comment

3A4 induction: Nelfinavir has only mild inhibitory effects on 3A4 and 1A2. However, nevirapine induces 3A4. Although the metabolism of doxepin has not been studied as well as the metabolisms of other tertiary tricyclics (amitriptyline and imipramine), the drug is probably metabolized similarly—primarily by 3A4 and secondarily by other enzymes. Nevirapine likely induced the metabolism of doxepin, causing low tricyclic levels despite a relatively high dose of doxepin. Nelfinavir is also metabolized at 3A4, and nevirapine was probably inducing the protease inhibitor, placing this patient at risk for viral resistance to all protease inhibitors.

References

Lemoine A, Gautier JC, Azoulay D, et al: Major pathway of imipramine metabolism is catalyzed by cytochromes P-450 1A2 and P-450 3A4 in human liver. Mol Pharmacol 43:827–832, 1993

Tseng AL, Foisy MM: Management of drug interactions in patients with HIV. Ann Pharmacother 31:1040–1058, 1997

Venkatakrishnan K, Greenblatt DJ, von Moltke LL, et al: Five distinct human cytochromes mediate amitriptyline N-demethylation in vitro: dominance of CYP 2C19 and 3A4. J Clin Pharmacol 38:112–121, 1998

Case 2

A 35-year-old HIV-positive African American man had been taking fluoxetine (20 mg/day) for several years and ritonavir for several months without problems. The patient tried his mother's zolpidem (10 mg) because of sleeplessness. He slept for 14 hours and had a "hangover" the next day.

Comment

3A4 inhibition: Zolpidem is metabolized by 3A4. Ritonavir potently inhibits 3A4, and fluoxetine also inhibits 3A4, though not as potently. It is likely that this inhibition caused a delay in zolpidem's clearance, leading to the enhanced effect.

References

Tseng AL, Foisy MM: Management of drug interactions in patients with HIV. Ann Pharmacother 31:1040–1058, 1997

von Moltke LL, Greenblatt DJ, Granda BW, et al: Zolpidem metabolism in vitro: responsible cytochromes, chemical inhibitors, and in vivo correlations. Br J Clin Pharmacol 48:89–97, 1999

Case 3

A 45-year-old Caucasian man with chronic schizophrenia was being treated with haloperidol decanoate at a stable dose of 200 mg/month. He developed a seizure disorder and was prescribed phenytoin by his neurologist. Within 2 months, the patient's psychotic symptoms worsened, and he required hospitalization. Although baseline haloperidol levels had not been obtained before initiation of phenytoin therapy, a haloperidol level obtained in the hospital while the patient was receiving both haloperidol and phenytoin was low (less than 2 ng/mL).

Comment

3A4 inhibition: Haloperidol is metabolized by several P450 enzymes, including 3A4, and by phase II enzymes. Phenytoin induces 3A4. It is likely that over several weeks, phenytoin induced 3A4 and decreased serum haloperidol levels, leading to a recurrence of psychotic symptoms.

References

Kudo S, Ishizaki T: Pharmacokinetics of haloperidol: an update. Clin Pharmacokinet 37:435–456, 1999

Linnoila M, Viukari M, Vaisanen K: Effect of anticonvulsants on plasma haloperidol and thioridazine levels. Am J Psychiatry 137:819–821,1980

Case 4

A teenage boy with Tourette's syndrome was treated with pimozide, 2 mg/day, by his psychiatrist. The primary care physician treated the patient's pharyngitis with clarithromycin. Twenty-four hours later, the patient developed heart palpitations.

Comment

3A4 inhibition: Clarithromycin is a potent inhibitor of 3A4. Pimozide needs 3A4 for clearance, and toxic cardiac side effects may occur when the drug's levels are increased. Deaths have been reported with coadministration of pimozide and erythromycin or clarithromycin. Other macrolides are not associated with this result.

References

Desta Z, Kerbusch T, Flockhart DA: Effect of clarithromycin on the pharmacokinetics and pharmacodynamics of pimozide in healthy poor and extensive metabolizers of cytochrome P450 2D6 (CYP2D6). Clin Pharmacol Ther 65:10–20, 1999

Food and Drug Administration: Report of pimozide and macrolide antibiotic interaction. FDA Medical Bulletin 26:3, 1996

■ DRUGS METABOLIZED BY 3A4

Antidepressants
Amitriptyline[1]
Citalopram[2]
Clomipramine[1]
Doxepin[2]
Fluoxetine[2]
Imipramine[1]
Mirtazapine[2]
Nefazodone
Paroxetine[2]
Reboxetine
Sertraline[2]
Trazodone[2,3]
Trimipramine[1]
Venlafaxine[2]

Antipsychotics
Aripiprazole
Chlorpromazine[2]
Clozapine[4]
Haloperidol[5]
Perphenazine[2]

Antipsychotics (continued)
Pimozide[6]
Quetiapine[2]
Risperidone[7]
Ziprasidone[2,6]

Sedative-hypnotics
Benzodiazepines
Clonazepam
Diazepam[2]
Flunitrazepam[2]
Nitrazepam[2]

Triazolobenzodiazepines
Alprazolam
Estazolam
Midazolam
Triazolam

Other sedative-hypnotics
Zaleplon
Zolpidem
Zopiclone[2]

Psychotropic drugs, other
Buspirone
Donepezil[2]
Galantamine[2]

Other drugs
Analgesics
Alfentanil
Buprenorphine
Codeine (10%, N-demethylated)
Fentanyl
Hydrocodone[2]
Meperidine[8]
Methadone
Propoxyphene[9]
Sufentanil
Tramadol[2]

Antiarrhythmics[6]
Amiodarone
Lidocaine
Mexiletine[2]
Propafenone[2]
Quinidine

■ DRUGS METABOLIZED BY 3A4 *(continued)*

Other drugs (continued)

Antibiotics (miscellaneous)
Ciprofloxacin
Rifabutin
Rifampin
Sparfloxacin[2,6,10]

Antiepileptics
Carbamazepine
Ethosuximide[2]
Felbamate[2]
Methsuximide[2]
Tiagabine[2]
Valproic acid[2]
Zonisamide[2]

Antihistamines
Astemizole[6,10]
Chlorpheniramine
Ebastine[6]
Loratadine[6,7]
Terfenadine[6,10]

Other drugs (continued)

Antimalarials
Chloroquine
Halofantrine[6]
Primaquine

Antineoplastics
Bulsulfan
Cyclophosphamide[2]
Daunorubicin
Docetaxel
Doxorubicin
Etoposide
Ifosfamide[2]
Paclitaxel[2]
Tamoxifen[2]
Teniposide
Trofosfamide
Vinblastine
Vincristine
Vindesine
Vinorelbine

Other drugs (continued)

Antiparkinsonian drugs
Bromocriptine
Pergolide[2]
Ropinirole[2]
Selegiline[2]
Tolcapone[2]

Antiprogesterone agents
Lilopristone
Mifepristone
Onapristone
Toremifene[2]

Antirejection drugs
Cyclosporine
Sirolimus (Rapamune)
Tacrolimus

β-Blockers
Metoprolol[2]
Propranolol[2]
Timolol[2]

■ DRUGS METABOLIZED BY 3A4 (continued)

Other drugs (continued)

Calcium-channel blockers
Amlodipine
Diltiazem[2]
Felodipine
Nicardipine
Nifedipine
Nimodipine[2]
Nitrendipine
Verapamil[2]

HMG-CoA reductase inhibitors[11]
Atorvastatin
Cerivastatin[10]
Lovastatin
Pravastatin
Simvastatin

Macrolide/ketolide antibiotics
Azithromycin
Clarithromycin
Dirithromycin
Erythromycin

Other drugs (continued)

Macrolide/ketolide antibiotics (continued)
Rokitamycin
Telithromycin
Troleandomycin

Nonnucleoside reverse transcriptase inhibitors
Delavirdine[2]
Efavirenz
Nevirapine[2]

Protease inhibitors (antivirals)
Amprenavir
Indinavir
Lopinavir
Nelfinavir
Ritonavir
Saquinavir

Proton pump inhibitors
Esomeprazole[11]
Lansoprazole[11]
Omeprazole[11]

Other drugs (continued)

Proton pump inhibitors (continued)
Pantoprazole[11]
Rabeprazole

Steroids
Cortisol
Dexamethasone
Estradiol
Gestodene
Hydrocortisone
Methylprednisolone
Prednisone
Progesterone
Testosterone

Triptans
Almotriptan[2]
Eletriptan

Miscellaneous drugs
Acetaminophen[2]
Carvedilol[2]
Cevimeline[2]

■ DRUGS METABOLIZED BY 3A4 *(continued)*

Other drugs **(continued)**	*Other drugs* **(continued)**	*Other drugs* **(continued)**
Miscellaneous drugs (continued)	*Miscellaneous drugs* (continued)	*Miscellaneous drugs* (continued)
Cilostazol[2]	Fluconazole	Miconazole
Cisapride[6,10]	Itraconazole	Montelukast
Colchicine	Ketoconazole	Ondansetron[2]
Cyclobenzaprine[12]	Levomethadyl[6]	Sildenafil
Dextromethorphan[13]	Meloxicam[2]	Sibutramine
Diclofenac[2]	Metoprolol[2]	Vesnarinone
Ergots		

Note. HMG-CoA = hydroxymethylglutaryl–coenzyme A.

[1]Tertiary tricyclics are metabolized preferentially by 3A4 but are also metabolized by 1A2, 2C19, 2D6, and uridine 5'-diphosphate glucuronosyltransferases.

[2]Also significantly metabolized by other P450 and/or phase II enzymes.

[3]Metabolized by 3A4 to *m*-chlorophenylpiperazine.

[4]Also metabolized by 1A2 and, to a lesser extent, 2D6.

[5]Also metabolized by 2D6 and 1A2.

[6]Potentially toxic to the cardiac conduction system at high levels and therefore should not be used with potent inhibitors of 3A4.

[7]Also metabolized by 2D6.

[8]Not confirmed but strongly suspected to be a primary metabolic pathway.

[9]3A4 activates to analgesic norpropoxyphene.

[10]No longer available in the United States. [11]Also metabolized by 2C19. [12]Also metabolized by 1A2.

[13]N-Demethylation specific for 3A4; reaction can be a probe for 3A4 activity.

■ INHIBITORS OF 3A4

Antidepressants

Selective serotonin reuptake inhibitors[1]

Fluoxetine
Fluvoxamine
Norfluoxetine
Paroxetine
Sertraline

Other antidepressants

Nefazodone

Antimicrobials

Antibiotics, other

Ciprofloxacin[2]
Norfloxacin[3]
Quinupristin/Dalfopristin
Sparfloxacin[3]

Azole antifungals

Fluconazole[4]
Itraconazole
Ketoconazole[5]
Miconazole

Antimicrobials (continued)

Macrolide and ketolide antibiotics

Clarithromycin
Erythromycin
Telithromycin
Troleandomycin

Nonnucleoside reverse transcriptase inhibitors

Delavirdine
Efavirenz

Protease inhibitors

Amprenavir
Indinavir
Lopinavir/Ritonavir[6]
Nelfinavir
Ritonavir[7]
Saquinavir

Antipsychotics

Haloperidol
Pimozide

Other inhibitors

Anastrozole
Androstenedione

Other inhibitors (continued)

Bromocriptine
Chloroquine
Cimetidine[8]
Cisapride
Cyclosporine
Diltiazem
Grapefruit juice[3]
Methadone
Methylprednisone
Mibefradil[9]
Mifepristone
Nifedipine
Omeprazole
Oral contraceptives
Phenobarbital
Primaquine
Propoxyphene
Tacrolimus
Tamoxifen
Valproic acid
Verapamil
Zafirlukast[10]

■ INHIBITORS OF 3A4 *(continued)*

Note. Names of potent inhibitors are in **bold** type.

[1]Also inhibit other P450 enzymes.

[2]Also a potent inhibitor of 1A2.

[3]Also an inhibitor of 1A2.

[4]Potent inhibitor of 2C9.

[5]Also an inhibitor of 2C19.

[6]Trade name **Kaletra**.

[7]Also a potent inhibitor of 2D6, 2C9, and 2C19.

[8]Also an inhibitor of 2D6, 1A2, and 2C9.

[9]Also a potent inhibitor of 2D6 and 1A2; no longer available in the United States.

[10]Also an inhibitor of 1A2 and 2C9.

■ INDUCERS OF 3A4

Antiepileptics	Other inducers
Carbamazepine[1]	Cisplatin
Felbamate	Cyclophosphamide
Oxcarbazepine	Dexamethasone
Phenobarbital[1]	Efavirenz
Phenytoin[1]	Ifosfamide
Primidone	Lopinavir/Ritonavir[2]
	Methadone
	Methylprednisolone
	Modafinil
	Nevirapine
	Pioglitazone
	Prednisone
	Rifabutin
	Rifampin[1]
	Rifapentine[1]
	Ritonavir[3]
	St. John's wort
	Troglitazone[4]

Note. Names of potent inhibitors are in **bold** type.
[1]"Pan-inducers"—also induce most other P450 enzymes. [2]Trade name Kaletra.
[3]Currently known to potently induce only 3A4. [4]Removed from the United States market.

7

1A2

■ WHAT DOES 1A2 DO?

1A2 is recognized as an important enzyme in human metabolism (Brosen 1995). 1A2's metabolic activity is primarily hydroxylation and demethylation of compounds through oxidative metabolism. It has long been identified as the primary enzyme involved in the oxidative metabolism of the methylxanthines, such as caffeine and theophylline.

1A2 metabolizes some endogenous compounds, such as estradiol-17β and uroporphyrinogen. Gender differences have been found in the Chinese population (Ou-Yang et al. 2000), with men having more 1A2 activity. 1A2 (along with 2E1 and the extrahepatic P450 enzymes 1A1 and 1B1) is also involved in the metabolism of many chemicals in the modern environment, including polycyclic aromatic hydrocarbons (PAHs). PAHs include many compounds found in tobacco smoke, gasoline and diesel fuels, and solvents (Yamazaki et al. 2000). Unfortunately, 1A2 (along with 2E1, 1A1, and 1B1) often metabolizes PAHs into carcinogenic compounds.

■ WHERE DOES 1A2 DO ITS WORK?

Unlike the other P450 enzymes described in this book, 1A2 is found exclusively in the liver. The enzyme accounts for 10%–15% of P450 activity in the liver. Like 3A4, 1A2 is a low-affinity/high-capacity enzyme in relation to 2D6, 2C9, and 2C19 in the metabolism of many medications (Zhang and Kaminsky 1995), including chlorpromazine. Although 2D6 represents only 1%–2% of liver P450 content by weight, it is believed to be high affinity/low capacity (Alam and Sharma 2001). At low concentrations, for medications that can be metabolized by either 2D6 or 1A2, 2D6 is the primary enzyme involved. At higher concentrations, 2D6 becomes overwhelmed (because it is high affinity/low capacity), and 1A2 takes over the bulk of the metabolic oxidative work for the particular drug. This can become a significant clinical issue if 1A2 is inhibited in a poor metabolizer at 2D6.

■ DOES 1A2 HAVE ANY POLYMORPHISMS?

The gene for 1A2 is found on chromosome 15 (see the *PubMed LocusLink* review at http://www.ncbi.nlm.nih.gov/LocusLink/LocRpt.cgi?l=1544). In 1998, Schrenk et al. identified slow metabolizers for caffeine (a 1A2 probe) among nonsmokers, but this apparent polymorphism has not been identified further. Alam and Sharma (2001) reported three known 1A2 alleles in addition to the wild type. One of these alleles involves exon 2, and its clinical relevance is unknown. A second polymorphism is from a point mutation change (a change from a guanine to an adenosine). So far, in two human drug studies, the clinical relevance of this change has been insignificant (Mihara et al. 2000, 2001).

The third variant is from a point mutation that replaces a cytosine with an adenosine ($C \rightarrow A$). This variation has led to intriguing clinical results. C/C homozygous smokers (but not nonsmokers) have a 40% reduction in 1A2 activity, perhaps because C/C resists induction (see "Are There Drugs That Induce 1A2 Activity?"). Basile et al. (2000) found that among 85 American smokers with schizophrenia, Abnormal Involuntary Movement Scale (AIMS) scores were four to five times higher among C/C patients than among A/A patients. The investigators suggested that because smoking does not induce 1A2 as much in C/C patients, their antipsychotic levels might be chronically higher and therefore lead to the risk of tardive dyskinesia. However, Schulze et al. (2001) found no correlation between the genotype and AIMS scores in a similar study involving German patients.

Currently, it is not clear how frequently the $C \rightarrow A$ variant occurs. Nevertheless, the clinical implications of the $C \rightarrow A$ variant may still be of importance to psychiatry. If smoking does induce 1A2 more in patients with the A/A (or A/C) genotype, it is possible that these individuals would have lower therapeutic levels of and poorer responses to medications (such as clozapine and olanzapine) whose oxidative metabolism is mediated in great part by 1A2 (Ozdemir et al. 2001). This hypothesis requires further testing (see "Are There Drugs That Induce 1A2 Activity?").

■ ARE THERE DRUGS THAT INHIBIT 1A2 ACTIVITY?

Yes. Fluvoxamine (Becquemont et al. 1998)—but not other selective serotonin reuptake inhibitors—and the fluoroquinolone antibiotic ciprofloxacin (Fuhr et al. 1990) are the two most common 1A2 inhibitors in use that have Ki values less than 1.0 μM. Other fluoroquinolone antibiotics, particularly enoxacin (Ki, 0.1–0.2 μM) and lomefloxacin (Ki, 1.2 μM), inhibit 1A2 potently (Fuhr et al. 1990), and evidence indicates that norfloxacin may inhibit theophylline clearance by 1A2 as potently as ciprofloxacin does (Davis et al. 1995). Indeed, it appears that nearly all fluoroquinolones inhibit 1A2 to a some extent (Kinzig-Schippers et al. 1999; Markowitz et al. 1997; Mizuki et al. 1996), but not as much as ciprofloxacin, enoxacin, lomefloxacin, and norfloxacin. The antiarrhythmic drugs mexiletine (Wei et al. 1999) and propafenone (Kobayashi et al. 1998) also have been shown to inhibit 1A2 potently, with Ki values less than 1.0 μM; other antiarrhythmics are less potent. A chemical in grapefruit juice also inhibits 1A2, but through a different process than its inhibition of 3A4 (Fuhr 1998). The antiandrogen flutamide is a weak inhibitor of 1A2, but the metabolite of flutamide from 1A2 (2-hydroxyflutamide) is a potent inhibitor of 1A2 (Shet et al. 1997).

Such inhibition may have clinical significance if the aforementioned are given with drugs with relatively narrow therapeutic windows. Drugs known to have 50% or more of their oxidative metabolic clearance by 1A2 include clozapine (to active norclozapine [Eiermann et al. 1997]), cyclobenzaprine (Wang et al. 1996), flutamide (Shet et al. 1997), frovatriptan (Frova 2001), melatonin (Hartter et al. 2001), mirtazapine (Stormer et al. 2000), methylxanthines (such as theophylline and caffeine [Miners and Birkett 1996]), naproxen (Miners et al. 1996), ropivacaine (Naropin 2001), riluzole (Rilutek 2001), tacrine (Cognex 2000), the tertiary tricyclics (particularly if 3A4 is inhibited), and zolmitriptan (Zomig 2001). When any of these drugs is used with a 1A2 inhibitor, serum levels of the former may increase, and toxicity may result. The consequences of inhibiting the metabolism of these drugs can range from clinically insignificant (in the case of melatonin) to life threatening (in the case of theophylline, clozapine, cyclobenzaprine, and other tertiary tricyclics). Caffeine, theophylline, and melatonin have been used as probes for 1A2 activity because so much (90%) of their oxidative metabolism is mediated by 1A2 (Hartter et al. 2001).

Fluvoxamine is the most potent psychotropic inhibitor of this enzyme. Haloperidol, clozapine, imipramine, and theophylline levels have all been reported to increase three to six times above baseline (Brosen 1995). When given with clozapine, fluvoxamine must be used very cautiously, because it inhibits 1A2, 2C9, and 2C19 potently and 3A4 and 2D6 moderately. Fluvoxamine inhibits each major route of clozapine's metabolism. Wetzel et al. (1998) demonstrated a threefold increase in clozapine or norclozapine levels when only 50 mg of fluvoxamine was administered per day.

One study of fluvoxamine 100 mg/day for 6 days followed by a single 40-mg dose of tacrine revealed a decrease in oral clearance of tacrine of 730% (Becquemont et al. 1997). Caution is of course advised, because tacrine's main route of elimination is through 1A2.

Theophylline's dependence on 1A2 for metabolism is behind reports of a 70% decrease in clearance (Rasmussen et al. 1997) and resulting toxicity when the drug is administered with fluvoxamine (DeVane et al. 1997) or ciprofloxacin (Batty et al. 1995). The anti-arrhythmics that potently inhibit 1A2—mexiletine (multiple cases, first reported by Ueno et al. [1990]) and propafenone (Spinler et al. 1993)—have been shown to increase theophylline levels to the point of toxicity. And although zafirlukast's inhibition of 1A2 is not considered as strong as the inhibition by fluvoxamine, ciprofloxacin, mexiletine, or propafenone, the leukotriene antagonist increased theophylline concentrations to the point of toxicity in one case (Katial et al. 1998).

We suspect that caffeine, which depends primarily on 1A2 for oxidative clearance, is inhibited more often than is recognized. Caffeine toxicity associated with concomitant use of 1A2 inhibitors is in all probability underreported because clinicians and patients alike do not recognize that patients' "jitters" are caused by increased levels of caffeine and are not a side effect of the therapeutic drug. The half-life of caffeine was increased from 5 to 31 hours with fluvoxamine coadministration (Jeppesen et al. 1996).

Ciprofloxacin also potently inhibits 1A2, and several case reports confirm that it can increase clozapine levels significantly (Markowitz et al. 1997; Raaska and Neuvonen 2000). Although clozapine's metabolism is complicated, 1A2 seems to metabolize much of clozapine to its active metabolite, desmethyl(nor)clozapine. Other enzymes are also involved in clozapine's metabolism, including 3A4, 2D6, and perhaps 2C19 and 2C9 (Olesen and Linnet 2001). These other enzymes, however, oxidize clozapine to an inactive clozapine-*N*-oxide. Therefore, when 1A2 is inhibited, one would expect a higher-than-baseline ratio of clozapine to norclozapine, which normally ranges from 1.0 to 3.4, with an average of 1.7 (Dumortier et al. 1998).

Oral contraceptives seem to be moderate inhibitors of 1A2, decreasing the clearance of caffeine, clozapine, and chlorpromazine (see Chapter 12 ["Gynecology: Oral Contraceptives"]).

■ ARE THERE DRUGS THAT INDUCE 1A2 ACTIVITY?

Yes. The most important inducer of 1A2 with clinical significance is tobacco smoke, which probably induces through stimulation of PAHs in the smoke (Schrenk et al. 1998; Zevin and Benowitz 1999). 1A2 is not unique in this property; 2E1 also appears to be induced by smoking. Any drug metabolized by 1A2 will be used at higher doses in smokers, because the enzyme is already induced. We suspect that this fact is usually not recognized by the clinician. However, there may be a polymorphic variation in 1A2 that "resists" smoking's induction, as noted in "Does 1A2 Have Any Polymorphisms?"

Nevertheless, when a patient stops smoking (an action that is often encouraged), drug toxicity may occur. Because it takes a few weeks for induction (and, conversely, dissipation of induction) to occur, cessation of smoking may result in increased drug levels several weeks later. Levels of drugs such as theophylline, clozapine, and olanzapine may reach the point of toxicity when smoking is stopped. Monitoring serum levels of drugs such as theophylline and clozapine during these transition periods is strongly recommended. Olanzapine is metabolized by 1A2 (30%–40%) and, to a minor degree, 2D6, and is glucuronidated by the glucuronosyltransferase (UGT) 1A4 (Calleghan et al. 1999). Studies have indicated that smokers may need higher doses to achieve desired effects, because smoking increases clearance of olanzapine by as much as 40%.

We wonder whether it is wise for psychiatric facilities and hospitals to require smoking cessation in the case of long inpatient stays. Most psychiatric patients resume smoking when discharged, which may lead to decreased serum levels of newly prescribed drugs several weeks later. As their clozapine or olanzapine levels decrease, these patients may become symptomatic. One state hospital that implemented a no-smoking policy found that clozapine levels increased an average of 57% in 10 inpatients, and levels of another patient at the hospital increased dramatically (to 3,066 ng/mL, more than three times the threshold value for toxicity) and resulted in aspiration pneumonia (Meyer 2001).

Some inducers of 1A2 are not medications. Brussels sprouts, broccoli, cabbage, and other cruciferous vegetables, if eaten daily, will induce this enzyme (Jefferson 1998; Jefferson and Griest 1996; Kall et al. 1996), and cooking does not negate the effect. In addition, daily consumption of charbroiled foods (burned meats) will result in induction of this enzyme. The average American diet will typically not lead to induction of 1A2.

■ REFERENCES

Alam DA, Sharma RP: Cytochrome enzyme genotype and the prediction of therapeutic response to psychotropics. Psychiatric Annals 31:715–722, 2001

Basile VS, Ozdemir V, Maseelis M, et al: A functional polymorphism of the cytochrome P450 *1A2 (CYP1A2)* gene: association with tardive dyskinesia in schizophrenia. Mol Psychiatry 5:410–417, 2000

Batty KT, Davis TM, Ilett KF, et al: The effect of ciprofloxacin on theophylline pharmacokinetics in healthy subjects. Br J Clin Pharmacol 39:305–311, 1995

Becquemont L, Ragueneau I, Le Bot MA, et al: Influence of the CYP1A2 inhibitor fluvoxamine on tacrine pharmacokinetics in humans. Clin Pharmacol Ther 61:619–627, 1997

Becquemont L, Le Bot MA, Riche C, et al: Use of heterologously expressed human cytochrome P450 1A2 to predict tacrine-fluvoxamine drug interaction in man. Pharmacogenetics 8:101–108, 1998

Bloomer JC, Clarke SE, Chenery RJ: In vitro identification of the P450 enzymes responsible for the metabolism of ropinirole. Drug Metab Dispos 25:1–11, 1997

Brosen K: Drug interactions and the cytochrome P450 system: the role of cytochrome P450 1A2. Clin Pharmacokinet 29 (suppl 1):20–25, 1995

Calleghan JT, Bergstrom RF, Ptak LR, et al: Olanzapine: pharmacokinetic and pharmacodynamic profile. Clin Pharmacokinet 37:177–193, 1999

Cognex (package insert). Vega Baja, Puerto Rico, Parke Davis Pharmaceuticals Ltd., 2000

Davis JD, Aarons L, Houston JB: Effect of norfloxacin on theophylline clearance: a comparison with other fluoroquinolones. Pharm Res 12:257–262, 1995

116

DeVane CL, Markowitz JS, Hardesty SJ, et al: Fluvoxamine-induced theophylline toxicity. Am J Psychiatry 154:1317–1318, 1997

Dumortier G, Lochu A, Zerrouk A, et al: Whole saliva and plasma levels of clozapine and desmethylclozapine. J Clin Pharm Ther 32:35–40, 1998

Eiermann B, Engel G, Johansson I, et al: The involvement of CYP1A2 and CYP3A4 in the metabolism of clozapine. Br J Clin Pharmacol 44:439–446, 1997

Frova (package insert). San Diego, CA, Elan Pharmaceuticals Ltd., 2001

Fuhr U: Drug interactions with grapefruit juice: extent, probable mechanism and clinical relevance. Drug Saf 18:251–272, 1998

Fuhr U, Wolff T, Harder S, et al: Quinolone inhibition of cytochrome P-450-dependent caffeine metabolism in human liver microsomes. Drug Metab Dispos 18:1005–1010, 1990

Hartter S, Ursing C, Morita S, et al: Orally given melatonin may serve as a probe drug for cytochrome P450 1A2 activity in vivo: a pilot study. Clin Pharmacol Ther 70:10–16, 2001

Jefferson JW: Drug and diet interactions: avoiding therapeutic paralysis. J Clin Psychiatry 59 (suppl 16):31–39, 1998

Jefferson JW, Griest JH: Brussels sprouts and psychopharmacology: understanding the cytochrome P450 enzyme system. Psychiatry Clin North Am: Annual on Drug Therapy 3:205–222, 1996

Jeppesen U, Loft S, Poulson HE, et al: A fluvoxamine-caffeine interaction study. Pharmacogenetics 6:213–222, 1996

Kall MA, Vang O, Clausen J: Effects of dietary broccoli on human in vivo drug metabolizing enzymes: evaluation of caffeine, oestrone and chlorzoxazone metabolism. Carcinogenesis 17:793–799, 1996

Katial RK, Stelzle RC, Bonner MW, et al: A drug interaction between zafirlukast and theophylline. Arch Intern Med 158:1713–1715, 1998

Kinzig-Schippers M, Fuhr U, Zaigler M, et al: Interaction of pefloxacin and enoxacin with the human cytochrome P450 enzyme CYP1A2. Clin Pharmacol Ther 65:262–274, 1999

Kobayashi K, Nakajima M, Chiba K, et al: Inhibitory effects of antiarrhythmic drugs on phenacetin O-demethylation catalysed by human CYP1A2. Br J Clin Pharmacol 45:361–368, 1998

Markowitz JS, Gill HS, DeVane CL, et al: Fluoroquinolone inhibition of clozapine metabolism (letter). Am J Psychiatry 154:881, 1997

Meyer JM: Individual changes in clozapine levels after smoking cessation: results and a predictive model. J Clin Psychopharmacol 21:569–574, 2001

Mihara K, Suzuki A, Kondo T, et al: Effect of a genetic polymorphism of CYP1A2 inducibility on the steady state plasma concentrations of haloperidol and reduced haloperidol in Japanese patients with schizophrenia. Ther Drug Monit 22:245–249, 2000

Mihara K, Kondo T, Suzuki A, et al: Effects of genetic polymorphism of CYP1A2 inducibility on the steady state plasma concentrations of trazodone and its active metabolite *m*-chlorophenylpiperazine in depressed Japanese patients. Pharmacol Toxicol 88:267–270, 2001

Miners JO, Birkett DJ: The use of caffeine as a metabolic probe for human drug metabolizing enzymes. Gen Pharmacol 27:245–249, 1996

Miners JO, Couler S, Tukey RH, et al: Cytochromes P450, 1A2, and 2C9 are responsible for the human hepatic O-demethylation of *R*- and *S*-naproxen. Biochem Pharmacol 51:1003–1008, 1996

Mizuki Y, Fujiwara I, Yamaguchi T: Pharmacokinetic interactions related to the chemical structures of fluoroquinolones. J Antimicrob Chemother 37 (suppl A):41–55, 1996

Nakajima M, Kobayashi K, Shimada N, et al: Involvement of CYP1A2 in mexiletine metabolism. Br J Clin Pharmacol 46:55–62, 1998

Naropin (package insert). Wilmington, DE, AstraZeneca Pharmaceuticals LP, 2001

Olesen OV, Linnet K: Contribution of five human cytochrome P450 isoforms to the N-demethylation of clozapine in vitro at low and high concentrations. J Clin Pharmacol 41:923–932, 2001

Ou-Yang DS, Huang SL, Wang W, et al: Phenotypic polymorphism and gender-related differences of CYP1A2 activity in a Chinese population. Br J Clin Pharmacol 49:145–151, 2000

Ozdemir V, Kalow W, Okey AB, et al: Treatment resistance to clozapine in association with ultrarapid CYP1A2 activity and the C → A polymorphism in intron 1 of the *CYP1A2* gene: effect of grapefruit juice and low-dose fluvoxamine. J Clin Psychopharmacol 21:603–607, 2001

Raaska K, Neuvonen PJ: Ciprofloxacin increases serum clozapine and *N*-desmethylclozapine: a study in patients with schizophrenia. Eur J Clin Pharmacol 56:585–589, 2000

Rasmussen BB, Jeppesen U, Gaist D, et al: Griseofulvin and fluvoxamine interactions with the metabolism of theophylline. Ther Drug Monit 19:56–62, 1997

Rilutek (package insert). Bridgewater, NJ, Aventis Pharmaceuticals Products Inc., 2001

Schrenk D, Brockmeier D, Morike K, et al: A distribution study of CYP1A2 phenotypes among smokers and non-smokers in a cohort of healthy Caucasian volunteers. Eur J Clin Pharmacol 53:361–367, 1998

Schulze TG, Schumacher J, Muller DJ, et al: Lack of association between a functional polymorphism of the cytochrome P450 1A2 (CYP1A2) gene and tardive dyskinesia in schizophrenia. Am J Med Genet 105:498–501, 2001

Shet MS, McPhaul M, Fisher CW, et al: Metabolism of the antiandrogenic drug (flutamide) by human CYP1A2. Drug Metab Dispos 25:1298–1303, 1997

Spinler SA, Gammaitoni A, Charland SL, et al: Propafenone-theophylline interaction. Pharmacotherapy 13:68–71, 1993

Stormer E, von Moltke LL, Shader RI, et al: Metabolism of the antidepressant mirtazapine in vitro: contribution of cytochromes P-450 1A2, 2D6, and 3A4. Drug Metab Dispos 28:1168–1175, 2000

Ueno K, Miyai K, Seki T, et al: Interaction between theophylline and mexiletine. DICP 24:471–472, 1990

Wang RW, Liu L, Cheng H: Identification of human liver cytochrome P450 isoforms involved in the in vitro metabolism of cyclobenzaprine. Drug Metab Dispos 24:786–791, 1996

Wei X, Dai R, Zhai S, et al: Inhibition of human liver cytochrome P-450 1A2 by the class IB antiarrhythmics mexiletine, lidocaine, and tocainide. J Pharmacol Exp Ther 289:853–858, 1999

Wetzel H, Anghelescu I, Szegedi A, et al: Pharmacokinetic interactions of clozapine with selective serotonin reuptake inhibitors: differential effects of fluvoxamine and paroxetine in a prospective study. J Clin Psychopharmacol 18:2–9, 1998

Yamazaki H, Hatanaka N, Kizu R, et al: Bioactivation of diesel exhaust particle extracts and their major nitrated aromatic hydrocarbon components, 1-nitropyrene and dinitropyrenes, by human cytochromes P450 1A1, 1A2, and 1B1. Mutat Res 472:129–138, 2000

Zevin S, Benowitz NL: Drug interactions with tobacco smoking: an update. Clin Pharmacokinet 36:425–438, 1999

Zhang ZY, Kaminsky LS: Characterization of human cytochromes P450 involved in theophylline 8-hydroxylation. Biochem Pharmacol 50:205–211, 1995

Zomig (package insert). Wilmington, DE, AstraZeneca Pharmaceuticals LP, 2001

■ STUDY CASES

Case 1

A 35-year-old Caucasian woman with major depression and/or bipolar disorder and multiple psychiatric hospitalizations failed to respond to numerous treatments, including electroconvulsive therapy. Her fluvoxamine dose was titrated to 300 mg/day, without much benefit. Psychotic symptoms began to predominate. Her clozapine dose was titrated to 200 mg/day over several weeks. The patient began to complain of dizziness and had mild hypotension. Her serum clozapine level was 1,950 ng/mL, and a confirmatory measurement revealed a level of 2,040 ng/mL. Fluvoxamine therapy was discontinued, and clozapine levels were closely monitored. Three days after discontinuation of fluvoxamine therapy, the clozapine level had decreased to 693 ng/mL, and on the fifth day after cessation of treatment with fluvoxamine, the level was 175 ng/mL. The aforementioned side effects disappeared.

Comment

1A2 inhibition: Fluvoxamine potently inhibits several P450 enzymes, including 1A2, 2C9, and 2C19. It also moderately inhibits 3A4. Clozapine is metabolized by 1A2 and, to some extent, 3A4 and 2D6. This case and others reported in the literature indicate just how much fluvoxamine can increase clozapine levels. The case also illustrates how quickly inhibition can be reversed when treatment with the offending inhibitor (here, fluvoxamine) is discontinued.

References

Armstrong SC, Stephans JR: Blood clozapine levels elevated by fluvoxamine: potential for side effects and lower clozapine dosage (letter). J Clin Psychiatry 58:499, 1997

Wetzel H, Anghelescu I, Szegedi A, et al: Pharmacokinetic interactions of clozapine and selective serotonin reuptake inhibitors: differential effects of fluvoxamine and paroxetine in a prospective study. J Clin Psychopharmacol 18:2–9, 1998

Case 2

A 48-year-old Caucasian man with schizophrenia was effectively treated with clozapine 500 mg/day. The patient was a longtime smoker but was able to spontaneously stop smoking 2 years after the clozapine dose was established. Several weeks after smoking cessation, the patient complained of some side effects (attributed to clozapine therapy), including sedation and constipation. Serum clozapine levels were found to be more than 700 ng/mL, nearly twice what the clozapine levels had been when the patient was smoking.

Comment

1A2 induction: The major P450 enzyme involved in metabolism of clozapine is 1A2, although 3A4 and 2D6 are also involved. Smoking induces 1A2. When smoking ceases, 1A2 activity returns to normal after 3–6 weeks. Patients taking drugs such as clozapine have increased serum levels several weeks after cessation of smoking.

Reference

Seppala NH, Leinonen EV, Lehtonen ML, et al: Clozapine serum concentrations are lower in smoking than non-smoking schizophrenic patients. Pharmacol Toxicol 85:244–246, 1999

Case 3

After multiple trials of other antipsychotics over many years, a 64-year-old Caucasian woman with chronic undifferentiated schizophrenia responded best to clozapine. Her condition was stable when she was given 125 mg twice a day. No baseline measurements of clozapine or norclozapine levels were obtained. Her primary care physician began ciprofloxacin 500 mg twice a day for a urinary tract infection. Near the end of the 10-day course of antibiotic treatment, the patient was lethargic and drooled profusely. Her psychiatrist checked serum clozapine and norclozapine levels, which were 1,043 and 432 ng/mL, respectively—indicating mild to moderate toxicity. Clozapine therapy was temporarily discontinued; it was restarted soon after treatment with ciprofloxacin had been stopped.

Comment

1A2 inhibition: Ciprofloxacin is a commonly used antibiotic that potently inhibits 1A2, which clozapine preferentially uses to metabolize to active norclozapine (*N*-desmethylclozapine). In this case, because baseline levels were not available, one cannot prove that this exact interaction occurred. However, the relatively high ratio of clozapine to norclozapine (2.4:1) suggests that 1A2 was inhibited.

References

Dumortier G, Lochu A, Zerrouk A et al: Whole saliva and plasma levels of clozapine and desmethylclozapine. J Clin Pharm Ther 32:35–40, 1998

Raaska K, Neuvonen PJ: Ciprofloxacin increases serum clozapine and *N*-desmethylclozapine: a study in patients with schizophrenia. Eur J Clin Pharmacol 56:585–589, 2000

■ DRUGS METABOLIZED BY 1A2

Antidepressants	Antipsychotics	Other drugs	
Amitriptyline[1,2]	Chlorpromazine[3]	Acetaminophen	Phenacetin
Clomipramine[1]	**Clozapine**[5]	**Caffeine**	Propafenone[9]
Fluvoxamine[3]	Fluphenazine	**Cyclobenzaprine**	Propranolol[9]
Imipramine[1]	Haloperidol[3]	Dacarbazine	**Riluzole**
Mirtazapine[4]	Mesoridazine[3]	**Flutamide**	**Ropinirole**
	Olanzapine[6]	**Frovatriptan**	**Ropivacaine**
	Perphenazine	Grepafloxacin[8]	**Tacrine**
	Thioridazine[3]	**Melatonin**	**Theophylline**
	Thiothixene[3]	Mexiletine	Toremifene
	Trifluoperazine[3]	Mibefradil[8]	Verapamil[9]
	Ziprasidone[7]	Naproxen	R-Warfarin[10]
		Ondansetron	**Zolmitriptan**
			Zolpidem[9]

Note. Names of drugs are in **bold** type if there is evidence that in normal human use of the drugs, at least 50% of enzymatic metabolism is through 1A2.

[1]Tertiary tricyclic antidepressants (TCAs) are demethylated by 1A2 and 3A4. 2D6, 2C9, and 2C19 also metabolize tertiary TCAs. [2]N-Demethylation may be preferentially done by 2C19. [3]Metabolized by other P450 enzymes as well. [4]Also metabolized by 3A4. [5]Demethylated by 1A2 to norclozapine. Clozapine is metabolized to clozapine-N-oxide by 3A4 and, to a lesser extent, 2D6 and others. [6]Metabolized 30%–40% by 1A2 and some by 2D6, glucuronidated by the glucuronosyltransferase (UGT) 1A4. [7]1A2 is a minor route of metabolism. [8]Removed from the United States market. [9]Contribution of 1A2 metabolism is small. [10]Weaker pharmacological isomer of racemic warfarin (see Chapter 8 ["2C9"]).

■ INHIBITORS OF 1A2

Fluoroquinolone antibiotics	SSRIs	Other drugs	
Ciprofloxacin	**Fluvoxamine**	Anastrozole	Phenacetin
Enoxacin		Caffeine	**Propafenone**
Grepafloxacin		Cimetidine	Ranitidine[2]
Lomefloxacin		Fluphenazine	Rifampin
Norfloxacin		**Flutamide**[1]	Ropinirole[3]
Ofloxacin		Grapefruit juice	Tacrine
Sparfloxacin		Lidocaine	Ticlopidine
		Mexiletine	Tocainide
		Mibefradil	Verapamil
		Nelfinavir	Zafirlukast
		Oral contraceptives	
		Perphenazine	

Note. Names of drugs are in **bold** type if there is evidence that in normal human use, the drugs are **potent** inhibitors. SSRI = selective serotonin reuptake inhibitor.

[1]Flutamide's primary metabolite is a potent inhibitor of 1A2. [2]Scant evidence of 1A2 inhibition. [3]Weak inhibitor.

■ INDUCERS OF 1A2

Drugs	Foods	Other inducers
Caffeine	Broccoli	Chronic smoking[2]
Carbamazepine	Brussels sprouts	
Esomeprazole	Cabbage	
Griseofulvin	Cauliflower	
Lansoprazole	Charbroiled foods[1]	
Moricizine		
Omeprazole		
Rifampin		
Ritonavir		

[1]Possibly induce through stimulation of polycyclic aromatic hydrocarbons (PAHs).
[2]Induces through stimulation of PAHs.

8

2C9

2C9 is a relatively minor P450 enzyme with regard to oxidative metabolism of psychotropic medications, yet its effects merit attention. The list of drugs metabolized by 2C9 is not overwhelming (Miners and Birkett 1998; see also the table "Drugs Metabolized by 2C9" at the end of this chapter) but does contain several important medications, including many nonsteroidal anti-inflammatory drugs (NSAIDs) and oral hypoglycemic agents. Older literature often refers to 2C10, but 2C10 is now considered a variant of 2C9. There are other closely related P450 enzymes with different (but at times overlapping) functions in humans—in particular, 2C8 (see Chapter 11 ["Other Relevant P450 Enzymes"]), 2C18, and 2C19 (see Chapter 9 ["2C19"]). Indeed, all these enzymes are coded in the same region of chromosome 10 (see the *PubMed LocusLink* review at http://www.ncbi.nlm.nih.gov/LocusLink/LocRpt.cgi?l=1559).

■ WHAT DOES 2C9 DO?

2C9's actions, like those of other P450 enzymes, include hydroxylation, demethylation, and dealkylation of endogenous and exogenous compounds. 2C9 (and 2C8) also metabolizes liver arachidonic acid (Rifkind et al. 1995).

■ WHERE IS 2C9?

2C9 is found in many tissues; 2C9 messenger RNA has been detected in the kidney, testes, adrenal gland, prostate, ovary, and duodenum (Klose et al. 1999). Most of 2C9's activity in terms of drug metabolism appears to occur in the liver, and 2C9 (along with 2C19) accounts for about 18% of P450 content in the liver (DeVane and Nemeroff 2002).

■ DOES 2C9 HAVE ANY POLYMORPHISMS?

Yes. Alam and Sharma (2001) reported that there are five known different 2C9 alleles in addition to the wild type. Four of the five alleles create an enzyme with reduced function, whereas the fifth polymorphism's phenotype is unclear. Therefore, persons who are heterozygous or homozygous for the polymorphisms could have reduced 2C9 function.

Recently, Lee et al. (2002) determined that two of the non-wild-type alleles, *2 and *3, are found in 35% of Caucasians. These alleles are present much less frequently in African Americans and Asians. Evidence suggests that people who are heterozygous for these alleles and the wild type have a reduced ability to metabolize drugs dependent on 2C9. For example, two separate studies have shown that phenytoin metabolism is reduced by a third in patients with at least one 2C9*2 or 2C9*3 allele (Odani et al. 1997; van der Weide et al. 2001). These studies indicate that poor metabolizers (PMs) of some drugs may be found among heterozygous individuals (wild type with mutant type) and are most certainly found among homozygous individuals (roughly 10% of Caucasians).

It becomes apparent, then, that this variability can have effects on drugs that are dependent on 2C9 for their oxidative clearance. PMs at 2C9 may have increased levels of drugs with narrow safety or therapeutic windows to include oral hypoglycemics, phenytoin, and S-warfarin (the more active isomer of racemic warfarin) (see "Drugs Metabolized by 2C9," the first table at the end of this chapter). Some drugs, such as tolbutamide (Miners and Birkett 1996) and phenytoin (Aynacioglu et al. 1999), have been used as probes for 2C9 activity. As with 2D6, we suspect that most clinicians never consider the possibility that a patient may be a PM at 2C9. Many would attribute unusually high levels of phenytoin, or the hypoglycemia with tolbutamide, to some other clinically unpredictable variation. We believe that in the near future, microarray chip technology for determining polymorphisms of P450 and other enzymes may become inexpensive enough to use with all patients (de Longueville et al. 2002).

■ ARE THERE DRUGS THAT INHIBIT 2C9 ACTIVITY?

Yes. In vitro human liver microsome studies suggest that the most potent inhibitors of 2C9 are the protease inhibitor ritonavir (Ki, 0.02 μM [Warrington et al. 2000]) and the little-used agent sulfaphenazole (Ki, 0.07 μM [Tracy et al. 1996]). However, the more commonly prescribed azole antifungal fluconazole (Niemi et al. 2001) and the selective serotonin reuptake inhibitor (SSRI) fluvoxamine (Facciola et al. 2001; Niemi et al. 2001) may also be categorized as potent 2C9 inhibitors, although their Ki values vary widely in published reports. The other SSRIs minimally inhibit 2C9 (Hemeryck et al. 1999). Inhibitors are listed in the table "Inhibitors of 2C9" at the end of the chapter.

In the sections that follow, we discuss substrates that produce adverse outcomes if inhibited at 2C9.

Warfarin

S-Warfarin is the more active isomer of the racemic mix of warfarin. S-Warfarin is metabolized primarily by 2C9, and R-warfarin is metabolized by 1A2. Although the literature indicates that hundreds of drugs have the potential to interact pharmacokinetically and/or pharmacodynamically with warfarin, it has been established that the following drugs increase S-warfarin levels through inhibition of 2C9: amiodarone's metabolite desethylamiodarone (Naganuma et al. 2001), fluconazole (Black et al. 1996), fluvoxamine (data on file, Solvay Pharmaceuticals, Inc., Marietta, GA), modafinil (Provigil

1999), ritonavir (Newshan and Tsang 1999), and zafirlukast (Dekhuijzen and Koopmans 2002). Clearly the concern regarding concomitant use of these 2C9 inhibitors and warfarin is the risk of increased bleeding times caused by warfarin levels that are too high. Other drugs that increase warfarin levels through this mechanism may be the SSRIs fluoxetine, paroxetine, and sertraline. However, these agents are all fairly modest 2C9 inhibitors, and it is unclear whether their effect on bleeding times in warfarin-treated patients is through 2C9 inhibition or some other mechanism.

Phenytoin

Phenytoin's metabolism is complicated, but 2C9 and 2C19 appear to play the major roles in metabolism. It is well established that fluconazole (Cadle et al. 1994) and fluoxetine (Nelson et al. 2001; Nightingale 1994) increase phenytoin levels through 2C9 inhibition. Although one would expect there to be ample clinical evidence that the addition of other potent inhibitors of 2C9, such as fluvoxamine and ritonavir, increases phenytoin levels, few reports have been published. Nevertheless, careful monitoring of phenytoin levels is warranted during treatment with these drugs (Barry et al. 1997; Schmider et al. 1997). Finally, although no cases are currently found in the literature, the package insert for Provigil (modafinil) warns that the agent might increase phenytoin levels through 2C9 inhibition (Provigil 1999).

The lack of case reports on 2C9 inhibition of phenytoin with administration of other drugs is curious, because phenytoin is still widely used. We suspect that many cases are missed because toxic levels are not reached, or if they are reached, the clinician is not aware of the drug-drug interaction that caused the high phenytoin level, and simply decreases the phenytoin dose.

Oral Hypoglycemics

The oral hypoglycemic class of drugs known as thiazolidinediones (the "glitazones"—troglitazone, rosiglitazone, and pioglitazone) are metabolized by 2C8 and 3A4 (Lebovitz 2002; see section on oral hypoglycemics in Chapter 13 ["Internal Medicine"]). Another class of oral hypoglycemics, the sulfonylureas (tolbutamide, glipizide, glyburide), are primarily metabolized by 2C9. 2C9 inhibitors might increase concentrations of oral hypoglycemics, perhaps leading to decreases in serum glucose levels. Indeed, tolbutamide's half-life increased threefold, and the area under the curve increased by 66%, in seven nondiabetic control subjects when the drug was used with ketoconazole, a 2C9 inhibitor (Krishnaiah et al. 1994). All seven individuals experienced decreases in serum glucose levels, and five had symptoms of mild hypoglycemia. Although this type of drug-drug interaction has not been reported with other oral hypoglycemics and potent inhibitors of 2C9, we suspect that it occurs more often and is not recognized by the pharmacist or clinician.

Nonsteroidal Anti-Inflammatory Drugs

Although multiple studies have indicated that many NSAIDs (including the newer cyclooxygenase-2 [Cox-2] inhibitors) depend on 2C9 for their metabolism, it is difficult to find reports of adverse outcomes in PMs at 2C9 or in patients receiving 2C9 inhibitors concomitantly. This lack of reports may be due to the fact that NSAIDs have wide therapeutic windows and are metabolized by uridine 5'-diphosphate glucuronosyltransferases (UGTs). For more details on NSAID-drug interactions, see Chapter 17 ("Pain Management I: Nonnarcotic Analgesics").

■ ARE THERE DRUGS THAT INDUCE 2C9 ACTIVITY?

Yes. The only clearly recognized inducer is rifampin. This drug was recognized as an inducer in the 1970s, although it was not until the mid-1990s that the actual enzyme induced was found to be 2C9 (its cousin 2C19 is also induced by rifampin). Rifampin has been shown to reduce, by induction, serum levels of warfarin (Heimark et al. 1987), tolbutamide (Zilly et al. 1977), and phenytoin (Kay et al. 1985)—all drugs very dependent on 2C9. Other drugs may induce 2C9 as well (see "Inducers of 2C9," a table at the end of this chapter).

■ REFERENCES

Alam DA, Sharma RP: Cytochrome enzyme genotype and the prediction of therapeutic response to psychotropics. Psychiatric Annals 31:715–722, 2001

Aynacioglu AS, Brackmoller J, Bauer S, et al: Frequency of cytochrome P450 CYP2C9 variants in a Turkish population and the functional relevance for phenytoin. Br J Clin Pharmacol 48:409–415, 1999

Baldwin SJ, Bloomer JC, Smith GJ, et al: Ketoconazole and sulphaphenazole as the respective selective inhibitors of P4503A and 2C9. Xenobiotica 25:261–270, 1995

Barry M, Gibbons S, Back D, et al: Protease inhibitors in patients with HIV disease: clinically important pharmacokinetic considerations. Clin Pharmacokinet 32:194–209, 1997

Black DJ, Kunze KL, Wienkers LC, et al: Warfarin-fluconazole, II: a metabolically based drug interaction—in vivo studies. Drug Metab Dispos 24:422–428, 1996

Cadle RM, Zenon GJ 3rd, Rodriguez-Barradas MC, et al: Fluconazole-induced symptomatic phenytoin toxicity. Ann Pharmacother 28:191–195, 1994

Dekhuijzen PN, Koopmans PP: Pharmacokinetic profile of zafirlukast. Clin Pharmacokinet 41:105–114, 2002

de Longueville F, Surry D, Meneses-Lorente G, et al: Gene expression profiling of drug metabolism and toxicology markers using a low-density DNA microarray. Biochem Pharmacol 64:137–149, 2002

DeVane CL, Nemeroff CB: 2002 guide to psychotropic drug interactions. Primary Psychiatry 9:28–57, 2002

Facciola G, Hidestrand M, von Bahr C, et al: Cytochrome P450 isoforms involved in melatonin metabolism in human liver microsomes. Eur J Pharmacol 56:881–888, 2001

Heimark LD, Gibaldi M, Trager WF, et al: The mechanism of the warfarin-rifampin drug interaction. Clin Pharmacol Ther 42:388–394, 1987

Hemeryck A, De Vriendt C, Belpaire FM: Inhibition of CYP2C9 by selective serotonin reuptake inhibitors: in vitro studies with tolbutamide and (S)-warfarin using human liver microsomes. Eur J Clin Pharmacol 54: 947–951, 1999

Kay L, Kampmann JP, Svendsen TL, et al: Influence of rifampicin and isoniazid on the kinetics of phenytoin. Br J Clin Pharmacol 20:323–326, 1985

Klose TS, Blaisdell JA, Goldstein JA: Gene structure of CYP2C8 and extrahepatic distribution of human CYP2Cs. J Biochem Mol Toxicol 13: 289–295, 1999

Krishnaiah YS, Satyanarayana S, Visweswaram D: Interaction between tolbutamide and ketoconazole in healthy subjects. Br J Clin Pharmacol 37: 205–207, 1994

Lebovitz HE: Differentiating members of the thiazolidinedione class: focus on safety. Diabetes Metab Res Rev 18 (suppl 2):S23–S29, 2002

Lee CR, Goldstein JA, Pieper JA: Cytochrome P450 2C9 polymorphisms: a comprehensive review of the in-vitro and human data. Pharmacogenetics 12:251–263, 2002

Miners JO, Birkett DJ: Use of tolbutamide as a substrate probe for human hepatic cytochrome P450 2C9. Methods Enzymol 272:139–145, 1996

Miners JO, Birkett DJ: Cytochrome P4502C9: an enzyme of major importance in human drug metabolism. Br J Clin Pharmacol 45:525–538, 1998

Moody GC, Griffin SJ, Mather AN, et al: Fully automated analysis of activities catalysed by the major human liver cytochrome P450 (CYP) enzymes: assessment of human CYP inhibition potential. Xenobiotica 29: 53–75, 1999

Naganuma M, Shiga T, Nishikata K, et al: Role of desethylamiodarone in the anticoagulant effect of concurrent amiodarone and warfarin therapy. J Cardiovasc Pharmacol Ther 6:363–367, 2001

Nelson MH, Birnbaum AK, Remmel RP: Inhibition of phenytoin hydroxylation in human liver microsomes by several selective serotonin reuptake inhibitors. Epilepsy Res 44:71–82, 2001

Newshan G, Tsang P: Ritonavir and warfarin interaction (letter). AIDS 13: 1788–1789, 1999

Niemi M, Backman JT, Neuvonen M, et al: Effects of fluconazole and fluvoxamine on the pharmacokinetics and pharmacodynamics of glimepiride. Clin Pharmacol Ther 69:194–200, 2001

Nightingale SL: From the Food and Drug Administration. JAMA 271:1067, 1994

Odani A, Hashimoto Y, Otsuki Y, et al: Genetic polymorphism of the CYP2C subfamily and its effect on the pharmacokinetics of phenytoin in Japanese patients with epilepsy. Clin Pharmacol Ther 62:287–292, 1997

Provigil (package insert). West Chester, PA, Cephalon, Inc., 1999

Rifkind AB, Lee C, Chang TK, et al: Arachidonic acid metabolism by human cytochrome P450s 2C8, 2C9, 2E1, and 1A2: regioselective oxygenation and evidence for a role for CYP2C enzymes in arachidonic acid epoxygenation in human liver microsomes. Arch Biochem Biophys 320:380–389, 1995

Schmider J, Greenblatt DJ, von Moltke LL, et al: Inhibition of CYP2C9 by selective serotonin reuptake inhibitors in vitro: studies of phenytoin p-hydroxylation. Br J Clin Pharmacol 44:495–498, 1997

Scripture CD, Pieper JA: Clinical pharmacokinetics of fluvastatin. Clin Pharmacokinet 49:263–281, 2001

Tracy TS, Marra C, Wrighton SA, et al: Studies of flurbiprofen 4′-hydroxylation: additional evidence suggesting the sole involvement of cytochrome P450 2C9. Biochem Pharmacol 52:1305–1309, 1996

van der Weide J, Steijns LS, van Weelden MJ, et al: The effect of genetic polymorphism of cytochrome P4502C9 on phenytoin dose requirement. Pharmacogenetics 11:287–291, 2001

Warrington JS, Shader RI, von Moltke LL, et al: In vitro biotransformation of sildenafil (Viagra): identification of human cytochromes and potential drug interactions. Drug Metab Dispos 28:392–397, 2000

Wen X, Wang JS, Backman JT, et al: Trimethoprim and sulfamethoxazole are selective inhibitors of CYP2C8 and CYP2C9, respectively. Drug Metab Dispos 30:631–635, 2002

Zilly W, Breimer DD, Richter E: Stimulation of drug metabolism by rifampicin in patients with cirrhosis or cholestasis measured by increased hexobarbital and tolbutamide clearance. Eur J Clin Pharmacol 11:287–293, 1977

■ STUDY CASES

Case 1

An 83-year-old man with dementia of the Alzheimer's type and behavioral disturbances was receiving 5 mg of oral glipizide twice a day for non-insulin-dependent diabetes mellitus. He was prescribed valproic acid (250 mg orally three times a day) for his behavioral problems. The drug appeared to have a positive effect, and his valproic acid level was an acceptable 51 ng/mL. However, his serum glucose level, which had been 120–140 mg/dL before initiation of valproic acid therapy, became consistently low in the morning, ranging from 48 to 60 mg/dL. The glipizide dose was reduced to compensate.

Comment

2C9 inhibition: Valproic acid modestly inhibits 2C9, and in this case it caused the patient's glipizide levels to increase, which decreased serum glucose levels significantly. Instead of abandoning one of the drugs (both of which seemed effective), the clinician decreased the glipizide dose.

References

Wen X, Wang J-S, Kivisto KT, et al: In vitro evaluation of valproic acid as an inhibitor of human cytochrome P450 isoforms: preferential inhibition of cytochrome P450 2C9 (CYP2C9). Br J Clin Pharmacol 52:547–533, 2001

Case 2

A 40-year-old Caucasian woman was prescribed fluoxetine 20 mg/day for anxiety and depressive symptoms. She had been treated for many years with phenytoin 300 mg/day for a seizure disorder, without significant side effects. After 1 week of fluoxetine therapy, she complained of dizziness and somnolence. Serum phenytoin levels were 30 μg/mL (reference range, 10–20 μg/mL).

Comment

2C9 and 2C19 inhibition: Phenytoin is metabolized by 2C9, 2C19, and phase II conjugation enzymes. Although not a potent inhibitor of 2C9 and 2C19, fluoxetine does inhibit these enzymes and most certainly was the cause of the increase in phenytoin levels found in this woman.

References

Nelson MH, Birnbaum AK, Remmel RP: Inhibition of phenytoin hydroxylation in human liver microsomes by several selective serotonin re-uptake inhibitors. Epilepsy Res 44:71–82, 2001

Nightingale SL: From the Food and Drug Administration. JAMA 271:1067, 1994

DRUGS METABOLIZED BY 2C9

Angiotensin II blockers	Hypoglycemics, oral[2]	NSAIDs[3]	Other drugs
Irbesartan	*Sulfonylureas*	Celecoxib	Carmustine
Losartan	Glimepiride	Diclofenac	Dapsone
Valsartan	Glipizide	Flurbiprofen	Fluvastatin[4]
	Glyburide	Ibuprofen	Mestranol[5]
Antidepressants	Tolbutamide	Indomethacin	Paclitaxel[1]
Fluoxetine[1]		Ketoprofen	Phenytoin
Sertraline[1]		Mefenamic acid	Tamoxifen
		Meloxicam	Tetrahydrocannabinol
		Naproxen	Torsemide
		Piroxicam	S-Warfarin[6]
		Valdecoxib	Zafirlukast
			?Zolpidem[7]

Note. NSAID=nonsteroidal anti-inflammatory drug.
[1]Metabolized by other P450 enzymes as well.
[2]"Glitazones" are metabolized by 2C8 and 3A4.
[3]Also metabolized extensively by phase II enzymes (see Chapter 17 ["Pain Management I: Nonnarcotic Analgesics"]).
[4]The exception to the "statins," most of which are oxidatively metabolized in part or in full by 3A4.
[5]Metabolized by 2C9 to active 17-hydroxyethinylestradiol.
[6]*S*-Warfarin is the more active isomer of warfarin. *R*-warfarin is metabolized by 1A2.
[7]Metabolized mainly by 3A4 and 1A2.

■ INHIBITORS OF 2C9

Selective serotonin reuptake inhibitors		*Other inhibitors*
Fluoxetine	Amiodarone[1]	Modafinil
Fluvoxamine	Anastrozole	Phenylbutazone
Paroxetine	Cimetidine	Ranitidine
Sertraline	Clopidogrel	**Ritonavir**
	Delavirdine	Sulfamethoxazole
	Efavirenz	**Sulfaphenazole**
	Fluconazole	Sulfinpyrazone
	Fluvastatin	Valproic acid
	Isoniazid	Zafirlukast

Note. Names of potent inhibitors are in **bold** type.
[1]Amiodarone, an inhibitor of 1A2 and 3A4, is an insignificant 2C9 inhibitor. However, its metabolite, desmethylamiodarone, is a clinically relevant 2C9 inhibitor.

■ INDUCERS OF 2C9

Carbamazepine	Phenobarbital	Rifapentine
Cyclophosphamide	Phenytoin	Ritonavir
Ethanol	Rifabutin	Secobarbital
Ifosfamide	Rifampin	?Valproic acid

2C19

2C19 differs from 2C9 by only 43 of 490 amino acids (Jung et al. 1998). Although some similarities in their substrates exist (e.g., both 2C9 and 2C19 are involved in phenytoin and indomethacin oxidative metabolism), there are many differences with regard to genetic variability, substrates, and inhibitors.

■ WHAT DOES 2C19 DO?

2C19 is involved in phase I metabolism of substances. Its actions, like those of other P450 enzymes, include hydroxylation, demethylation, and dealkylation of compounds.

■ WHERE IS 2C19?

2C19 is found in many tissues, but it plays its role in the metabolism of drugs in the liver. Together, 2C19 and 2C9 are responsible for approximately 20% of P450 activity in the liver.

■ DOES 2C19 HAVE ANY POLYMORPHISMS?

Yes. The gene for 2C19 is located on chromosome 10 and is close to its related P450 enzymes—2C8, 2C9, and 2C18 (see the *PubMed LocusLink* review at http://www.ncbi.nlm.nih.gov/LocusLink/LocRpt.cgi?l=1557). Alam and Sharma (2001) described seven different alleles in addition to the normal wild type. Six of the seven alleles are from single nucleotide changes, and the other is from an inversion of a base pair. All seven of these variant alleles lead to reduced or no enzyme function. Hence, as with 2D6, there are two possible phenotypes: the poor metabolizer (PM) phenotype and the extensive (average) metabolizer (EM) phenotype. In general, studies have revealed that 2%–6% of Caucasians, 15%–20% of Japanese, and 10%–20% of Africans are PMs (Flockhart 1995). But there is wide variability among populations. For example, the percentage of Polynesians who are PMs ranges from 38% to 79%, depending on the location within Polynesia. This variability was discovered somewhat accidentally; patients from the Vanuatu Islands were reported to have high or toxic levels of proguanil, the antimalarial agent metabolized by 2C19 (side effects were nausea, vomiting, and diarrhea) (Kaneko et al. 1999). This polymorphism is also unfortunate because proguanil is a pro-drug that is metabolized by 2C19 to its active antimalarial compound, cycloguanil (Funck-Brentano et al. 1997).

S-Mephenytoin has long been used in the laboratory as a substrate probe for 2C19 activity (Wedlund et al. 1984; Wrighton et al. 1993). In fact, older literature often referred to 2C19 as the S-*mephenytoin enzyme.* Measuring the clearance of *S*-mephenytoin can help to establish whether a patient is a 2C19 PM.

2C19's phenotypic variability has clinical implications. For example, Jiang et al. (2002) demonstrated that the area under the curve (AUC) of amitriptyline (which is N-demethylated by 2C19) was significantly higher in PMs than in EMs. By contrast, the AUC of nortriptyline, which is metabolized primarily by 2D6, did not differ between PMs and EMs. This study, along with others (e.g., Venkatakrishnan et al. 1998), indicates that 2C19 plays a role in amitriptyline's metabolism, despite the fact that other P450 enzymes (such as 1A2, 3A4, and 2C9) are involved as well.

Aoyama et al. (1999) discovered that patients with *Helicobacter pylori* gastritis who were PMs at 2C19 responded better to treatment with the proton pump inhibitor omeprazole, in terms of both amelioration of symptoms and eradication of *H. pylori*. This outcome is thought to be due to the higher exposure to serum omeprazole in PMs. The EMs in the study had poorer outcomes at all dose ranges. In subsequent studies, some investigators have confirmed the findings (Inaba et al. 2002); others have not (Dojo et al. 2001). Nevertheless, Desta et al. (2002) suggested that in Asian populations, which include more PMs than do Caucasian populations, routine 2C19 polymorphic testing could save $5,000 (U.S.) per 100 patients tested. Such testing can aid in determining optimal duration of treatment with and dosages of proton pump inhibitors. Determining metabolizer phenotype might also help in the case of treatment with other drugs that rely on 2C19, including phenytoin, diazepam, cyclophosphamide, and ifosfamide.

Although phenytoin levels have been shown to be higher in PMs at 2C19, the enzyme 2C9 seems to play a more important role in phenytoin's metabolism (Mamiya et al. 1998). Other investigators have noted that at higher concentrations of phenytoin, 2C19 becomes more significant in phenytoin's clearance (Ninomiya et al. 2000).

Diazepam is preferentially demethylated by 2C19 (Ono et al. 1996). Therefore, it is possible that PMs at 2C19 could have higher serum diazepam levels, but we are not aware of any attempts to determine the clinical relevance (if any) of such a result. However, inhibition of 2C19 by other drugs has been found to lead to higher diazepam levels (see "Are There Drugs That Inhibit 2C19 Activity?").

Chang et al. (1997) demonstrated that the antitumor agents cyclophosphamide and ifosfamide are 4-hydroxylated to their more active forms by 2C9 and 2C19. However, these pro-drugs are also 4-hydroxylated and activated by 2B6 (Roy et al. 1999) and by 3A4, so it is unclear whether determining that a patient is a PM at 2C19 would be helpful in treatment with these alkylating agents.

■ ARE THERE DRUGS THAT INHIBIT 2C19 ACTIVITY?

Yes. The SSRI fluvoxamine is the most potent 2C19 inhibitor, with an in vivo Ki of 0.69 μM (Rasmussen et al. 1998). Subtherapeutic doses of fluvoxamine inhibit 2C19 (Christensen et al. 2002). Ticlopidine is the other potent inhibitor of 2C19, with a Ki of 1.2 μM (Ko

et al. 2000). Other drugs with the potential for potent inhibition of
2C19 include omeprazole (Ki, 7.1 μM [Furuta et al. 2001]); fluoxetine (Harvey and Preskorn 2001) and its metabolite, norfluoxetine
(Ki, 7.1 μM [Rasmussen et al. 1998]); ritonavir (von Moltke et al.
1998); and possibly paroxetine (Fogelman et al. 1999). *S*-Omeprazole
(esomeprazole) appears to inhibit 2C19 as strongly as the racemic
mix of omeprazole. Concurrent use of *S*-omeprazole and diazepam
leads to an 81% increase in the AUC of diazepam and an increase
from 43 to 86 hours in diazepam's elimination half-life (Andersson
et al. 2001). Oral contraceptives are moderate inhibitors of 2C19
and may cause phenytoin toxicity as phenytoin is inducing the metabolism of oral contraceptives. (See Chapter 12 ["Gynecology:
Oral Contraceptives"] for a complete review of oral contraceptive
inhibition of 1A2.)

■ ARE THERE DRUGS THAT INDUCE 2C19 ACTIVITY?

Yes. Rifampin has been known to induce 2C19 as well as 2C9
(Zhou et al. 1990). Other drugs (such as anticonvulsants and steroids) that typically induce other P450 enzymes may also induce
2C19, but to a lesser extent than they induce 2C9 and 3A4 (Gerbal-
Chaloin et al. 2001).

■ REFERENCES

Alam DA, Sharma RP: Cytochrome enzyme genotype and the prediction of
therapeutic response to psychotropics. Psychiatric Annals 31:715–722,
2001

Andersson T, Hassan-Alin M, Hasselgren G, et al: Drug interaction studies
with esomeprazole, the *(S)*-isomer of omeprazole. Clin Pharmacokinet
40:523–537, 2001

Aoyama N, Tanigawara Y, Kita T, et al: Sufficient effect of 1-week omeprazole and amoxicillin dual treatment for *Helicobacter pylori* eradication
in cytochrome P450 2C19 poor metabolizers. J Gastroenterol 34 (suppl
11):80–83, 1999

Chang TK, Yu L, Goldstein JA, et al: Identification of the polymorphically expressed CYP2C19 and the wild-type CYP2C9-ILE359 allele as low-Km catalysts of cyclophosphamide and ifosfamide. Pharmacogenetics 7:211–221, 1997

Christensen M, Tybring G, Mihara K, et al: Low daily 10-mg and 20-mg doses of fluvoxamine inhibit the metabolism of both caffeine (cytochrome P4501A2) and omeprazole (cytochrome P4502C19). Clin Pharmacol Ther 71:141–152, 2002

Desta Z, Zhao X, Shin JG, et al: Clinical significance of the cytochrome P450 2C19 genetic polymorphism. Clin Pharmacokinet 41:913–958, 2002

Dojo M, Azuma T, Saito T, et al: Effects of CYP2C19 gene polymorphism on cure rates for *Helicobacter pylori* infection by triple therapy with proton pump inhibitor (omeprazole or rabeprazole), amoxycillin and clarithromycin in Japan. Dig Liver Dis 33:671–675, 2001

Flockhart DA: Drug interactions and the cytochrome P450 system: a role of cytochrome P450 2C19. Clin Pharmacokinet 29 (suppl 1):45–52, 1995

Fogelman SM, Schmider J, Venkatakrishnan K, et al: O- and N-demethylation of venlafaxine in vitro by human liver microsomes and by microsomes from cDNA-transfected cells: effect of metabolic inhibitors and SSRI antidepressants. Neuropsychopharmacology 20:480–490, 1999

Funck-Brentano C, Becquemont L, Lenevu A, et al: Inhibition by omeprazole of proguanil metabolism: mechanism of the interaction in vitro and prediction of in vivo results from the in vitro experiments. J Pharmacol Exp Ther 280:730–738, 1997

Furuta S, Kamada E, Suzuki T, et al: Inhibition of drug metabolism in human liver microsomes by nizatidine, cimetidine and omeprazole. Xenobiotica 31:1–10, 2001

Gerbal-Chaloin S, Pascussi JM, Pichard-Garcia L, et al: Induction of *CYP2C* genes in human hepatocytes in primary culture. Drug Metab Dispos 29:242–251, 2001

Glue P, Banfield CR, Perhach JL, et al: Pharmacokinetic interactions with felbamate: in vitro-in vivo correlation. Clin Pharmacokinet 33:214–224, 1997

Harvey AT, Preskorn SH: Fluoxetine pharmacokinetics and effect on CYP2C19 in young and elderly volunteers. J Clin Psychopharmacol 21:161–166, 2001

Inaba T, Mizuno M, Kawai K, et al: Randomized open trial for comparison of proton pump inhibitors in triple therapy for *Helicobacter pylori* infection in relation to CYP2C19 genotype. J Gastroenterol Hepatol 17:748–753, 2002

142

Jiang ZP, Shu Y, Chen XP, et al: The role of CYP2C19 in amitriptyline N-demethylation in Chinese subjects. Eur J Clin Pharmacol 58:109–113, 2002

Jung F, Griffin KJ, Song W, et al: Identification of amino acid substitutions that confer a high affinity for sulfaphenazole binding and a high catalytic efficiency for warfarin metabolism to P450 2C19. Biochemistry 37:16270–16279, 1998

Kaneko A, Lum JK, Yaviong L, et al: High and variable frequencies of CYP2C19 mutations: medical consequences of poor metabolism in Vanuatu and other Pacific islands. Pharmacogenetics 9:581–590, 1999

Ko JW, Desta Z, Soukhova NV, et al: In vitro inhibition of the cytochrome P450 (CYP450) system by the antiplatelet drug ticlopidine: potent effect on CYP2C19 and CYP2D6. Br J Clin Pharmacol 49:343–351, 2000

Mamiya K, Ieiri I, Shimamoto J, et al: The effects of genetic polymorphisms of CYP2C9 and CYP2C19 on phenytoin metabolism in Japanese adult patients with epilepsy: studies in stereoselective hydroxylation and population pharmacokinetics. Epilepsia 39:1317–1323, 1998

Ninomiya H, Mamiya K, Matsuo S, et al: Genetic polymorphism of the CYP2C subfamily and excessive serum phenytoin concentration with central nervous system intoxication. Ther Drug Monit 22:230–232, 2000

Ono S, Hatanaka T, Miyazawa S, et al: Human liver microsomal diazepam metabolism using cDNA-expressed cytochrome P450s: role of CYP2B6, 2C19 and the 3A subfamily. Xenobiotica 26:1155–1166, 1996

Rasmussen BB, Nielsen TL, Brosen K: Fluvoxamine inhibits the CYP2C19-catalysed metabolism of proguanil in vitro. Eur J Clin Pharmacol 54: 735–740, 1998

Roy P, Yu LJ, Crespi CL, et al: Development of a substrate-activity based approach to identify the major human liver P-450 catalysts of cyclophosphamide and ifosfamide activation based on cDNA-expressed activities and liver microsomal P-450 profiles. Drug Metab Dispos 27:655–666, 1999

Venkatakrishnan K, Greenblatt DJ, von Moltke LL, et al: Five distinct human cytochromes mediate amitriptyline N-demethylation in vitro: dominance of CYP 2C19 and 3A4. J Clin Pharmacol 38:112–121, 1998

von Moltke LL, Greenblatt DJ, Grassi JM, et al: Protease inhibitors as inhibitors of human cytochromes P450: high risk associated with ritonavir. J Clin Pharmacol 38:106–111, 1998

Wedlund PJ, Aslanian WS, McAllister CB, et al: Mephenytoin hydroxylation deficiency in Caucasians: frequency of a new oxidative drug metabolism polymorphism. Clin Pharmacol Ther 36:773–780, 1984

Wrighton SA, Stevens JC, Becker GW, et al: Isolation and characterization of human liver cytochrome P450 2C19: a correlation between 2C19 and *S*-mephenytoin 4′-hydroxylation. Arch Biochem Biophys 306:240–245, 1993

Zhou HH, Anthony LB, Wood AJ, et al: Induction of polymorphic 4′-hydroxylation of *S*-mephenytoin by rifampicin. Br J Clin Pharmacol 30: 471–475, 1990

■ STUDY CASE

A 42-year-old Caucasian businessman had been taking diazepam (5 or 10 mg prn) once or twice a week for several years to treat anxiety associated with his work. It generally calmed him, and he did not experience sedation or light-headedness. His physician prescribed omeprazole 40 mg/day for relief of gastroesophageal reflux. The patient reported that the next time he had taken 10 mg of diazepam, he felt dizzy and lethargic the entire day.

Comment

2C19 inhibition: Omeprazole inhibits 2C19. Diazepam has a complicated metabolism, but 2C19 appears to be the primary enzyme involved in its oxidative demethylation. Both racemic omeprazole and *S*-omeprazole can inhibit diazepam's metabolism.

References

Andersson T, Andren K, Cederberg C, et al: Effect of omeprazole and cimetidine on plasma diazepam levels. Eur J Clin Pharmacol 39:51–54, 1990

Andersson T, Hassan-Alin M, Hasselgren G, et al: Drug interaction studies with esomeprazole, the *(S)*-isomer of omeprazole. Clin Pharmacokinet 40:523–537, 2001

■ DRUGS METABOLIZED BY 2C19

Antidepressants	Barbiturates	Proton pump inhibitors	Other drugs
Amitriptyline[1]	Hexobarbital	Esomeprazole[5]	Alprazolam[6]
Citalopram[2]	Mephobarbital	Lansoprazole[5]	Cilostazol
Clomipramine[3]		Omeprazole[5]	Cyclophosphamide[7]
Fluoxetine[3]		Pantoprazole[5]	Diazepam[8]
Imipramine[3]		Rabeprazole[5]	Flunitrazepam[5]
Moclobemide			Ifosfamide[7]
Sertraline[3]			Indomethacin[9]
Trimipramine[3]			Mephenytoin
Venlafaxine[4]			Nelfinavir[5]
			Phenytoin[9]
			Proguanil[10]
			Propranolol
			Teniposide
			Tolbutamide[9]

[1]Amitriptyline is also metabolized by 1A2, 3A4, and 2C19. Poor metabolizers at 2C19 have been shown to have higher amitriptyline levels. [2]Also metabolized by 2D6 and 3A4. [3]Also metabolized by other P450 enzymes. [4]2C19 is a minor enzyme in venlafaxine's metabolism. 2D6 and 3A4 are the major enzymes. [5]Also metabolized by 3A4. [6]2C19 is a minor enzyme in alprazolam's metabolism. 3A4 is the major enzyme. [7]Also metabolized by 2B6 and 3A4. [8]Diazepam is demethylated by 2C19, but other P450 enzymes and conjugation enzymes are also involved in clearance. Diazepam is also metabolized by 3A4. [9]2C9 is the major route of metabolism. [10]Metabolized by 2C19 to the active compound cycloguanil.

■ INHIBITORS OF 2C19

Selective serotonin reuptake inhibitors

	Other drugs	
Fluoxetine	Cimetidine	Oral contraceptives
Fluvoxamine	Delavirdine	Oxcarbazepine
Norfluoxetine	Efavirenz	Ranitidine
Paroxetine	**Esomeprazole**	**Ritonavir**
	Felbamate	Sulfaphenazole
Other antidepressants	Fluconazole	**Ticlopidine**
Amitriptyline	Indomethacin	Topiramate
Imipramine	Lansoprazole	Tranylcypromine
	Modafinil	Valdecoxib
	Omeprazole	

Note. Names of drugs are in **bold** type if there is evidence of potent inhibition.

■ INDUCERS OF 2C19

Carbamazepine	Phenytoin	Rifampin
?Norethindrone	Prednisone	Ritonavir
Phenobarbital	Rifabutin	?Valproic acid

10

2E1

■ WHAT DOES 2E1 DO?

2E1 is unique among the P450 enzymes in its enzymatic reactions. Although it shares with 1A1 and 1A2 (see Chapter 7 ["1A2"]) the role of metabolizing polycyclic aromatic hydrocarbons (Desai et al. 2001), it can also oxidize or reduce compounds and create free radicals, which can be cytotoxic and cause tissue damage (Meskar et al. 2001). Because of its ability to metabolize numerous organic chemicals with very simple structures, such as benzene and nitrosamines (in cigarette smoke), 2E1 is believed to contribute to the risk of cancer by creating mutagens (Tanaka et al. 2000).

■ WHERE IS 2E1?

2E1 is found almost exclusively in the liver and accounts for about 5%–7% of all hepatic cytochrome activity (DeVane and Nemeroff 2002). The gene, like the genes of the 2C subfamily, is located on chromosome 10 (see the *PubMed LocusLink* review at http://www.ncbi.nlm.nih.gov/LocusLink/LocRpt.cgi?l=1571).

■ DOES 2E1 HAVE ANY POLYMORPHISMS?

Yes, but the significance of these polymorphisms is unclear (Zhang and Bian 2001). 2E1's link to liver, stomach, and esophageal cancer, through its metabolic activity of creating carcinogens, has led to intense research into the significance of polymorphisms. There may also be a relationship to polymorphisms of 2E1 and the risk of alcohol dependence (Harada 2001) or alcoholic liver disease (Ingelman-Sundberg et al. 1994).

Phenotypic variability of this enzyme has important clinical implications. For example, if organic compounds such as nitrosamines are metabolized to carcinogenic compounds by 2E1, then having more or less 2E1 activity may affect the risk of cancer.

Unfortunately, the application of bench research data to clinical practice has been difficult. Environmental factors greatly change 2E1's activity, so the importance of 2E1 polymorphisms can be difficult to measure—particularly when cancers take years to develop. For example, 2E1 activity is induced by chronic alcohol consumption (Lieber 1997b), poorly controlled diabetes (Lieber 1997a), and obesity (Kotlyar and Carson 1999). It is also inhibited by acute alcohol (Lieber 1997a), disulfiram (Emery et al. 1999), and even a single serving of watercress (Leclercq et al. 1998). Determining the significance of being a poor metabolizer, extensive metabolizer, or ultra-extensive metabolizer at this enzyme is difficult in clinical practice (Carriere et al. 1996; Itoga et al. 1998). Although different alleles have been found in Mexican Americans (Wan et al. 1998), Japanese (Sun et al. 1999), and Caucasians (Grove et al. 1998), clinical conclusions regarding 2E1 polymorphisms should not be drawn at this time.

■ ARE THERE DRUGS THAT INHIBIT 2E1 ACTIVITY?

Yes. Disulfiram may be the best-known and most potent inhibitor of 2E1. In six healthy volunteers, concomitant use of disulfiram (a single 500-mg dose) and chlorzoxazone (which is 6-hydroxylated by 2E1) increased chlorzoxazone's elimination half-life fivefold and its peak plasma levels twofold (Kharasch et al. 1993). The drug's metabolite diethylcarbamate also inhibits 2E1 (Guengerich et al. 1991). Disulfiram inhibits only 2E1, not the other P450 enzymes (Kharasch et al. 1999).

Isoniazid both inhibits and induces 2E1 (Zand et al. 1993). When treatment with isoniazid is initiated, the drug immediately inhibits 2E1 (competitive inhibition), increasing levels of other compounds dependent on 2E1 for metabolism. After isoniazid therapy has continued for several weeks, the drug decreases the serum levels of the same compounds. Induction by isoniazid may be the reason its use with acetaminophen is associated with hepatotoxicity (Self et al. 1999).

■ ARE THERE DRUGS THAT INDUCE 2E1 ACTIVITY?

Yes. The best-known chronic inducer of 2E1 is ethyl alcohol (Seitz and Csomos 1992), when used chronically. Alcohol can increase 2E1 activity 10-fold. Of course, alcohol has many other undesired effects on the liver (Lieber 1997b), and other enzymes are induced, but it appears that 2E1 is the only P450 enzyme that is induced by alcohol. The other inducers of 2E1 are isoniazid (which, as noted in the previous paragraph, both inhibits and induces 2E1), obesity (Kotlyar and Carson 1999), uncontrolled diabetes (Lieber 1997a) and smoking (Desai et al. 2001). Obesity induces none of the other P450 enzymes; however, obesity appears to be associated with some decrease in function (by an unclear mechanism) of 3A4. It is unclear why uncontrolled diabetes can induce 2E1 (Lieber 1997a), but it is believed that starvation and chronic ketone formation are involved. Smoking appears to induce 2E1 (and 1A2), probably through chronic exposure to polycyclic aromatic hydrocarbons in the smoke.

■ MISCELLANEOUS ISSUES

Chlorzoxazone (Parafon Forte), a skeletal muscle relaxant, is metabolized to 6-hydroxychlorzoxazone strictly by 2E1, which makes it an ideal probe for 2E1 activity in helping identify poor metabolizers or drugs that inhibit or induce 2E1 (Lucas et al. 1999).

Usually, 2E1's role in the metabolism of acetaminophen is minimal. 2E1 creates N-acetyl-p-benzoquinone imine (NAPQI) when it metabolizes acetaminophen, a hepatotoxic drug (Manyike et al. 2000); 3A4 and 2A6 contribute slightly to NAPQI formation as well. In normal circumstances, the liver metabolizes acetaminophen through conjugates of glucuronidation and sulfation, and very little NAPQI is produced by 2E1. The small amounts of NAPQI made are quickly conjugated with glutathione in a phase II reaction. Unfortunately, glutathione exists in relatively small quantities. When the usual hepatic metabolism of acetaminophen is overwhelmed, either by an acetaminophen overdose or by induction of 2E1 through chronic alcohol use (thereby increasing the percentage of acetaminophen being metabolized by 2E1), clinical hepatotoxic effects are possible owing to the creation of NAPQI. Although NAPQI is metabolized by phase II glutathione conjugation during an overdose, glutathione stores are rapidly depleted. The accepted clinical response is the emergent use of N-acetylcysteine, which allows glutathione stores to regenerate by competitive inhibition with NAPQI at 2E1 (McClain et al. 1999). N-Acetylcysteine then prevents further formation of NAPQI and buys time for the NAPQI created by 2E1 to be metabolized by the glutathione (Kozer and Koren 2001).

Alcoholic individuals have a higher risk of developing hepatotoxicity from therapeutic doses of acetaminophen (Seeff et al. 1986), partly because of induction of 2E1. Administration of 2E1 inhibitors (such as disulfiram) to alcoholic patients might protect these patients from acetaminophen hepatotoxicity (Hazai et al. 2002; Manyike et al. 2000). However, no definitive studies have shown that routine use of disulfiram can reduce the risk of hepatotoxicity from acetaminophen overdose or in alcoholic patients with 2E1 induction (Manyike et al. 2000).

■ REFERENCES

Carriere V, Berthou F, Baird S, et al: Human cytochrome P450 2E1 (CYP2E1): from genotype to phenotype. Pharmacogenetics 6:203–211, 1996

Desai HD, Seabolt J, Jann MW: Smoking in patients receiving psychotropic medications: a pharmacokinetic perspective. CNS Drugs 15:469–494, 2001

DeVane CL, Nemeroff CB: 2002 guide to psychotropic drug interactions. Primary Psychiatry 9:28–57, 2002

Emery MG, Jubert C, Thummel KE, et al: Duration of cytochrome P-450 2E1 (CYP2E1) inhibition and estimation of functional CYP2E1 enzyme half-life after single-dose disulfiram administration in humans. J Pharmacol Exp Ther 291:213–219, 1999

Grove J, Brown AS, Daly AK, et al: The RsaI polymorphism of CYP2E1 and susceptibility to alcoholic liver disease in Caucasians: effect on age of presentation and dependence on alcohol dehydrogenase genotype. Pharmacogenetics 8:335–342, 1998

Guengerich FP, Kim DH, Iwasaki M: Role of human cytochrome P-450 IIE1 in the oxidation of many low molecular weight cancer suspects. Chem Res Toxicol 4:168–179, 1991

Harada S: Classification of alcohol metabolizing enzymes and polymorphisms—specificity in Japanese (in Japanese). Nihon Arukoru Yakubutsu Igakkai Zasshi 36:85–106, 2001

Hazai E, Vereczkey L, Monostory K: Reduction of toxic metabolite formation of acetaminophen. Biochem Biophys Res Commun 291:1089–1094, 2002

Ingelman-Sundberg M, Ronis MJ, Lindros KO, et al: Ethanol-inducible cytochrome P4502E1: regulation, enzymology and molecular biology. Alcohol Alcohol Suppl 2:131–139, 1994

Itoga S, Harada S, Nomura F, et al: Genetic polymorphism of human CYP2E1: new alleles detected in exons and exon-intron junctions (in Japanese). Nihon Arukoru Yakubutsu Igakkai Zasshi 33:56–64, 1998

Kharasch ED, Thummel KE, Mhyre J, et al: Single-dose disulfiram inhibition of chlorzoxazone metabolism: a clinical probe for P450 2E1. Clin Pharmacol Ther 53:643–650, 1993

Kharasch ED, Hankins DC, Jubert C, et al: Lack of single-dose disulfiram effects on cytochrome P-450 2C9, 2C19, 2D6, and 3A4 activities: evidence for specificity toward P-450 2E1. Drug Metab Dispos 27:717–723, 1999

Kotlyar M, Carson SW: Effects of obesity on the cytochrome P450 enzyme system. Int J Clin Pharmacol Ther 37:8–19, 1999

Kozer E, Koren G: Management of paracetamol overdose: current controversies. Drug Saf 24:503–512, 2001

Leclercq I, Desager JP, Horsmans Y: Inhibition of chlorzoxazone metabolism, a clinical probe for CYP2E1, by a single ingestion of watercress. Clin Pharmacol Ther 64:144–149, 1998

Lieber CS: Cytochrome P-4502E1: its physiological and pathological role. Physiol Rev 77:517–544, 1997a

Lieber CS: Ethanol metabolism, cirrhosis and alcoholism. Clin Chim Acta 257:59–84, 1997b

Lucas D, Ferrara R, Gonzalez E, et al: Chlorzoxazone, a selective probe for phenotyping CYP2E1 in humans. Pharmacogenetics 9:377–388, 1999

Manyike PT, Kharasch ED, Kalhorn TF, et al: Contribution of CYP2E1 and CYP3A to acetaminophen reactive metabolite formation. Clin Pharmacol Ther 67:275–282, 2000

McClain CJ, Price S, Barve S, et al: Acetaminophen hepatotoxicity: an update. Curr Gastroenterol Rep 1:42–49, 1999

Meskar A, Plee-Gautier E, Amet Y, et al: Alcohol-xenobiotic interactions: role of cytochrome P450 2E1 (in French). Pathol Biol (Paris) 49:696–702, 2001

Novak RF, Woodcroft KJ: The alcohol-inducible form of cytochrome P450 (CYP 2E10): role in toxicology and regulation of expression. Arch Pharm Res 23:267–282, 2000

Seeff LB, Cuccherini BA, Zimmerman HJ, et al: Acetaminophen hepatotoxicity in alcoholics: a therapeutic misadventure. Ann Intern Med 104:399–404, 1986

Seitz HK, Csomos G: Alcohol and the liver: ethanol metabolism and the pathomechanism of alcoholic liver damage (in Hungarian). Orv Hetil 133:3183–3189, 1992

Self TH, Chrisman CR, Baciewicz AM, et al: Isoniazid drug and food interactions. Am J Med Sci 317:304–311, 1999

Sun F, Tsuritani I, Honda R, et al: Association of genetic polymorphisms of alcohol-metabolizing enzymes with excessive alcohol consumption in Japanese men. Hum Genet 105:295–300, 1999

Tanaka E, Terada M, Misawa S: Cytochrome P450 2E1: its clinical and toxicological role. J Clin Pharm Ther 25:165–175, 2000

Wan YJ, Poland RE, Lin KM: Genetic polymorphism of CYP2E1, ADH2, and ALDH2 in Mexican-Americans. Genet Test 2:79–83, 1998

Zand R, Nelson SD, Slattery JT, et al: Inhibition and induction of cytochrome P4502E1-catalyzed oxidation by isoniazid in humans. Clin Pharmacol Ther 54:142–149, 1993

Zhang Z, Bian J: Progress in researches on the relationship between genetic polymorphisms of alcohol-metabolizing enzymes and cancers (in Chinese). Zhonghua Yi Xue Yi Chuan Xue Za Zhi 18:62–65, 2001

Ziment I: Acetylcysteine: a drug that is much more than a mucokinetic. Biomed Pharmacother 42:513–519, 1988

■ STUDY CASE

A 26-year-old Caucasian man who had been binge drinking for several weeks decided to stop drinking. After 2 days of abstinence, he took five 650-mg tablets of acetaminophen. Forty-eight hours later, he was brought to the emergency room with symptoms of hepatitis.

Comment

2E1 induction: The patient's 2E1 enzymes were induced by the chronic, heavy ethanol consumption. When a large dose of acetaminophen is taken, the enhanced 2E1 enzymes metabolize acetaminophen into the hepatotoxic metabolite NAPQI. A theoretical therapeutic option is to give the patient a potent 2E1 inhibitor, such as disulfiram, to stop the metabolism of acetaminophen by 2E1.

Reference

Manyike PT, Kharasch ED, Kalhorn TF, et al: Contribution of CYP2E1 and CYP3A to acetaminophen reactive metabolite formation. Clin Pharmacol Ther 67:275–282, 2000

■ DRUGS METABOLIZED BY 2E1

Anesthetics[1]	Other drugs and chemicals
Enflurane	Acetaminophen[2]
Halothane	Aniline
Isoflurane	Benzene
Methoxyflurane	Capsaicin
Sevoflurane	Carbon tetrachloride[3]
	Chlorzoxazone[4]
	Dacarbazine[3]
	Ethanol[5]
	Ethylene glycol
	Ketones
	Nitrosamines
	Verapamil[6]

[1] 2E1 defluorinates these anesthetics.

[2] 2E1 is a minor substrate in normal circumstances. In cases of overdose or induction of 2E1, the hepatotoxic metabolite N-acetyl-p-benzoquinone imine (NAPQI) is created.

[3] Metabolism by 2E1 leads to production of a hepatotoxic metabolite.

[4] Used as a probe for 2E1 activity.

[5] Metabolized by other hepatic and extrahepatic enzymes.

[6] 2E1 is a minor enzyme in verapamil's metabolism. 3A4 and 2C8 are more important.

■ INHIBITORS OF 2E1

Diethylcarbamate
Disulfiram
Isoniazid
Watercress[1]

Note. Names of drugs are in **bold** type if there is evidence of clinically potent inhibition.
[1]Inhibition possibly due to phenyl isothiocyanate.

■ INDUCERS OF 2E1

Ethanol[1]
Isoniazid
Obesity
Retinoids

Smoking
Starvation
Uncontrolled diabetes

[1]Chronic ethanol use induces 2E1.

11

2A6, 2B6, AND 2C8

■ 2A6

The gene for 2A6 is located on chromosome 19 (see the *PubMed LocusLink* review at http://www.ncbi.nlm.nih.gov/LocusLink/LocRpt.cgi?l=1548). It accounts for approximately 4% of the total liver P450 content, but it has only a few clinically relevant substrates (DeVane and Nemeroff 2002). Polymorphisms have been identified with 2A6 (Nakajima et al. 2001) and may relate to the risk of cancers (Tsukino et al. 2002), perhaps because 2A6 is involved in oxidation of many precarcinogens, such as nitrosamines and aflatoxin B_1 (Oscarson 2001).

2A6 is the major enzyme involved in C-oxidation of nicotine (Yamazaki et al. 1999); 2B6 is secondarily involved in this reaction. Studies of the polymorphic nature of this enzyme and the risk of smoking behavior because of its importance in nicotine clearance have yielded conflicting results. Theoretically, a poor metabolizer (PM) would smoke less because the high nicotine levels achieved in a person with poor metabolism at this enzyme would be a deterrent to continued smoking.

2A6 specifically 7-hydroxylates coumarin, and thus 2A6 is referred to as the *coumarin* or *7-hydroxycoumarin enzyme.* This reaction may be used as a probe for 2A6 activity. Warfarin is a coumarin glycoside (dicumarol), and therefore some of warfarin's metabolism probably occurs at 2A6 along with 1A2, 2C9, and 2C19. 2A6 also appears to be the major P450 enzyme involved in metabolism of alkoxy ethers, such as methyl *tert*-butyl ether (MTBE), which have been used to decrease carbon monoxide emissions in automobile exhaust (Le Gal et al. 2001).

Potent inhibitors of 2A6 have been identified and include the monoamine oxidase inhibitor tranylcypromine (Zhang et al. 2001). Methoxsalen and tryptamine were also found to inhibit 2A6; they moderately inhibit 1A2 as well. The fact that tranylcypromine can inhibit 2A6 (Ki, 0.05–2.0 μM, depending on whether the drug is a racemic mix or an isomer) has led some to propose that using tranylcypromine or methoxsalen can reduce smoking. These drugs could functionally create PMs at 2A6, which would lead individuals to smoke less, presumably because of higher—and unpleasant—nicotine levels (Sellers et al. 2000).

References

DeVane CL, Nemeroff CB: 2002 guide to psychotropic drug interactions. Primary Psychiatry 9:28–57, 2002

Le Gal A, Dreano Y, Gervasi PG, et al: Human cytochrome P450 2A6 is the major enzyme involved in the metabolism of three alkoxyethers used in oxyfuels. Toxicol Lett 124:47–58, 2001

Kharasch ED, Hankins DC, Fenstamaker K, et al: Human halothane metabolism, lipid peroxidation, and cytochromes P(450)2A6 and P(450)3A4. Eur J Clin Pharmacol 55:853–859, 2000

Nakajima M, Kwon JT, Tanaka N, et al: Relationship between interindividual differences in nicotine metabolism and CYP2A6 genetic polymorphism in humans. Clin Pharmacol Ther 69:72–78, 2001

Niemela O, Parkkila S, Juvonen RO, et al: Cytochromes P450 2A6, 2E1, and 3A and the production of protein-aldehyde adducts in the liver of patients with alcoholic and non-alcoholic liver diseases. J Hepatol 33:893–901, 2000

Oscarson M: Genetic polymorphisms in the cytochrome P450 2A6 (CYP2A6) gene: implications for interindividual differences in nicotine metabolism. Drug Metab Dispos 29:91–95, 2001

Satarug S, Lang MA, Yongvanit P, et al: Induction of cytochrome P450 2A6 expression in humans by the carcinogenic parasite infection, opisthorchiasis viverrini. Cancer Epidemiol Biomarkers Prev 5:795–800, 1996

Sellers EM, Kaplan HL, Tyndale RF: Inhibition of cytochrome P450 2A6 increases nicotine's oral bioavailability and decreases smoking. Clin Pharmacol Ther 68:35–43, 2000

Tsukino H, Kuroda Y, Qiu D, et al: Effects of cytochrome P450 (CYP) 2A6 gene deletion and CYP2E1 genotypes on gastric adenocarcinoma. Int J Cancer 100:425–428, 2002

Yamazaki H, Inoue K, Hashimoto M, et al: Roles of CYP2A6 and CYP2B6 in nicotine C-oxidation by human liver microsomes. Arch Toxicol 73: 65–70, 1999

Zhang W, Kilicarslan T, Tyndale RF, et al: Evaluation of methoxsalen, tranylcypromine, and tryptamine as specific and selective CYP2A6 inhibitors in vitro. Drug Metab Dispos 29:897–902 2001

■ 2A6 SUBSTRATES, INHIBITORS, AND INDUCERS

Substrates	Inhibitors	Inducers
Aflatoxin B_1	Methoxsalen	Alcohol
Coumarin[1]	Tranylcypromine	?Fibrosis of the
Cyclophosphamide[2]	Tryptamine	intrahepatic bile duct
ETBE		
Halothane[3]		
Ifosfamide[2]		
MTBE		
Nicotine[4]		
Nitrosamines[5]		
TAME		

Note. ETBE=ethyl *tert*-butyl ether; MTBE=methyl *tert*-butyl ether; TAME= *tert*-amyl methyl ether.
[1]2A6 specifically 7-hydroxylates coumarin.
[2]2B6 and 3A4 are more important in the metabolism of this alkylating agent.
[3]Metabolized more by 2E1.
[4]Also metabolized by 2B6.
[5]Also metabolized by 2E1 and 1A2.

■ 2B6

The gene for 2B6 is located on chromosome 19 (see the *PubMed LocusLink* review at http://www.ncbi.nlm.nih.gov/LocusLink/LocRpt.cgi?l=1555). It accounts for less than 1% of hepatic P450 activity (DeVane and Nemeroff 2002). Genetic variability has been reported, but clear functional polymorphisms have not yet been fully elucidated.

Several important drugs are substrates of 2B6. The alkylating cancer chemotherapy agents cyclophosphamide and ifosfamide are pro-drugs and are bioactivated by 2B6 (2A6 and 3A4 also participate in metabolism) to their active phosphoramide mustards, which cross-link DNA and lead to cell death (Kan et al. 2001). (See Chapter 16: "Oncology," for more complete discussion of alkylating agents.)

Bupropion, a widely used antidepressant, is hydroxylated by 2B6 (Faucette et al. 2000), its primary oxidative route (Hesse et al. 2000). However, bupropion has alternate sites of metabolism (including 1A2, 2A6, 2C9, 2E1, and 3A4), and it is a potent inhibitor of 2D6 (Wellbutrin 2002).

The anesthetic propofol is hydroxylated by 2B6 (Court et al. 2001), and tamoxifen is metabolized to the potent antiestrogen Z-4-hydroxytamoxifen in part by 2B6 (and by 2C9 and 2D6) (Coller et al. 2002).

Potent inhibitors of 2B6 have been described, but none (except perhaps thiotepa) are specific inhibitors of 2B6 alone. The search for a specific 2B6 inhibitor will produce additional data on this enzyme. Known 2B6 inhibitors include the following:

- *The antiretrovirals ritonavir, efavirenz, and nelfinavir* (Hesse et al. 2001), which have Ki values ranging from 2.2 to 5.5 μM. Each of these drugs in the study by Hesse et al. (2001) significantly decreased hydroxylation of bupropion, whereas other antiretrovirals (indinavir, saquinavir, delavirdine, and nevirapine) had little effect on 2B6 activity of bupropion.
- *Thiotepa, an alkylating agent.* This drug has been shown to be a specific and potent 2B6 inhibitor (Rae et al. 2002). Hence, its use with cyclophosphamide and ifosfamide could lead to reduced efficacy.
- *Orphenadrine, a central nervous system active muscle relaxant* (Guo et al. 1997).
- *Fluvoxamine.* This agent was shown to inhibit bupropion's hydroxylation at 2B6 (Ki, 6 μM) (Hesse et al. 2000).

Induction of 2B6 does occur. Phenobarbital and cyclophospha-mide are the two most potent inducers found in cultured human hepatocytes (Gervot et al. 1999).

References

Coller JK, Krebsfaenger N, Klein K, et al: The influence of CYP2B6, CYP2C9 and CYP2D6 genotypes on the formation of the potent anti-estrogen Z-4-hydroxy-tamoxifen in human liver. Br J Clin Pharmacol 54:157–167, 2002

Court MH, Duan SX, Hesse LM, et al: Cytochrome P-450 2B6 is responsible for interindividual variability of propofol hydroxylation by human liver microsomes. Anesthesiology 94:110–119, 2001

DeVane CL, Nemeroff CB: 2002 guide to psychotropic drug interactions. Primary Psychiatry 9:28–57, 2002

Faucette SR, Hawke RL, Lecluyse EL, et al: Validation of bupropion hydroxylation as a selective marker of human cytochrome P450 2B6 catalytic activity. Drug Metab Dispos 28:1222–1230, 2000

Gervot L, Rochat B, Gautier JC, et al: Human CYP2B6: expression, inducibility and catalytic activities. Pharmacogenetics 9:295–306, 1999

Guo Z, Raeissi S, White RB, et al: Orphenadrine and methimazole inhibit multiple cytochrome P450 enzymes in human liver microsomes. Drug Metab Dispos 25:390–393, 1997

Hesse LM, Venkatakrishnan K, Court MH, et al: CYP2B6 mediates the in vitro hydroxylation of bupropion: potential drug interactions with other antidepressants. Drug Dispos Metab 28:1176–1183, 2000

Hesse LM, von Moltke LL, Shader RI, et al: Ritonavir, efavirenz, and nelfinavir inhibit CYP2B6 activity in vitro: potential drug interactions with bupropion. Drug Metab Dispos 29:100–102, 2001

Kan O, Griffiths L, Bathan D, et al: Direct retroviral delivery of human cytochrome P450 2B6 for gene-directed enzyme prodrug therapy in cancer. Cancer Gene Ther 8:473–482, 2001

Rae JM, Soukhova NV, Flockhart DA, et al: Triethylenethiophosphoramide is a specific inhibitor of cytochrome P450 2B6: implications for cyclophosphamide metabolism. Drug Metab Dispos 30:525–530, 2002

Wellbutrin (package insert). Research Triangle, NC, GlaxoSmithKline, 2002

Yamazaki H, Inoue K, Hashimoto M, et al: Roles of CYP2A6 and CYP2B6 in nicotine C-oxidation by human liver microsomes. Arch Toxicol 73: 65–70, 1999

■ 2B6 SUBSTRATES, INHIBITORS, AND INDUCERS

Substrates	Inhibitors	Inducers
Bupropion	Efavirenz	Cyclophosphamide
Cyclophosphamide[1]	Fluoxetine	Phenobarbital
Diazepam[2]	Fluvoxamine	
Ifosfamide[1]	Nelfinavir	
Nicotine[3]	Orphenadrine	
Propofol	**Paroxetine**	
Sertraline	Ritonavir	
Tamoxifen[4]	Thiotepa	

Note. **Bold** type indicates potent inhibitor.
[1]2B6 metabolizes this alkylating agent to its active drug.
[2]2B6 is a minor enzyme; other P450 enzymes and phase II are more important.
[3]2B6 is secondary to 2A6 in C-oxidation.
[4]Metabolized by 2B6, 2C9, and 2D6 to a potent active antiestrogenic compound.

■ 2C8

2C8 is a minor hepatic P450 enzyme that is closely related to 2C9 and 2C19. The genes for all three of these enzymes are located on chromosome 10 (see the *PubMed LocusLink* review of 2C8 at http://www.ncbi.nlm.nih.gov/LocusLink/LocRpt.cgi?l=1558). Although 2C8 plays a relatively minor role in drug metabolism, a few drugs rely on 2C8 activity for oxidative metabolism:

- *The thiazolidinediones, or "glitazones."* These oral hypoglycemic agents rely to some extent on 2C8 for clearance. Troglitazone, which was removed from the United States market because its use resulted in liver toxicity, is metabolized by 2C8 and 3A4 (Yamazaki et al. 1999). Pioglitazone (Actos 2002) and rosiglitazone (Malinowski and Bolesta 2000) are also metabolized by 2C8 and 3A4, although rosiglitazone appears to utilize 2C8 much more than 3A4.
- *Cerivastatin.* This agent is unique among the group of cholesterol-lowering agents known as hydroxymethylglutaryl–coenzyme A reductase inhibitors (or "statins"), in that it is metabolized by

2C8 as well as by 3A4 (Muck 2000). Other statin drugs are metabolized by 3A4 alone or by 2C9 (fluvastatin). Cerivastatin, however, is no longer available in the United States, because of the increased risk of death from rhabdomyolysis.

- *The anticancer drug paclitaxel.* This taxane relies on 2C8 for clearance (Cresteil et al. 2002). The related drug docetaxel relies on 3A4 instead. Dai et al. (2001) measured paclitaxel metabolism in polymorphic PMs at 2C8 and found that metabolism was reduced sixfold. The clinical implications of this finding are not yet known.

- *Verapamil.* This agent was found to be metabolized by 2C8 in addition to 3A4 (Tracy et al. 1999). Other P450 enzymes (2D6 and 2E1) may be involved in its metabolism, but they were determined to be of minor importance.

- *Retinoic acid.* 4-Hydroxylation of both isomers of retinoic acid was found to be performed by 2C8 and 3A4 (Marill et al. 2002; Nadin and Murray 1999).

- *Amiodarone.* N-demethylation of amiodarone is catalyzed by 2C8 and 3A4, with other P450 enzymes performing only a small part of this reaction (Ohyama et al. 2000).

References

Actos (package insert). Indianapolis, IN, Eli Lilly and Company, 2002

Cresteil T, Monsarrat B, Dubois J, et al: Regioselective metabolism of taxoids by human CYP3A4 and 2C8: structure-activity relationship. Drug Metab Dispos 39:438–445, 2002

Dai D, Zeldin DC, Blaisdell JA, et al: Polymorphisms in human CYP2C8 decrease metabolism of the anticancer drug paclitaxel and arachidonic acid. Pharmacogenetics 11:597–607, 2001

Malinowski JM, Bolesta S: Rosiglitazone in the treatment of type 2 diabetes mellitus: a critical review. Clin Ther 22:1151–1168, 2000

Marill J, Capron CC, Idres N, et al: Human cytochrome P450s involved in the metabolism of 9-*cis*- and 13-*cis*-retinoic acids. Biochem Pharmacol 63:933–943, 2002

Muck W: Clinical pharmacokinetics of cerivastatin. Clin Pharmacokinet 39: 99–116, 2000

Nadin L, Murray M: Participation of CYP2C8 in retinoic acid 4-hydroxylation in human hepatic microsomes. Biochem Pharmacol 58:1201–1208, 1999

Ohyama K, Nakajima M, Nakamura S, et al: A significant role of human cytochrome P450 2C8 in amiodarone N-demethylation: an approach to predict the contribution with relative activity factor. Drug Metab Dispos 28:1303–1310, 2000

Tracy TS, Korzekwa KR, Gonzalez FJ, et al: Cytochrome P450 isoforms involved in metabolism of the enantiomers of verapamil and norverapamil. Br J Clin Pharmacol 47:545–552, 1999

Yamazaki H, Shibata A, Suzuki M, et al: Oxidation of troglitazone to a quinone-type metabolite catalyzed by cytochrome P-450 2C8 and P-450 3A4 in human liver microsomes. Drug Metab Dispos 27:1260–1266, 1999

■ 2C8 SUBSTRATES

Amiodarone	Thiazolidinediones ("glitazones")
Cerivastatin	Pioglitazone
Naproxen	Rosiglitazone
Paclitaxel	Troglitazone
Retinoic acid	Verapamil
	Zopiclone

Note. Most of these drugs are metabolized by other P450 enzymes as well.

Part III

Drug Interactions by Medical Specialty

12

GYNECOLOGY: ORAL CONTRACEPTIVES

Forty years ago, the introduction of Enovid (norethynodrel 10 mg and mestranol 150 µg), which provided convenient and reliable contraception, revolutionized birth control. Reports of interactions between oral contraceptives (OCs) and other drugs began to trickle into the literature. At first, these drug interactions appeared to be random and unrelated. Increased understanding of P450 enzymes and phase II reactions of sulfation and glucuronidation has permitted preliminary categorization and assessment of the clinical relevance of these drug interactions.

> **Reminder:** This chapter is dedicated primarily to metabolic interactions. Interactions due to displaced protein-binding, alterations in absorption or excretion, and pharmacodynamics are not covered.

■ ORAL CONTRACEPTIVES

Most OCs contain both estrogen and progestin. The estrogen suppresses ovulation, and the progestin suppresses luteinizing hormone, to create an environment unreceptive to sperm. In addition, progestins limit endometrial hyperplasia and decrease the likeli-

Portions of this chapter are adapted from Shader RI, Oesterheld JR: "Contraceptive Effectiveness: Cytochromes and Induction." *Journal of Clinical Psychopharmacology* 20:119–121, 2000.

hood of endometrial carcinoma. There has been a strong trend in recent years toward using lower-dose estrogen preparations, to reduce the likelihood of estrogen-related complications (e.g., headache and thromboembolic disorders). Most OCs contain between 35 and 50 mg of estrogen, usually in the form of 17α-ethinylestradiol. Very low dose OCs contain only 20 μg of ethinyl estradiol (EE) (e.g., Alesse, Levlite, Loestrin 1/20, and Mircette). Only a few OCs contain the original estrogen, mestranol, the 3-methyl ether of EE (e.g., Genora 1/50, Nelova 1/50M, Norinyl 1+50, and Ortho-Novum 1/50).

Several formulations of OCs are available. Monophasic preparations contain the same amount of EE and progestin and are taken for 21 days in each 28-day cycle. Biphasic and triphasic preparations take the form of two or three types of pills, with varying amounts of active ingredients. Biphasic and triphasic OCs have been formulated so that the amount of progestin is reduced and the effects correspond more closely to hormonal influences during natural menstrual cycles. There are a limited number of progestin-only contraceptives. These contraceptives are the minipill, which contains 350 μg of norethindrone or 75 μg of norgestrel; a subdermal implant of norgestrel (Norplant); an intramuscular preparation of medroxyprogesterone acetate (Depo-Provera), administered every 3 months; and an intrauterine device (Progestasert).

Metabolism of Oral Contraceptives

The metabolism of OCs, which is very complicated, is incompletely understood. Mestranol is first metabolized by 2C9 to EE. After first-pass metabolism, about half of EE reaches the systemic circulation unchanged; the remainder is metabolized in the liver and gut wall. Although a variety of metabolic pathways exist, the major route of inactivation of EE is via 3A4 (Guengerich 1990b). An enterohepatic recirculation is also postulated for conjugated EE (but is not important for progestins). EE is hydrolyzed by gut bacteria (principally clostridia) back to free EE. Further metabolic steps include formation of estrone, estratriol, and catechol estrogens. Each estrogen is glucuronidated and sulfated via unique or overlapping conjugates (see Raftogianis et al. 2000 for an excellent review of estrogen metabolism). Sulfated estrone, the major circulating form of estrogen, is desulfated, metabolized, and transported to free EE to act at estrogen receptors (Song 2001). Transformation of EE and estrone to catechol estrogens and to quinones can result in DNA adducts that are genotoxins and that may be very important in the development of breast and other cancers (Adjei and Weinshilboum 2002). The possible genetic polymorphisms at each "node" of this complex metabolic "web" may account for the enormous interindividual variations of each estrogen.

Progestins are also metabolized via 3A4, with the exception of progestins containing desogestrel, a pro-drug that must be metabolized via 2C9 to the active form of progestin.

3A4 and UGT Induction of Oral Contraceptives

Induction of 3A4 or uridine 5'-diphosphate glucuronosyltransferase UGT 1A1 (and others) may lead to increased clearance of EE and/ or progestins and loss of clinical efficacy. Drug interactions resulting in spotting, breakthrough bleeding, or unwanted pregnancy have occurred in women taking OCs and griseofulvin (van Dijke and Weber 1984), rifampin (Joshi et al. 1980), rifabutin (Barditch-Crovo et al. 1999), troglitazone (Loi et al. 1999), or enzyme-inducing anticonvulsants (phenobarbital, primidone, phenytoin [Baciewicz 1985], or oxcarbazepine [Fattore et al. 1999]). Carbamazepine can both render OCs ineffective and cause fetal neural tube defects. Topiramate and felbamate may also induce 3A4. These two drugs increase clearance of EE (Rosenfeld et al. 1997; Saano et al. 1995), and it is possible that they also cause contraceptive failure.

Chronic use of ritonavir may induce metabolism of EE (Ouellet et al. 1998). A combination human immunodeficiency virus drug, a protease inhibitor containing lopinavir and ritonavir, carries a manufacturer's warning about lopinavir/ritonavir's ability to induce metabolism of EE. This drug induces glucuronidation and may also induce metabolism of EE at 3A4 (Abbott Laboratories, Products Division, personal communication, December 2000). Nevirapine has been shown to affect EE similarly (Mildvan et al. 2002), and it is likely that efavirenz also has the same action.

St. John's wort has recently been shown to induce 3A4 (Moore et al. 2000; Roby et al. 2000), and the herbal preparation is likely to cause contraceptive failure, although formal case reports have not yet entered the literature. Clinicians should ask their patients about use of St. John's wort. Modafinil has also been shown to decrease the maximum observed plasma concentration of EE (Robertson et al. 2002). Some anticonvulsants/mood stabilizers (valproate [Crawford et al. 1986], gabapentin [Eldon et al. 1998], lamotrigine [Holdich et al. 1991; Hussein and Posner 1997], and vigabatrin [Bartoli et al. 1997]) have been shown *not* to increase OC clearance. (However, lamotrigine concentrations are reduced by OC induction.)

3A4 or UGT inducers also increase clearance of progestin-only contraceptives, substrates of 3A4. Although not as well documented as interactions involving EE, contraceptive failure of levonorgestrel has been reported in women given phenobarbital (Shane-McWhorter et al. 1998) or phenytoin (Haukkamaa 1986; Odlind and Olsson 1986).

There are reports of women becoming pregnant while taking both EE or progestin-only preparations and other drugs, but it is not known how common such pregnancies are. Pharmacokinetic interactions between OCs and 3A4 or UGT inducers do occur, but how often do clinically significant pharmacodynamic outcomes result? Given the wide interindividual variation of 3A4 and UGTs, some women may be vulnerable to these drug interactions. A recent small clinical study of rifampin, rifabutin, and OCs substantiated the ability of rifampin and rifabutin to increase clearance of OCs, although none of the 12 women in the study ovulated (Barditch-Crovo et al. 1999). Currently, lower and lower dosing of EE is being used, and women who take OCs with only 20 µg of EE may be especially vulnerable. It is recommended that until clinicians can identify women at risk, patients taking enzyme-inducing anticonvulsants (except phenytoin [see the discussion in "1A2, 2C19, and 3A4 Inhibition by Oral Contraceptives" later in the chapter]) with OCs take the former with 50–100 µg of EE. Another option is more frequent dosing of

■ DRUGS, HERBS, AND FOODS THAT AFFECT ORAL CONTRACEPTIVES

Some drugs and herbal preparations that induce 3A4 and can cause contraceptive failure	*Some drugs and foods that may increase or prolong oral contraceptive activity*
Carbamazepine (Tegretol and others)	Acetaminophen (Tylenol)
?Efavirenz (Sustiva)	Fluconazole (Diflucan)
Felbamate (Felbatol)	Dapsone
Griseofulvin (Fulvicin and others)	Erythromycin, other macrolides
Modafinil (Provigil)	Fluoxetine (Prozac)
Nevirapine (Viracept)	Fluvoxamine (Luvox)
Oxcarbazepine (Trileptal)	?Gestodene
Phenobarbital (Luminal and others)	Grapefruit juice
Phenytoin (Dilantin)	Itraconazole (Sporanox)
Primidone (Mysoline)	Ketoconazole (Nizoral)
Rifabutin (Mycobutin)	Nefazodone (Serzone)
Rifampin (Rifadin and others)	Ritonavir (Norvir)
Ritonavir (Norvir)	Vitamin C
St. John's wort	
Topiramate (Topamax)	
Troglitazone (Rezulin)	

DRUGS WHOSE CLEARANCE IS CHANGED BY ORAL CONTRACEPTIVES

Drugs whose clearance is decreased by oral contraceptives	*Drugs whose clearance is increased by oral contraceptives*
Amitriptyline (Elavil, Endep)	Acetaminophen (Tylenol)
Caffeine	Clofibrate (Atromid-S)
Chlordiazepoxide (Librium)	Diflunisal (Dolobid)
Chlorpromazine (Thorazine)	Lamotrigine (Lamictal)
Clozapine (Clozaril)	?Lorazepam (Ativan)
?Cyclooxygenase-2 inhibitors	?Oxazepam (Serax)
Cyclosporine (Neoral and others)	Phenprocoumon
Diazepam (Valium)	?Temazepam (Restoril)
Imipramine (Tofranil)	
?Olanzapine (Zyprexa)	
Phenytoin (Dilantin)	
Prednisolone	
?Proton pump inhibitors	
Selegiline (Deprenyl and others)	
?Tacrine (Cognex)	
Theophylline (Slo-Bid and others)	

intramuscular preparations of progestin-only OCs. In addition to either of these approaches, women taking enzyme-inducing drugs along with OCs should also be instructed to use barrier contraceptives midcycle to prevent pregnancy (Crawford et al. 1990). Replacement of 3A4-inducing anticonvulsants with noninducing alternatives should also be considered (Guberman 1999). An enzyme inducer's effects can continue after administration of the inducer has ceased. As has been recommended with rifampin use ("Use of Rifampin and Contraceptive Steroids" 1999), after short-term treatments with 3A4 or UGT inducers are discontinued, patients taking OCs need to take extra contraceptive precautions for up to 4 weeks.

3A4 Inhibition of Oral Contraceptives

Because EE is a 3A4 substrate, potent inhibitors of 3A4 can decrease EE clearance and increase or prolong estrogenic activity. Although not likely to impair contraceptive efficacy, potent 3A4 inhibitors can be expected to increase estrogen-related side effects (e.g., migraine headaches or thromboembolic events) in susceptible women. Well-described drugs known to increase EE levels include the antifungals ketoconazole, itraconazole, and fluconazole (Hilbert et al. 2001; Sinofsky and Pasquale 1998); antivirals such as ritonavir; and potent macrolides (Meyer et al. 1990; Pessayre 1983; Wermeling et al. 1995). Dapsone has been shown to increase peak EE concentration (Joshi et al. 1984). Even grapefruit juice is known to increase EE levels (Weber et al. 1996). Although gestodene has been shown to increase EE in vitro (Guengerich 1990a), this interaction may not be clinically significant (Lawrenson and Farmer 2000). It is likely that psychotropics (e.g., nefazodone, fluvoxamine, and fluoxetine) known to potently inhibit 3A4 will also be shown to affect EE clearance. If these 3A4 inhibitors are added to OCs that contain only 20 µg of EE, the low-dose OCs may become higher-dose OCs and cause adverse events (e.g., breast tenderness, bloating, weight gain). In one case, these symptoms occurred when nefazodone was added to Mircette (Adson and Kotlyar 2001).

2C9 Inhibition of Oral Contraceptives

Mestranol is demethylated to EE by 2C9, so potent inhibitors of 2C9 may lessen the likelihood of adequate EE levels in OCs such as Genora 1/50, Nelova 1/50M, Norinyl 1+ 50 and Ortho-Novum 1/50. Examples of 2C9 inhibitors are sulfaphenazole and other sulfonamide antibiotics, valproate, and fluconazole (see Chapter 8 ["2C9"]). Once demethylated, mestranol is as susceptible to induction or inhibition as any EE.

OCs containing desogestrel (e.g., Mircette, Ortho-Cept) are also vulnerable to 2C9 inhibitors because such OCs are metabolized to their active forms by 2C9 (and other enzymes [Gentile et al. 1998]). Long-term use of OCs that do not contain progestin may have deleterious effects (Adson and Kotlyar 2001). When these OCs are used, potent 2C9 inhibitors should be avoided.

1A2, 2C19, and 3A4 Inhibition by Oral Contraceptives

Not only is clearance of OCs affected by other agents, but OCs can affect clearance of other drugs. Current evidence suggests that OCs are moderate inhibitors of 1A2 and 2C19 and mild inhibitors of 3A4. OCs decrease clearance of caffeine and theophylline, well-known substrates of 1A2 (Abernethy and Todd 1985; Gu et al. 1992; Roberts et al. 1983; Tornatore et al. 1982; Zhang and Kaminsky 1995). Because a 30% decrease in theophylline clearance occurs with OC use (Jonkman 1986), clinicians should decrease theophylline doses. Although the side-chain oxidation of propranolol is a 1A2 phenomenon (Yoshimoto et al. 1995) and is inhibited by OCs (Walle et al. 1996), nullifying effects of OCs on propranolol glucuronidation prevent significant interactions (Walle et al. 1989, 1996). Two cases of interactions between OCs and psychotropic 1A2 substrates have recently been reported. Clozapine levels were significantly increased with the addition of an OC (Gabbay et al. 2002), and chlorpromazine levels increased sixfold when an OC was added (Chetty and Miller 2001). No reports of drug interactions between olanzapine or tacrine with OCs are currently found in the literature, although these drug interactions are possible. Plasma concentrations of tacrine have been shown to be increased by hormone replacement therapy (which contains very low amounts of estrogen) (Laine et al. 1999b); therefore, tacrine levels are likely increased by OCs.

Support for OCs' inhibition of 2C19 was provided by three population studies (Hagg et al. 2001; Laine et al. 2000; Tamminga et al. 1999). The activity of 2C19 in women who used OCs was decreased by 68% compared with that in women who did not use OCs (Tamminga et al. 1999). Although the focus of interest in the interaction between OC and phenytoin has been on phenytoin's induction of OC metabolism, OCs have also been found to decrease clearance of phenytoin (De Leacy et al. 1979). Thus, increasing OC dosing to overcome phenytoin induction of EE can result in phenytoin toxicity, and this drug combination is best avoided. The concentration of selegiline (a substrate of 2C19 and 2B6) is increased more than 10-fold when OCs are added (Laine et al. 1999a). No information regarding other 2C19 substrates (e.g., proton pump inhibitors, cyclooxygenase-2 inhibitors, citalopram, proguanil) was found, but these drugs may be similarly affected.

Results of in vitro studies of EE effects are conflicting (Guengerich 1990a), but there is evidence to support the finding of very modest in vivo inhibition of 3A4 by EE (Belle et al. 2002; Palovaara et al. 2000). Although concentrations of EE are higher in women who take OCs for more than 6 months, clearance of EE in these women is reduced (Tornatore et al. 1982). Other inferential evidence comes from several interactions between OCs and drugs known to be substrates of 3A4: cyclosporine (Deray et al. 1987), prednisolone (Seidegard et al. 2000), and levonorgestrel (Fotherby 1991).

Inhibition by OCs of both 3A4 and 2C19 is likely responsible for several well-documented OC-drug interactions. Clearances of imipramine, amitriptyline, and diazepam are decreased by OCs (Abernethy et al. 1982, 1984; Edelbroek et al. 1987). 2C19 is a principal pathway for demethylation of these drugs; 3A4 is also involved (Jung et al. 1997; Koyama et al. 1997; Venkatakrishnan et al. 1998). Clearance of chlordiazepoxide may also be reduced by OCs (Patwardhan et al. 1983). Chlordiazepoxide's intermediate metabolite, nordiazepam, is known to be metabolized by 3A4 and 2C19 (Ono et al. 1996). Whether other benzodiazepines that are metabolized via this intermediate metabolite are also affected has not yet been investigated.

Glucuronidation Induction by Oral Contraceptives

Although the specific UGTs remain to be identified, OCs increase glucuronidation clearance of the following drugs: clofibrate (Miners et al. 1984), propranolol (Walle et al. 1996), phenprocoumon (Monig et al. 1990), diflunisal (Herman et al. 1994), and lamotrigine (Sabers et al. 2001). Data are conflicting with regard to lorazepam, oxazepam, and temazepam (Abernethy et al. 1983; Patwardhan et al. 1983; Stoehr et al. 1984).

Acetaminophen is conjugated by UGT1A1, UGT1A6, and UGT1A9 (Court et al. 2001), and OCs are known to increase glucuronidation of acetaminophen (Mitchell et al. 1983). EE clearance also decreases when vitamin C or acetaminophen is added. This interaction occurs because vitamin C and acetaminophen compete with EE in the gut wall (Rogers et al. 1987) for sulfation (via sulfotransferase SULT1A1 [Dooley 1998]).

■ CONCLUSION

When obtaining a woman's medication history, the clinician should inquire whether the patient is taking OCs. Clinicians often neglect to ask this question (Hocking and deMello 1997). Physicians need to be vigilant about drug interactions involving OCs, and they should be particularly alert at times of addition or subtraction of drugs in women taking OCs.

■ REFERENCES

Abernethy DR, Todd EL: Impairment of caffeine clearance by chronic use of low-dose oestrogen-containing oral contraceptives. Eur J Clin Pharmacol 28:425–428, 1985

Abernethy DR, Greenblatt DJ, Divoll M, et al: Impairment of diazepam metabolism by low-dose estrogen-containing oral-contraceptive steroids. N Engl J Med 306:791–792, 1982

Abernethy DR, Greenblatt DJ, Ochs HR, et al: Lorazepam and oxazepam kinetics in women on low-dose oral contraceptives. Clin Pharmacol Ther 33:628–632, 1983

Abernethy DR, Greenblatt DJ, Shader RI: Imipramine disposition in users of oral contraceptive steroids. Clin Pharmacol Ther 35:792–797, 1984

Adjei AA, Weinshilboum RM: Catecholestrogen sulfation: possible role in carcinogenesis. Biochem Biophys Res Commun 292:402–408, 2002

Adson DE, Kotlyar M: A probable interaction between a very low-dose oral contraceptive and the antidepressant nefazodone: a case report. J Clin Psychopharmacol 21:618–619, 2001

Baciewicz AM: Oral contraceptive drug interactions. Ther Drug Monit 7: 26–35, 1985

Barditch-Crovo P, Trapnell CB, Ette E, et al: The effects of rifampin and rifabutin on the pharmacokinetics and pharmacodynamics of a combination oral contraceptive. Clin Pharmacol Ther 65:428–438, 1999

Bartoli A, Gatti G, Cipolla G, et al: A double-blind, placebo-controlled study on the effect of vigabatrin on in vivo parameters of hepatic microsomal enzyme induction and on the kinetics of steroid oral contraceptives in healthy female volunteers. Epilepsia 38:702–707, 1997

Belle DI, Callaghan JT, Gorski JC, et al: The effects of an oral contraceptive containing ethinylestradiol and norgestrel on CYP3A activity. Br J Clin Pharmacol 53:67–74, 2002

Chetty M, Miller R: Oral contraceptives increase the plasma concentrations of chlorpromazine. Ther Drug Monit 23:556–558, 2001

Court MH, Duan SX, von Moltke LL, et al: Interindividual variability in acetaminophen glucuronidation by human liver microsomes: identification of relevant acetaminophen UDP-glucuronosyltransferase isoforms. J Pharmacol Exp Ther 299:998–1006, 2001

Crawford P, Chadwick D, Cleland P, et al: The lack of effect of sodium valproate on the pharmacokinetics of oral contraceptive steroids. Contraception 33:23–29, 1986

Crawford P, Chadwick DJ, Martin C, et al: The interaction of phenytoin and carbamazepine with combined oral contraceptive steroids. Br J Clin Pharmacol 30:892–896, 1990

De Leacy EA, McLeay CD, Eadie MJ, et al: Effects of subjects' sex, and intake of tobacco, alcohol and oral contraceptives on plasma phenytoin levels. Br J Clin Pharmacol 8:33–36, 1979

Deray G, le Hoang P, Cacoub P, et al: Oral contraceptive interaction with cyclosporin. Lancet 1:158–159, 1987

Dooley TP: Molecular biology of the human phenol sulfotransferase gene family. J Exp Zool 282:223–230, 1998

Edelbroek PM, Zitman FG, Knoppert-van der Klein EA, et al: Therapeutic drug monitoring of amitriptyline: impact of age, smoking and contraceptives on drug and metabolite levels in bulimic women. Clin Chim Acta 165:177–187, 1987

Eldon MA, Underwood BA, Randinitis EJ, et al: Gabapentin does not interact with a contraceptive regimen of norethindrone acetate and ethinyl estradiol. Neurology 50:1146–1148, 1998

Fattore C, Cipolla G, Gatti G, et al: Induction of ethinylestradiol and levonorgestrel metabolism by oxcarbazepine in healthy women. Epilepsia 40:783–787, 1999

Fotherby K: Intrasubject variability in the pharmacokinetics of ethinyloestradiol. J Steroid Biochem Mol Biol 38:733–736, 1991

Gabbay V, O'Dowd MA, Mamamtavrishvili M, et al: Clozapine and oral contraceptives: a possible drug interaction. J Clin Psychopharmacol 22:621–622, 2002

Gentile DM, Verhoeven CH, Shimada T, et al: The role of CYP2C in the in vitro bioactivation of the contraceptive steroid desogestrel. J Pharmacol Exp Ther 287:975–982, 1998

Gu L, Gonzalez FJ, Kalow W, et al: Biotransformation of caffeine, paraxanthine, theobromine and theophylline by cDNA-expressed human CYP1A2 and CYP2E1. Pharmacogenetics 2:73–77, 1992

Guberman A: Hormonal contraception and epilepsy. Neurology 53 (suppl 1):838–840, 1999

Guengerich FP: Inhibition of oral contraceptive steroid-metabolizing enzymes by steroids and drugs. Am J Obstet Gynecol 163:2159–2163, 1990a

Guengerich FP: Metabolism of 17 alpha-ethynylestradiol in humans. Life Sci 47:1981–1988, 1990b

Hagg S, Spigset O, Dahlqvist R: Influence of gender and oral contraceptives on CYP2D6 and CYP2C19 activity in healthy volunteers. Br J Clin Pharmacol 51:169–173, 2001

Haukkamaa M: Contraception by Norplant subdermal capsules is not reliable in epileptic patients on anticonvulsant treatment. Contraception 33:559–565, 1986

Herman RJ, Loewen GR, Antosh DM, et al: Analysis of polymorphic variation in drug metabolism, III: glucuronidation and sulfation of diflunisal in man. Clin Invest Med 17:297–307, 1994

Hilbert J, Messig M, Kuye O, et al: Evaluation of interaction between fluconazole and an oral contraceptive in healthy women. Obstet Gynecol 98:218–223, 2001

Hocking G, deMello WF: Taking a 'drugs' history. Anaesthesia 52:904–905, 1997

Holdich T, Whiteman P, Orme M, et al: Effect of lamotrigine on the pharmacology of the combined oral contraceptive pill (abstract). Epilepsia 32 (suppl 1):96, 1991

Hussein Z, Posner J: Population pharmacokinetics of lamotrigine monotherapy in patients with epilepsy: retrospective analysis of routine monitoring data. Br J Clin Pharmacol 43:457–465, 1997

Jonkman JH: Therapeutic consequences of drug interactions with theophylline pharmacokinetics. J Allergy Clin Immunol 78:736–742, 1986

Joshi JV, Joshi UM, Sankolli GM, et al: A study of interaction of a low-dose combination oral contraceptive with anti-tubercular drugs. Contraception 21:617–629, 1980

Joshi JV, Maitra A, Sankolli G, et al: Norethisterone and ethinyl estradiol kinetics during dapsone therapy. J Assoc Physicians India 32:191–193, 1984

Jung F, Richardson TH, Raucy JL, et al: Diazepam metabolism by cDNA-expressed human 2C P450s: identification of P4502C18 and P4502C19 as low K(M) diazepam N-demethylases. Drug Metab Dispos 25:133–139, 1997

Koyama E, Chiba K, Tani M, et al: Reappraisal of human CYP isoforms involved in imipramine N-demethylation and 2-hydroxylation: a study using microsomes obtained from putative extensive and poor metabolizers of S-mephenytoin and eleven recombinant human CYPs. J Pharmacol Exp Ther 281:1199–1210, 1997

Laine K, Anttila M, Helminen A, et al: Dose linearity study of selegiline pharmacokinetics after oral administration: evidence for strong drug interaction with female sex steroids. Br J Clin Pharmacol 47:249–254, 1999a

Laine K, Palovaara S, Tapanainen P, et al: Plasma tacrine concentrations are significantly increased by concomitant hormone replacement therapy. Clin Pharmacol Ther 66:602–608, 1999b

Laine K, Tybring G, Bertilsson L: No sex-related differences but significant inhibition by oral contraceptives of CYP2C19 activity as measured by the probe drugs mephenytoin and omeprazole in healthy Swedish white subjects. Clin Pharmacol Ther 68:151–159, 2000

Lawrenson R, Farmer R: Venous thromboembolism and combined oral contraceptives: does the type of progestogen make a difference? Contraception 62 (suppl 2):S21–S28, 2000

Liu HF, Magdalou J, Nicolas A, et al: Oral contraceptives stimulate the excretion of clofibric acid glucuronide in women and female rats. Gen Pharmacol 22:393–397, 1991

Loi CM, Stern R, Koup JR, et al: Effect of troglitazone on the pharmacokinetics of an oral contraceptive agent. J Clin Pharmacol 39:410–417, 1999

Meyer B, Muller F, Wessels P, et al: A model to detect interactions between roxithromycin and oral contraceptives. Clin Pharmacol Ther 47:671–674, 1990

Mildvan D, Yarish R, Marshak A, et al: Pharmacokinetic interaction between nevirapine and ethinylestradiol/norethindrone when administered concurrently to HIV-infected women. J Acquir Immune Defic Syndr 29:471–477, 2002

Miners JO, Robson RA, Birkett DJ: Gender and oral contraceptive steroids as determinants of drug glucuronidation: effects on clofibric acid elimination. Br J Clin Pharmacol 18:240–243, 1984

Mitchell MC, Hanew T, Meredith CG, et al: Effects of oral contraceptive steroids on acetaminophen metabolism and elimination. Clin Pharmacol 34:48–53, 1983

Monig H, Baese C, Heidemann HT, et al: Effect of oral contraceptive steroids on the pharmacokinetics of phenprocoumon. Br J Clin Pharmacol 30:115–118, 1990

Moore LB, Goodwin B, Jones SA, et al: St. John's wort induces hepatic drug metabolism through activation of the pregnane X receptor. Proc Natl Acad Sci USA 97:7500–7502, 2000

Odlind V, Olsson SE: Enhanced metabolism of levonorgestrel during phenytoin treatment in a woman with Norplant implants. Contraception 33:257–261, 1986

Ono S, Hatanaka T, Miyazawa S, et al: Human liver microsomal diazepam metabolism using cDNA-expressed cytochrome P450s: role of CYP2B6, 2C19 and the 3A subfamily. Xenobiotica 26:1155–1166, 1996

Ouellet D, Hsu A, Qian J, et al: Effect of ritonavir on the pharmacokinetics of ethinyl oestradiol in healthy female volunteers. Br J Clin Pharmacol 46:111–116, 1998

Palovaara S, Kivisto KT, Tapanainen P, et al: Effect of an oral contraceptive preparation containing ethinylestradiol and gestodene on CYP3A4 activity as measured by midazolam 1'-hydroxylation. Br J Clin Pharmacol 50:333–337, 2000

Patwardhan RV, Mitchell MC, Johnson RF, et al: Differential effects of oral contraceptive steroids on the metabolism of benzodiazepines. Hepatology 3:248–253, 1983

Pessayre D: Effects of macrolide antibiotics on drug metabolism in rats and in humans. Int J Clin Pharmacol Res 3:449–458, 1983

Raftogianis R, Creveling C, Weinshilboum R, et al: Estrogen metabolism by conjugation. J Natl Cancer Inst Monogr 27:113–124, 2000

Roberts RK, Grice J, McGuffie C, et al: Oral contraceptive steroids impair the elimination of theophylline. J Lab Clin Med 101:821–825, 1983

Robertson P Jr, Hellriegel ET, Arora S, et al: Effect of modafinil on the pharmacokinetics of ethinyl estradiol and triazolam in healthy volunteers. Clin Pharmacol Ther 71:46–56, 2002

Roby CA, Anderson GD, Kantor E, et al: St John's wort: effect on CYP3A4 activity. Clin Pharmacol Ther 67:451–457, 2000

Rogers SM, Back DJ, Stevenson PJ, et al: Paracetamol interaction with oral contraceptive steroids: increased plasma concentrations of ethinyloestradiol. Br J Clin Pharmacol 23:721–725, 1987

Rosenfeld WE, Doose DR, Walker SA, et al: Effect of topiramate on the pharmacokinetics of an oral contraceptive containing norethindrone and ethinyl estradiol in patients with epilepsy. Epilepsia 38:317–323, 1997

Saano V, Glue P, Banfield CR, et al: Effects of felbamate on the pharmacokinetics of a low-dose combination oral contraceptive. Clin Pharmacol Ther 58:523–531, 1995

Sabers A, Buckholt JM, Uldall P, et al: Lamotrigine plasma levels reduced by oral contraceptives. Epilepsy Res 47:151–154, 2001

Seidegard J, Simonsson M, Edsbacker S: Effect of an oral contraceptive on the plasma levels of budesonide and prednisolone and the influence on plasma cortisol. Clin Pharmacol Ther 67:373–381, 2000

Shane-McWhorter L, Cerveny JD, MacFarlane LL, et al: Enhanced metabolism of levonorgestrel during phenobarbital treatment and resultant pregnancy. Pharmacotherapy 18:1360–1364, 1998

Sinofsky FE, Pasquale SA: The effect of fluconazole on circulating ethinyl estradiol levels in women taking oral contraceptives. Am J Obstet Gynecol 178:300–304, 1998

Song WC: Biochemistry and reproductive endocrinology of estrogen sulfotransferase. Ann N Y Acad Sci 948:43–50, 2001

Stoehr GP, Kroboth PD, Juhl RP, et al: Effect of oral contraceptives on triazolam, temazepam, alprazolam, and lorazepam kinetics. Clin Pharmacol Ther 36:683–690, 1984

Tamminga WJ, Wemer J, Oosterhuis B, et al: CYP2D6 and CYP2C19 activity in a large population of Dutch healthy volunteers: indications for oral contraceptive-related gender differences. Eur J Clin Pharmacol 55: 177–184, 1999

Tornatore KM, Kanarkowski R, McCarthy TL, et al: Effect of chronic oral contraceptive steroids on theophylline disposition. Eur J Clin Pharmacol 23:129–134, 1982

Use of rifampin and contraceptive steroids. Br J Fam Plann 24:169–170, 1999

van Dijke CP, Weber JC: Interaction between oral contraceptives and griseofulvin. Br Med J (Clin Res Ed) 288:1125–1126, 1984

Venkatakrishnan K, Greenblatt DJ, von Moltke LL, et al: Five distinct human cytochromes mediate amitriptyline N-demethylation in vitro: dominance of CYP 2C19 and 3A4. J Clin Pharmacol 38:112–121, 1998

Walle T, Walle UK, Cowart TD, et al: Pathway-selective sex differences in the metabolic clearance of propranolol in human subjects. Clin Pharmacol Ther 46:257–263, 1989

Walle T, Fagan TC, Walle UK, et al: Stimulatory as well as inhibitory effects of ethinyloestradiol on the metabolic clearances of propranolol in young women. Br J Clin Pharmacol 41:305–309, 1996

Weber A, Jager R, Borner A, et al: Can grapefruit juice influence ethinylestradiol bioavailability? Contraception 53:41–47, 1996

Wermeling DP, Chandler MH, Sides GD, et al: Dirithromycin increases ethinyl estradiol clearance without allowing ovulation. Obstet Gynecol 86:78–84, 1995

Yoshimoto K, Echizen H, Chiba K, et al: Identification of human CYP isoforms involved in the metabolism of propranolol enantiomers—N-desisopropylation is mediated mainly by CYP1A2. Br J Clin Pharmacol 39: 421–431, 1995

Zhang Z-Y, Kaminsky LS: Characterization of human cytochromes P450 involved in theophylline 8-hydroxylation. Biochem Pharmacol 50:205–211, 1995

13

INTERNAL MEDICINE

Updated by Gary H. Wynn, M.D.

A complete discussion of drugs used in general medicine would be impossible in this Concise Guide, and in fact, most drugs have not been fully studied. This chapter contains an in-depth examination of drugs that affect other drugs (i.e., inhibit or induce the metabolism of other drugs), along with some discussion of the P450 metabolic sites for drugs with narrow therapeutic windows. P-glycoprotein information is presented as well.

Cardiovascular drugs (antiarrhythmics, anticoagulants, antihyperlipidemics [hydroxymethylglutaryl–coenzyme A [HMG-CoA] reductase inhibitors], calcium-channel blockers [CCBs], and β-blockers), gastrointestinal drugs, and antidiabetic agents are well covered. Antimicrobials, which are used across medical and surgical specialties and produce the greatest number of P450-mediated drug interactions, have earned their own chapter (Chapter 14 ["Infectious Diseases"]). Analgesics are covered in Chapters 17 ("Pain Management I: Nonnarcotic Analgesics") and 18 ("Pain Management II: Narcotic Analgesics"). The chapter opens with a historical review of allergy medications, the drugs where the quest for more information about the P450 system really began.

> **Reminder:** This chapter is dedicated primarily to metabolic and P-glycoprotein interactions. Interactions due to displaced protein-binding, alterations in absorption or excretion, and pharmacodynamics are not covered.

■ ALLERGY DRUGS

The specialty of allergy and immunology involves management of some of the world's most frequent ailments: asthma and allergic rhinitis or hay fever. Antihistamines are among the most widely prescribed medications in the world (Woosley 1996). Theophylline is still a common element in the treatment of asthma and chronic obstructive pulmonary disease, and its sensitivity to metabolism inhibition by other drugs has made it an important tool in the study of drug interactions as a probe drug. Many of the toxic nonsedating antihistamines have been removed from the market or reformulated. Here, a review of allergy medications past and present serves as a way to discuss how an understanding of drug-drug interactions developed.

Histamine, Subtype 1 (H_1), Receptor Blockers and Leukotriene D_4/E_4 Receptor Antagonists

First-Generation H_1-Receptor Blockers

Diphenhydramine (Benadryl), an over-the-counter antihistamine used for allergic rhinitis, urticaria, and insomnia and found in multiple combination preparations, was recently shown to be a potent 2D6 inhibitor. Lessard et al. (2001) studied 15 healthy men—nine extensive metabolizers and six poor metabolizers at 2D6—and found that diphenhydramine alters the disposition of venlafaxine (Effexor) via 2D6 inhibition. (This article clearly reveals how dextromethorphan and polymerase chain reaction are used to determine phenotypic and genotypic variability in a study population.) Diphenhydramine given at therapeutic doses inhibited metabolism of venlafaxine, yet appeared not to be metabolized itself at 2D6. The authors warned that some drugs with narrow therapeutic windows are dependent on 2D6 for metabolism (tricyclic antidepressants [TCAs], antiarrhythmics, β-blockers, tramadol (Ultram), and some antipsychotics, to name a few). Although diphenhydramine in vitro and in vivo seems to be a less potent inhibitor than quinidine (Quinidex) at

■ ALLERGY DRUGS

Drug	Metabolism site(s)	Enzyme(s) inhibited
H[1]-receptor antagonists		
Astemizole (Hismanal)[1,2]	3A4[1]	None known
Cetirizine (Zyrtec)	3A4	None known
Chlorpheniramine	2D6, 3A4	None known
Desloratadine (Clarinex)	3A4, 2D6	None known
Diphenhydramine (Benadryl)[3]	Unknown	2D6
Ebastine (Bastel)[1]	3A4[1]	None known
Fexofenadine (Allegra)[4]	None	None known
Levocetirizine (Xyzal)	None	None known
Loratadine (Claritin)	3A4, 2D6	None known
Terfenadine (Seldane)[1,2]	3A4[1]	None known
Leukotriene D[4]/E[4] receptor antagonists		
Montelukast (Singulair)	3A4, 2C9	None known
Zafirlukast (Accolate)	2C9	2C9, 3A4, 1A2
Xanthines		
Theophylline	1A2	None known

Note. H[1]=histamine, subtype 1. [1]Arrhythmogenic parent compounds. [2]No longer marketed in the United States. [3]May be representative of all first-generation H[1]-receptor antagonists (including chlorpheniramine, tripelennamine, promethazine, and hydroxyzine). [4]Active metabolite of terfenadine.

2D6 (Hamelin et al. 1998), the fact that it is sold over the counter and is found in multiple cold remedies suggests that patients should be warned about the potential for increased side effects and toxicities and should be monitored for such.

Second-Generation H_1-Receptor Blockers

Drug interactions involving second-generation H_1-receptor antagonists (or nonsedating antihistamines) were one of the first-studied drug-drug interactions relating to the P450 system. (Interactions involving fluoxetine (Prozac) and TCAs were noted earlier but were not associated with lethal or severe arrhythmias.) These newer antihistamines do not cross the blood-brain barrier and are more H_1 selective than the older drugs, resulting in less sedation, less weight gain, and fewer other antihistaminic side effects. The first report of life-threatening cardiac arrhythmia associated with the use of terfenadine (Seldane) appeared in 1989, when a patient developed an arrhythmia after an intentional overdose (Davies et al. 1989). Monahan et al. (1990) wrote the first article on the cause of an arrhythmia in conjunction with terfenadine therapy. A woman taking terfenadine and cefaclor (Ceclor) developed Candida vaginitis and treated herself with ketoconazole (Nizoral) that she had remaining from treatment of a previous episode of vaginitis. She developed palpitations and later torsades de pointes, even though she was taking standard doses of all medications. These case reports led to in vivo studies involving healthy volunteers, which clearly demonstrated that the potent 3A4 inhibitor ketoconazole increases levels of unmetabolized terfenadine and is associated with QT interval prolongation (Woosley 1996; Yap and Camm 1999).

Terfenadine (Seldane) is a pro-drug that usually undergoes a rapid and nearly complete first-pass hepatic biotransformation, producing the active metabolite at 3A4. The parent or pro-drug is cardiotoxic in overdose or when its first-pass metabolism is impaired by another compound at the same hepatic enzyme (in this case, 3A4), causing prolongation of the QT interval. Terfenadine seems to block potassium channels and to be as potent as quinidine in inhibiting the delayed rectifier potassium channel in cardiac tissue (Yap and Camm 1999). Carboxyterfenadine (fexofenadine [Allegra]), terfenadine's active metabolite, is not cardiotoxic and has no known hepatic metabolism (it is eliminated unchanged in urine). Terfenadine was sold over the counter for a time. The pro-drug terfenadine has been voluntarily removed by the manufacturer from the United States market and has been replaced by fexofenadine. Even at 10 times the recommended dose, fexofenadine is not associated with the problems that occur with terfenadine use. Long-term postmarketing surveillance further indicated its safety, as did a recent observational cohort study (Craig-McFeely et al. 2001).

Astemizole (Hismanal) (which has also been taken off the United States market) and ebastine (Bastel) (which is available in Europe and is being considered for release in the United States) also are arrhythmogenic at high doses, and this effect may be heightened when either of these drugs is administered with potent inhibitors of 3A4, including nefazodone (Serzone), cyclosporine (Neoral), cimetidine (Tagamet), some macrolide antibiotics, azole antifungals, antiretrovirals, some selective serotonin reuptake inhibitors (SSRIs), and grapefruit juice (Renwick 1999; Slater et al. 1999; Woosley 1996; Yap and Camm 1999). (See the table entitled "Allergy drugs"; also see Chapter 6 ["3A4"].)

Cetirizine (Zyrtec) is the carboxylic acid metabolite of hydroxyzine (Atarax). With regard to cetirizine, there are no reports in the literature of QT interval prolongation or hepatic metabolism. In studies in which healthy volunteers were administered cetirizine at three times the recommended dose, no effect on QT interval was found. Cetirizine is a racemate with R and S enantiomers. Levocetirizine (Xyzal) is the eutomer of cetirizine. Eutomers are the active or more active enantiomers of a racemic compound. Levocetirizine seems to have a smaller volume of distribution than cetirizine, providing for better safety and efficacy. To date, there are no reports of cardiotoxicity or drug interactions associated with levocetirizine therapy (Baltes et al. 2001).

Loratadine (Claritin) is hepatically metabolized at 3A4 and 2D6 and was thought not to be associated with QT interval prolongation at high doses, even in in vivo drug interaction studies involving potent 3A4 inhibitors such as erythromycin (Renwick 1999; Woosley 1996; Yap and Camm 1999). The package insert states that 3A4 inhibitors can increase levels of loratadine but that 2D6 takes over when this occurs (Claritin 2002). The insert does not mention that the drug may affect the QTc.

Abernethy et al. (2001) studied healthy volunteers who received 300 mg of nefazodone (a potent 3A4 inhibitor) every 12 hours (a high dose, but it is the manufacturer's recommended maximum dose) plus either terfenadine 60 mg twice a day or loratadine 20 mg once a day. For comparison, each of the three drugs was also used alone. Blood levels of parent compounds and metabolites were measured, and electrocardiograms were obtained. As expected, terfenadine's levels increased and the average QTc increased 42.4 milliseconds (ms) when the drug was used with nefazodone. Interestingly, the QTc was unchanged when terfenadine was used alone. Concomitant use of nefazodone and loratadine yielded an average increase in QTc of 21.6 ms. Loratadine alone did not increase the QTc. The authors of this study noted that the change in QTc associated with the loratadine-nefazodone combination is similar to the change noted with ziprasidone (Geodon) alone. They pointed out that loratadine is often used at higher doses than 20 mg/day and that they studied only healthy volunteers.

In contrast, Kosoglou et al. (2000) reported that in healthy volunteers, coadministration of loratadine and the potent 3A4 inhibitor ketoconazole significantly increased plasma concentrations of loratadine and its major metabolite, desloratadine (Clarinex), without significantly affecting the QTc. Coadministration of cimetidine (a potent 3A4 and 2D6 inhibitor) and loratadine significantly increased plasma loratadine concentrations, but not those of desloratadine, and did not significantly alter the QTc. The investigators concluded that although a statistically significant drug interaction occurred, there were no clinically significant QTc changes in healthy adult volunteers.

These conflicting data suggest that when loratadine and potent 3A4 and 2D6 inhibitors are used, careful monitoring is required—

at a minimum, electrocardiograms at every dose change or whenever a new inhibitor or substrate is added. Loratadine may be an inhibitor of P-glycoprotein, causing an increase in adenosine triphosphatase activity to above baseline levels in vitro (by inhibiting the adenosine triphosphate–binding transporters), but it is less potent than verapamil (Calan) and cyclosporine (Wang et al. 2001).

Desloratadine (Clarinex), the orally active major metabolite of loratadine, is now available in the United States. Desloratadine is 15 times more potent than loratadine at the H_1 receptor, and it seems to have a more rapid onset of action (McClellan and Jarvis 2001). It is reported to have no adverse cardiac effects in healthy volunteers, even at 10 times the recommended dose. Like loratadine, desloratadine neither inhibits nor induces metabolism of other medications via the P450 system, and no clinically significant P450-mediated drug interactions have been reported to date. Desloratadine does not seem to have any action on P-glycoprotein (Geha and Meltzer 2001; Wang et al. 2001).

Leukotriene D_4/E_4 Receptor Antagonists

Zafirlukast (Accolate) is a leukotriene D_4/E_4 receptor antagonist and is used in prophylactic and chronic treatment of asthma. This drug antagonizes the contractile activity of leukotrienes. Zafirlukast suppresses airway responses to antigens such as pollen and cat dander and inhibits bronchoconstriction. It is a moderate inhibitor of 2C9 and possibly 3A4. In one case, zafirlukast's activity at 1A2 was implicated in increasing serum theophylline levels. The agent has also been reported to increase the half-life of warfarin (Coumadin) (Katial et al. 1998). In vitro studies of montelukast (Singulair) do not reveal this leukotriene D_4/E_4 receptor antagonist to be an inhibitor or inducer, but it is metabolized at 3A4 and 2C9. Clinical studies of montelukast are under way. Montelukast has been studied in healthy volunteers also taking warfarin (Van Hecken et al. 1999) or digoxin (Depre et al. 1999). No significant interactions with these two drugs were noted.

Summary

First-generation antihistamines, namely diphenhydramine, are inhibitors of 2D6 and may alter the metabolism of drugs dependent on 2D6 for metabolism, such as venlafaxine, TCAs, some antipsychotics, β-blockers, antiarrhythmics, and some opiates. Nonsedating antihistamines with cardiotoxic parent drugs include terfenadine, astemizole (Hismanal), and ebastine, which in overdose or when inhibited by other compounds at the 3A4 enzyme may lead to palpitations, syncope, or fatal arrhythmias. None of the H_1-receptor antagonist nonsedating antihistamines are inhibitors or inducers in the P450 system. Loratadine in combination with potent 3A4 inhibitors may increase the QTc interval, but more studies are needed before conclusions can be drawn. Zafirlukast inhibits several enzymes in vitro, and there are case reports of interactions involving warfarin and theophylline via 1A2 inhibition.

Xanthines

Aminophylline and its active metabolite theophylline are thought to cause bronchodilation, or smooth muscle relaxation, and suppression of airway response to antigens or irritants in asthmatic patients. Clinical efficacy is achieved at serum levels of 5–20 μg/mL. Serum concentrations greater than 20 μg/mL produce adverse reactions, including nausea, vomiting, headache, tremor, seizures, cardiac arrhythmias, and death. With such a narrow therapeutic window and such dangerous toxic adverse reactions, this hepatically metabolized compound is very susceptible to drug interactions.

Theophylline is known to be metabolized at 1A2. Inhibitors of 1A2 therefore have the potential to increase serum theophylline levels (see Chapter 7 ["1A2"]). Serum levels of theophylline also may be decreased by compounds that induce 1A2, such as omeprazole (Prilosec), rifampin (Rifadin), caffeine, cigarette smoke, and some foods (see Chapter 7 ["1A2"]). Some metabolism of theophylline occurs at 2E1 (Rasmussen et al. 1997). Because theophylline metabolism is so sensitive to inhibition and induction and theophylline levels are easily measured, the drug is used as a probe in determining whether other compounds are metabolized at 1A2.

Upton (1991) reviewed the pharmacokinetic interactions of theophylline. He noted that in the 1980s, numerous investigators reported theophylline toxicity when the drug was administered with fluoroquinolones and quinolones and that rifampin, carbamazepine (Tegretol), phenytoin (Dilantin), and barbiturates cause an increase in theophylline clearance, leading to subtherapeutic serum levels. Reports began appearing in 1991 of cases of theophylline toxicity when the agent was administered with fluvoxamine (Luvox) (Rasmussen et al. 1995). By the mid-1990s, it had been established—through in vitro human liver microsome studies as well as in vivo healthy volunteer pharmacokinetic studies—that theophylline metabolism is inhibited at 1A2 by fluvoxamine and most fluoroquinolones (Batty et al. 1995). Despite these findings, and warnings in package inserts, cases of theophylline toxicity are still reported. Andrews (1998) reported a case of theophylline toxicity in which the addition of ciprofloxacin (Cipro) to an asthmatic patient's regimen to treat productive cough resulted in hospitalization and hemodialysis. DeVane et al. (1997) reported that a patient at a residential-care facility who was being treated with fluvoxamine for depression with psychotic features was prescribed theophylline for chronic obstructive pulmonary disease by her primary care physician. The woman experienced confusion, lack of energy, reduced sleep, and nausea and vomiting, all leading to an acute hospital admission. The half-life of theophylline in this case was increased fivefold.

Zevin and Benowitz (1999), in their thorough review of tobacco smoking, reported on the effect of polycyclic hydrocarbons in tobacco smoke, which induce 1A2 and 2E1 and may result in a reduction in serum theophylline levels.

Summary

Theophylline is metabolized almost exclusively at 1A2 and has a narrow therapeutic index. Therefore, whenever possible, use of potent inhibitors of 1A2 (which include the fluoroquinolones [ciprofloxacin is the most potent] and the SSRI fluvoxamine) should be avoided. If it is necessary to administer a fluoroquinolone, the least-potent drug of that class must be chosen, and serum theophylline levels must be monitored (some clinicians suggest decreasing the theophylline daily dose by two-thirds).

■ CARDIOVASCULAR AGENTS

Antiarrhythmics

General Drug Interactions

2D6 inhibition *by* antiarrhythmics.   Quinidine is associated with multiple drug interactions of significance. Quinidine is not a 2D6 substrate (not metabolized by 2D6); rather, it is a potent inhibitor of 2D6. Full inhibition of the enzyme occurs when just one-sixth of the usual antiarrhythmic dose is given. Quinidine's potent inhibition of 2D6 can lead to toxic levels of digoxin, TCAs, and codeine (Trujillo and Nolan 2000). Quinidine's stereoisomer, quinine, is not an inhibitor of 2D6. (For an excellent review of this drug and a full table with references to pertinent literature, see Grace and Camm 1998.) Note that quinidine's metabolism is at 3A4. Inhibition at this site by drugs such as nefazodone, erythromycin, astemizole, ketoconazole, ritonavir (Norvir) (acutely), and clarithromycin (Biaxin) may lead to quinidine toxicity.

2D6 inhibition *of* antiarrhythmics.   Mexiletine (Mexitil), encainide (Enkaid), and propafenone (Rythmol) metabolism may be affected if a patient is administered a potent 2D6 inhibitor. When propafenone is administered with quinidine, propafenone toxicity may result, in the form of bradycardia, heart block, heart failure, or worsening arrhythmia (Labbe 2000). Other potent 2D6 inhibitors include the SSRIs, cimetidine, and ritonavir.

1A2 inhibition *by* antiarrhythmics.   Mexiletine and propafenone are potent 1A2 inhibitors and therefore may increase levels of theophylline, caffeine, warfarin (Konishi e al 1999; Wei et al. 1999), and tacrine.

■ ANTIARRHYTHMICS

Drug	Metabolism site(s)	Enzyme(s) inhibited	Enzyme(s) induced
Amiodarone (Cordarone)	3A4, 2C8	2D6	None known
Encainide (Enkaid)	2D6	None known	None known
Flecainide (Tambocor)[1]	2D6	None known	None known
Lidocaine (Xylocaine)	3A4	1A2[c]	None known
Mexiletine (Mexitil)[1]	2D6, 1A2	**1A2**[a]	None known
Moricizine (Ethmozine)[2]	None known	None known	1A2, 3A4, 2D6[3]
Propafenone (Rythmol)	2D6, 3A4	**1A2**[a]	None known
Quinidine (Quinidex)	3A4	**2D6**[a]	None known
Tocainide (Tonocard)	None known	1A2[c]	None known

[1] Also significant renal metabolism and elimination.
[2] Induces antipyrine metabolism and its own metabolism.
[3] Possible induction.

[a] Potent (**bold** type).
[b] Moderate.
[c] Mild.

Induction by antiarrhythmics.   Moricizine (Ethmozine) seems to induce its own metabolism and has been found to induce the metabolism of theophylline, diltiazem (Tiazac), and the probe antipyrine (Benedek et al. 1994; Pieniaszek et al. 1993; Shum et al. 1996). No newer studies (including human liver microsome studies or other probe studies of this drug) were found that indicated whether cytochrome induction or some other type of drug interaction occurs. These studies support the notion that moricizine induces 1A2. It may increase induction of 3A4 and 2D6.

Psychotropic Drug Interactions

Tricyclic antidepressants.   Antiarrhythmics should rarely be prescribed with TCAs, given TCAs' quinidine-like potential to prolong the QTc interval, as well as the potential for sudden death in post–myocardial infarction patients. Secondary amine tricyclics are metabolized at 2D6 and are strongly contraindicated with potent 2D6 inhibitors such as quinidine.

Antipsychotics.   The package insert for thioridazine (Mellaril) has a "black box" warning about the drug's potential to lengthen the QTc interval. Thioridazine is partially metabolized at 2D6. Olanzapine (Zyprexa) and clozapine (Clozaril) are both at least partially metabolized at 1A2. Therefore, administering olanzapine or clozapine with potent 1A2 inhibitors such as mexiletine or propafenone may result in increased side effects and/or toxicity.

Summary

The effectiveness of antiarrhythmics and the morbidity and mortality associated with their administration vary across patient groups. Very narrow therapeutic windows also make drug interactions all the more difficult to predict. Buchert and Woosley (1992) and Trujillo and Nolan (2000) carefully reviewed patient variability with regard to response to this group of drugs, as well as the genetically determined differences in metabolism. 2D6 and its genetic polymorphisms play a role in many interactions involving this class of drugs. Mexiletine and propafenone are potent inhibitors of 1A2, and caution should be used when these drugs are coadministered with 1A2-dependent drugs such as theophylline, tacrine, caffeine, and the newer atypical antipsychotics.

Anticoagulants

Warfarin is primarily metabolized at 2C9, with some contributions from 2C19, 2C8, 2C18, 1A2, and 3A4. The S-enantiomer of warfarin, the more active isomer, is metabolized at 2C9. R-Warfarin is metabolized at 1A2. It is because of this complicated metabolism (and because of the protein binding–vitamin K interrelationships and the drug's narrow therapeutic window) that warfarin is so sensitive to inhibition and induction by so many drugs. In the *Physicians' Desk Reference* (2002), the list of warfarin interactions takes up three columns. In general, if a patient is taking warfarin, careful monitoring of anticoagulation (prothrombin time and international normalized ratio) and levels of drugs coadministered is necessary. Nearly every psychotropic drug has been implicated in a warfarin interaction.

Antiplatelet Drugs

The thienopyridines ticlopidine (Ticlid) and clopidogrel (Plavix) are inhibitors of platelet function. These agents reduce the incidence of atherosclerotic events in patients with histories of myocardial infarction, peripheral vascular disease, or stroke. Ticlopidine is a potent, specific inhibitor of 2C19 and also inhibits 2D6. Donahue et al. (1999) reported on ticlopidine and its effects on phenytoin clearance via 2C19. Ha-Duong et al. (2001) showed that ticlopidine is a selective inhibitor of 2C19. Clopidogrel is an inhibitor of 2C9. No reports were found in the literature of in vivo randomized, double-blind pharmacokinetic studies of clopidogrel. In theory, clopidogrel could increase serum concentrations, and hence side-effect profiles, of phenytoin, tamoxifen, tolbutamide, warfarin, fluvastatin, zafirlukast, oral hypoglycemics, and many nonsteroidal anti-inflammatory drugs (Plavix 1997).

Calcium-Channel Blockers

General Drug Interactions

3A4 inhibition *of* calcium-channel blockers (CCBs).   All CCBs are substrates of 3A4 (Katoh et al. 2000). Caution is prudent whenever a CCB is administered with potent 3A4 inhibitors, especially erythromycin, clarithromycin, ketoconazole, ritonavir, nefazodone, and grapefruit juice. For example, ketoconazole increased the mean area under the curve (AUC) and maximal drug concentration (C_{max}) of nisoldipine and its active metabolite in healthy volunteers in a randomized crossover trial (Heinig et al. 1999).

The dihydropyridine CCBs became available in the late 1980s, and by 1991, the first reports of interactions with orally administered drugs of this class and grapefruit juice appeared. Grapefruit juice causes an increase in the AUC and C_{max} of these drugs. Intravenous administration of CCBs in combination with grapefruit juice has no such effect, and compared with 3A4 inhibition by a potent inhibitor such as erythromycin, grapefruit juice does not prolong the half-lives of CCBs, indicating that there is no hepatic interaction and that the interaction may be entirely in the gut wall, likely through P-glycoprotein. Johnson et al. (2001) showed that P-glycoprotein efflux significantly affected the overall gut metabolism of CCBs (specifically verapamil) and greatly affected levels of medication available.

3A4 inhibition *by* CCBs.   Diltiazem (Tiazac) is the most potent 3A4 inhibitor of this class of drugs. There have been case reports of cisapride (Propulsid) toxicity with other CCBs as well (Posicor 1997; Thomas et al. 1998). Diltiazem also inhibits metabolism of "statins" (Azie et al. 1998; Mousa et al. 2000). Ocran et al. (1999) described tacrolimus (Prograf) toxicity in a renal transplant recipient being given mibefradil (Posicor), and CCB inhibition of 3A4 has been exploited to reduce the cost of cyclosporine therapy (see Chapter 20 ["Transplant Surgery and Rheumatology"]).

2D6 inhibition *by* CCBs.   Mibefradil, which is no longer on the United States market, is an example of an agent with potent inhibi-

■ CALCIUM-CHANNEL BLOCKERS

Drug	Metabolism site(s)	Enzyme(s) inhibited	Enzyme(s) induced
Amlodipine	3A4	None known	None known
Diltiazem	3A4, 2D6	**3A4**[a]	None known
Felodipine	3A4	None known	None known
Isradipine	None known	None known	None known
Mibefradil[1]	3A4	**3A4,**[a] **2D6**[a]	None known
Nicardipine	3A4	None known	None known
Nifedipine	3A4, ?2D6	None known	None known
Nimodipine	3A4	None known	None known
Nisoldipine	3A4, 2D6	None known	None known
Verapamil	3A4, 2C9, 2E1	3A4	None known

[1]No longer available because of adverse drug interactions based on inhibition of 2D6 and 3A4 substrates.

[a]Potent (**bold** type).
[b]Moderate.
[c]Mild.

tion at both 2D6 and 3A4. Mibefradil was voluntarily withdrawn in 1998 after multiple reports of life-threatening drug interactions. Mullins et al. (1998) reported one death and three survivals after cardiogenic shock associated with mibefradil administered with dihydropyridine CCBs and β-blockers (2D6).

Induction of CCBs.   Rifampin is a potent inducer of many P450 enzymes. Oral rifampin seems to have induced nifedipine (Adalat) metabolism in six healthy volunteers in a randomized, double crossover study, as evidenced by increased oral clearance and decreased bioavailability, with a calculated extraction of nifedipine in gut wall mucosa being significantly increased. Intravenous administration of nifedipine in the same subjects was not associated with altered nifedipine pharmacokinetics (Holtbecker et al. 1996). (See "Antimycobacterials and Antitubercular Agents" in Chapter 14 ["Infectious Diseases"]).

Psychotropic Interactions

Triazolobenzodiazepines.   Metabolism of all triazolobenzodiazepines is inhibited by the 3A4 inhibitors diltiazem and verapamil. In a randomized, three-phase crossover study in healthy volunteers, diltiazem increased the AUC, C_{max}, and half-life of triazolam (Halcion), which worsened triazolam's sedative effects (Kosuge et al. 1997). Ahonen et al. (1996) randomly assigned 30 patients who were to undergo coronary artery bypass surgery to treatment with diltiazem or placebo in addition to standard cardiac anesthesia with midazolam (Versed) and alfentanil (Alfenta). In this double-blind study, the researchers found that diltiazem increased the mean concentration-time curves of both midazolam and alfentanil and increased the half-lives of the drugs by 43% and 50%, respectively. Extubation of the patients who received diltiazem occurred 2.5 hours later than extubation of the control subjects, a significant difference.

Buspirone.   The CCBs verapamil and diltiazem increased the AUC of buspirone (BuSpar) in healthy volunteers, diltiazem to a greater degree than verapamil. Buspirone side effects were also greater in the patients given diltiazem than in the placebo group (Lamberg et al. 1998).

Summary

CCBs have noxious side effects that may be dose limiting. Inhibition of CCB metabolism by 3A4 inhibitors, including grapefruit juice, leads to orthostasis, hypotension, and tachycardia. Diltiazem and verapamil are inhibitors of 3A4 metabolism and cause increases in side effects of triazolobenzodiazepines, buspirone, alfentanil, and potentially any other 3A4 substrate.

β-Blockers

β-Blockers have multiple uses in current practice, from primary therapy for hypertension to pain management in patients with migraine headaches. The myriad β-blockers on the market include β-blockers metabolized by both the kidney and the liver. β-Blockers metabolized only by the liver, such as propranolol (Inderal) and metoprolol (Lopressor), are metabolized at 2D6. There is no evidence that CCBs are P450 inhibitors or inducers.

Hydroxymethylglutaryl–Coenzyme A Reductase Inhibitors ("Statins")

Hydroxymethylglutaryl–coenzyme A (HMG-CoA) reductase inhibitors decrease plasma cholesterol levels by inhibiting cholesterol synthesis in the liver. Toxicity may lead to myopathy, muscle toxicity, and rhabdomyolysis (Worz and Bottorff 2001). Lovastatin (Mevacor), simvastatin (Zocor), and atorvastatin (Lipitor) are 3A4 substrates. When these drugs are administered with potent 3A4 inhibitors, HMG-CoA toxicity may result. In contrast, fluvastatin (Lescol) is primarily metabolized by 2C9. Pravastatin (Pravachol) is only partially metabolized at 3A4, and most of the drug is eliminated by the kidney unchanged (Armstrong et al. 2002). Pravastatin metabolism seems to be less susceptible to potent inhibition by 3A4

■ HYDROXYMETHYLGLUTARYL–COENZYME A REDUCTASE INHIBITORS ("STATINS")

Drug	Metabolism site(s)	Enzyme(s) inhibited	Enzyme(s) induced
Atorvastatin (Lipitor)	3A4	None known	None known
Fluvastatin (Lescol)	2C9	None known	None known
Lovastatin (Mevacor)	3A4	None known	None known
Pravastatin (Pravachol)	3A4	None known	None known
Rosuvastatin (Crestor)	3A4[1]	None known	None known
Simvastatin (Zocor)	3A4	None known	None known

[1]Minimal metabolism at this site.

inhibitors because of these characteristics. The most recent statin, rosuvastatin (Crestor), shows low potential for P450-related interactions, with only minimal metabolism occurring at 3A4 in an initial study (White 2002). Current research does not indicate any significant inhibition or induction by HMG-CoA reductase inhibitors.

■ GASTROINTESTINAL AGENTS

General Drug Interactions

Metoclopramide

Metoclopramide is frequently prescribed for conditions previously treated with cisapride, which is now off the market. In a study using human liver microsomes and recombinant human cytochromes, Desta et al. (2002) showed that metoclopramide is both metabolized by and a potent inhibitor of 2D6.

Histamine Subtype 2 (H_2) Receptor Blockers

Cimetidine (Tagamet) is involved in numerous drug interactions at multiple enzyme sites. Because most of cimetidine's premarketing research was conducted in the early 1980s, microsomal and drug-interaction studies are incomplete and results are sometimes conflicting. Cimetidine has been documented as causing decreased clearance, unwanted side effects, and toxic levels of nonsteroidal anti-inflammatory drugs and warfarin (2C9), theophylline and olanzapine (1A2) (Szymanski et al. 1991), propranolol and other β-blockers (2D6), and tricyclics (2D6). Ranitidine (Zantac) is associated with almost none of these interactions, although there are case reports of interactions between ranitidine and phenytoin (Tse et al. 1993). Perhaps the greatest problem with cimetidine is its availability as an over-the-counter preparation. Physicians must ask patients about use of this drug before prescribing any drug with a narrow therapeutic window or when evaluating a potential adverse event. Famotidine (Pepcid) is associated with no reported metabolic interactions (Humphries 1987). H_2-receptor blockers also reduce

■ GASTROINTESTINAL AGENTS

Drug	Metabolism site(s)	Enzyme(s) inhibited	Enzyme(s) induced
Prokinetics			
Cisapride[1]	3A4	3A4	None known
H₂-receptor blockers			
Cimetidine	None known	3A4, 2D6, 1A2, 2C9	None known
Famotidine	None known	None known	None known
Metoclopramide	2D6	**2D6**[a]	None known
Nizatidine	None known	None known	None known
Ranitidine	None known	1A2, 2C9, 2C19[b]	None known
Proton pump inhibitors			
Esomeprazole	3A4, 2C19	None known	None known
Lansoprazole	3A4, 2C19	None known	1A2[c]
Omeprazole	3A4, 2C19	2C19	1A2
Pantoprazole	3A4, 2C19	None known	None known
Rabeprazole	3A4, 2C19	None known	None known

[1]Cardiotoxic pro-drug; removed from the United States market in July 2000.

[a]Potent (**bold** type).

[b]Moderate.

[c]Mild.

the plasma concentrations of ketoconazole, indomethacin (Indocin), and chlorpromazine (Thorazine) by altering their absorption. (For a full discussion of many of these interactions, see the review of antiulcer drugs by Negro [1998].)

Proton Pump Inhibitors

Proton pump inhibitors inhibit enzymes on the apical surface of parietal cells in the stomach, preventing secretion of gastric acid. Some of the agents in this class interfere with absorption of drugs such as digoxin and ketoconazole. All proton pump inhibitors are extensively metabolized via 2C19 and 3A4 (Stedman and Barclay 2000); the variation in potential for drug interactions is based on differences in enzyme inhibition and induction. A genetic polymorphism of 2C19 also affects the metabolism of proton pump inhibitors and thus their metabolic profiles (Ishizaki and Horai 1999; McColl and Kennerley 2002). 2C19 inhibition occurs with administration of omeprazole (Prilosec) and, more markedly, its *S*-enantiomer, esomeprazole (Nexium) (McColl 2002). Omeprazole and lansoprazole (Prevacid) *induce* 1A2 and may affect theophylline and caffeine levels. However, a study by Dilger and colleagues (1999) demonstrated no interactions with coadministration of omeprazole, pantoprazole (Protonix), or lansoprazole with theophylline. Newer agents in the class, rabeprazole and pantoprazole, seem to have none of these effects, a conclusion drawn from a review of the literature and findings of randomized studies involving healthy volunteers (Andersson et al. 2001; Hartmann et al. 1999; Humphries and Merritt 1999). Rabeprazole is free of interactions and is not affected by inhibition of either 3A4 or 2C19 because of its clearance by two enzymes (Robinson 2001).

Psychotropic Drug Interactions

H₂-Receptor Blockers

In a comparative study, Greenblatt et al. (1984) found no difference between subjects taking both diazepam and cimetidine and control subjects taking cimetidine only, in terms of cognitive and psycho-motor functions. Digit-symbol substitution, tracking, and self-reports of drowsiness and fatigue were used, and reaction time was also determined. Plasma concentrations were statistically significantly higher in the test group, however; levels were up to 57% higher than those in the control group. Klotz et al. (1985) also showed that there is an increase in plasma concentrations of midazolam when the drug is administered with cimetidine, but such coadministration has no cognitive or psychomotor effect. Sanders et al. (1993) conducted a head-to-head study of ranitidine and cimetidine. Midazolam was added to steady-state H_2-receptor blockers in a randomized, double-blind crossover study involving healthy volunteers. The investigators found a significant difference in impairment (pharmacodynamic effect; 2.5 hours) in the cimetidine treatment group compared with the ranitidine treatment group, and the decrement was evident in cognitive and psychomotor functions but was not subjectively reported by the subjects. Although Sanders et al. (1993) reported a cognitive effect, they also reported no subjective effect. Given the findings of these three studies, one can conclude that cimetidine affects plasma concentrations of benzodiazepines in healthy volunteers but the effect may be without clinical relevance.

Proton Pump Inhibitors

Omeprazole, and more markedly its S-enantiomer, esomeprazole, are inhibitors of 2C19. Omeprazole's effect on diazepam levels was studied in poor and extensive metabolizers of omeprazole. In a double-blind crossover study, diazepam was administered intravenously after steady state had been achieved with omeprazole therapy (Andersson et al. 1990). Diazepam metabolism was slowed significantly in the extensive metabolizers (i.e., the extensive metabolizers became phenotypic poor metabolizers) by omeprazole. The poor metabolizers showed no apparent interaction.

In a study of low-dose fluvoxamine administered with omeprazole, Christensen et al. (2002) found marked inhibition of omeprazole metabolism at 2C19 by fluvoxamine.

■ ORAL HYPOGLYCEMICS

Thiazolidinedione Agents

The thiazolidinedione antidiabetic agents have been designed to decrease insulin resistance in patients with type II diabetes (diabetes mellitus). Troglitazone (Rezulin) has been shown to decrease cyclosporine concentrations in renal transplant recipients (Kaplan et al. 1998). The drug is a known 3A4 inducer; it can decrease serum concentrations of 3A4 substrates, including protease inhibitors and oral contraceptives. Troglitazone hepatotoxicity was the primary reason for withdrawal from the U.S. market ("Rezulin to Be Withdrawn From the Market" 2000).

Rosiglitazone (Avandia), in the manufacturer's randomized, open-label, crossover study involving 28 healthy volunteers, produced no clinically significant decrease in nifedipine pharmacokinetics, nifedipine being a probe drug for 3A4 interactions. Baldwin et al. (1999) showed that rosiglitazone is primarily metabolized by 2C8 and, to a lesser degree, 2C9. Pioglitazone (Actos) is partially metabolized by 3A4 and 2C8, and drug interaction studies have not been conducted. Postmarketing surveillance revealed that pioglitazone is less hepatotoxic than others in this class.

Sulfonylureas

The oral hypoglycemics of the sulfonylurea class include tolbutamide (Orinase), glipizide (Glucotrol), glyburide (Glynase), and glimepiride (Amaryl). All of these drugs are primarily metabolized at 2C9. Coadministration with 2C9 inhibitors—fluvoxamine (Luvox), fluconazole (Diflucan), and ritonavir (Norvir), for example (see table "Inhibitors of 2C9" in Chapter 8)—may cause significant hypoglycemia (Kidd et al. 1999; Kirchheiner et al. 2002a, 2002b; Niemi et al. 2002). Some members of this class of drugs may induce 3A4, but the data are still scarce (van Giersbergen et al. 2002).

■ ORAL HYPOGLYCEMICS

Drug	Metabolism site(s)	Enzyme(s) inhibited	Enzyme(s) induced
Thiazolidinediones			
Pioglitazone (Actos)	2C8, 3A4	None known	None known
Rosiglitazone (Avandia)	2C8	None known	None known
Troglitazone (Rezulin)[1]	2C8, 3A4	None known	3A4
Sulfonylureas			
Tolbutamide	2C9	None known	None known
Glimepiride	2C9	None known	None known
Glipizide	2C9	None known	None known
Glyburide	2C9, 2C19, 3A4	None known	None known

[1]No longer available.

■ REFERENCES

Abernethy DR, Barbey JT, Franc J, et al: Loratadine and terfenadine interaction with nefazodone: both antihistamines are associated with QTc prolongation. Clin Pharmacol Ther 69:96–103, 2001

Ahonen J, Olkkola KT, Salmenpera M, et al: Effect of diltiazem on midazolam and alfentanil disposition in patients undergoing coronary artery bypass grafting. Anesthesiology 85:1246–1252, 1996

Andersson T, Cederberg C, Edvardsson G, et al: Effect of omeprazole treatment on diazepam plasma levels in slow versus normal rapid metabolizers of omeprazole. Clin Pharmacol Ther 47:79–85, 1990

Andersson T, Hassan-Alin M, Hasselgren G, et al: Drug interaction studies with esomeprazole, the (S)-isomer of omeprazole. Clin Pharmacokinet 40:523–537, 2001

Andrews PA: Interactions with ciprofloxacin and erythromycin leading to aminophylline toxicity. Nephrol Dial Transplant 13:1006–1008, 1998

Armstrong SC, Cozza KL, Oesterheld JR: Med-psych drug-drug interactions update. Psychosomatics 43:79–81, 2002

Azie NE, Brater DC, Becker PA, et al: The interaction of diltiazem with lovastatin and pravastatin. Clin Pharmacol Ther 64:369–377, 1998

Bailey DG, Bend JR, Arnold JM, et al: Erythromycin-felodipine interaction: magnitude, mechanism, and comparison with grapefruit juice. Clin Pharmacol Ther 60:25–33, 1996

Bailey DG, Kreeft JH, Munoz C, et al: Grapefruit juice-felodipine interaction: effect of naringin and 6′,7′-dihydroxybergamottin in humans. Clin Pharmacol Ther 64:248–256, 1998

Baldwin SJ, Clarke SE, Chenery RJ: Characterization of the cytochrome P450 enzymes involved in the in vitro metabolism of rosiglitazone. Br J Clin Pharmacol 48:424–432, 1999

Baltes E, Coupez R, Giezek H, et al: Absorption and disposition of levocetirizine, the eutomer of cetirizine, administered alone or as cetirizine to healthy volunteers. Fundam Clin Pharmacol 15:269–277, 2001

Batty KT, Davis TM, Ilett KF, et al: The effect of ciprofloxacin on theophylline pharmacokinetics in healthy subjects. Br J Clin Pharmacol 39:305–311, 1995

Benedek IH, Davidson AF, Pieniaszek HJ Jr: Enzyme induction by moricizine: time course and extent in healthy subjects. J Clin Pharmacol 34:167–175, 1994

Bloch A, Ben-Chetrit E, Muszkat M, et al: Major bleeding caused by warfarin in a genetically susceptible patient. Pharmacotherapy 22:97–101, 2002

Boberg M, Angerbauer R, Fey P, et al: Metabolism of cerivastatin by human liver microsomes in vitro: characterization of primary metabolic pathways and of cytochrome P450 isozymes involved. Drug Metab Dispos 25:321–331, 1997

Buchert E, Woosley RL: Clinical implications of variable antiarrhythmic drug metabolism. Pharmacogenetics 2:2–11, 1992

Chong PH, Seeger JD, Franklin C: Clinically relevant differences between the statins: implications for therapeutic selection. Am J Med 111:390–400, 2001

Christensen M, Tybring G, Mihara K, et al: Low daily 10-mg and 20-mg doses of fluvoxamine inhibit the metabolism of both caffeine (cytochrome P4501A2) and omeprazole (cytochrome P4502C19). Clin Pharmacol Ther 71:141–152, 2002

Craig-McFeely PM, Acharya NV, Shakir SA: Evaluation of the safety of fexofenadine from experience gained in general practice use in England in 1997. Eur J Clin Pharmacol 57:313–320, 2001

Davies AJ, Harindra V, McEwan A, et al: Cardiotoxic effect with convulsions in terfenadine overdose. BMJ 298:325, 1989

Depre M, Van Hecken A, Verbesselt R, et al: Effect of multiple doses of montelukast, a CysLT1 receptor antagonist, on digoxin pharmacokinetics in healthy volunteers. J Clin Pharmacol 39:941–944, 1999

Desta Z, Wu GM, Morocho AM, et al: The gastroprokinetic and antiemetic drug metoclopramide is a substrate and inhibitor of cytochrome P450 2D6. Drug Metab Dispos 30:336–343, 2002

DeVane CL, Markowitz JS, Hardesty SJ, et al: Fluvoxamine-induced theophylline toxicity. Am J Psychiatry 154:1317–1318, 1997

Dilger K, Zheng Z, Klotz U: Lack of drug interaction between omeprazole, lansoprazole, pantoprazole and theophylline. Br J Clin Pharmacol 48:438–444, 1999

Donahue S, Flockhart DA, Abernethy DR: Ticlopidine inhibits phenytoin clearance. Clin Pharmacol Ther 66:563–568, 1999

Ferron GM, Preston RA, Noveck RJ, et al: Pharmacokinetics of pantoprazole in patients with moderate and severe hepatic dysfunction. Clin Ther 23:1180–1192, 2001

Flockhart DA, Desta Z, Mahal SK: Selection of drugs to treat gastro-esophageal reflux disease: the role of drug interactions. Clin Pharmacokinet 39:295–309, 2000

Food and Drug Administration: Janssen Pharmaceutica stops marketing cisapride in the US (Talk Paper T00–14). Rockville, MD, National Press Office, March 23, 2000

Fuhr U, Maier-Bruggemann A, Blume H, et al: Grapefruit juice increases oral nimodipine bioavailability. Int J Clin Pharmacol Ther 36:126–132, 1998

Geha RS, Meltzer EO: Desloratadine: a new, nonsedating, oral antihistamine. J Allergy Clin Immunol 107:751–762, 2001

Grace AA, Camm AJ: Quinidine. N Engl J Med 338:35–44, 1998

Greenblatt DJ, Abernethy DR, Morse DS, et al: Clinical importance of the interaction of diazepam and cimetidine. N Engl J Med 310:1639–1643, 1984

Gruer PJ, Vega JM, Mercuri MF, et al: Concomitant use of cytochrome P450 3A4 inhibitors and simvastatin. Am J Cardiol 84:811–815, 1999

Ha-Duong NT, Dijols S, Macherey AC, et al: Ticlopidine as a selective mechanism-based inhibitor of human cytochrome P450 2C19. Biochemistry 40:12112–12122, 2001

Hamelin BA, Bouayad A, Drolet B, et al: In vitro characterization of cytochrome P450 2D6 inhibition by classic histamine H_1 receptor antagonists. Drug Metab Dispos 26:536–539, 1998

Hartmann M, Zech K, Bliesath H, et al: Pantoprazole lacks induction of CYP1A2 activity in man. Int J Clin Pharmacol Ther 37:159–164, 1999

Heinig R, Adelmann HG, Ahr G: The effect of ketoconazole on the pharmacokinetics, pharmacodynamics and safety of nisoldipine. Eur J Clin Pharmacol 55:57–60, 1999

Holtbecker N, Fromm MF, Kroemer HK, et al: The nifedipine-rifampin interaction: evidence for induction of gut wall metabolism. Drug Metab Dispos 24:1121–1123, 1996

Hsyu PH, Schultz-Smith MD, Lillibridge JH, et al: Pharmacokinetic interactions between nelfinavir and 3-hydroxy-3-methylglutaryl coenzyme A reductase inhibitors atorvastatin and simvastatin. Antimicrob Agents Chemother 45:3445–3450, 2001

Humphries TJ: Famotidine: a notable lack of drug interactions. Scand J Gastroenterol Suppl 134:55–60, 1987

Humphries TJ, Merritt GJ: Review article: drug interactions with agents used to treat acid-related diseases. Aliment Pharmacol Ther 13 (suppl 3):18–26, 1999

Igel M, Sudhop T, von Bergmann K: Metabolism and drug interactions of 3-hydroxy-3-methylglutaryl coenzyme A-reductase inhibitors (statins). Eur J Clin Pharmacol 57:357–364, 2001

Ishizaki T, Horai Y: Review article: cytochrome P450 and the metabolism of proton pump inhibitors—emphasis on rabeprazole. Aliment Pharmacol Ther 13 (suppl 3):27–36, 1999

Johnson BM, Charman WN, Porter CJ: The impact of P-glycoprotein efflux on enterocyte residence time and enterocyte-based metabolism of verapamil. J Pharm Pharmacol 53:1611–1619, 2001

Kaplan B, Friedman G, Jacobs M, et al: Potential interaction of troglitazone and cyclosporine. Transplantation 27:1399–1400, 1998

Katial RK, Stelzle RC, Bonner MW, et al: A drug interaction between zafirlukast and theophylline. Arch Intern Med 158:1713–1715, 1998

Katoh M, Nakajima M, Yamazaki H, et al: Inhibitory potencies of 1,4-dihydropyridine calcium antagonists to P-glycoprotein-mediated transport: comparison with the effects on CYP3A4. Pharm Res 17:1189–1197, 2000

Kidd RS, Straughn AB, Meyer MC, et al: Pharmacokinetics of chlorpheniramine, phenytoin, glipizide and nifedipine in an individual homozygous for the *CYP2C9*3* allele. Pharmacogenetics 9:71–80, 1999

Kirchheiner J, Bauer S, Meineke I, et al: Impact of CYP2C9 and CYP2C19 polymorphisms on tolbutamide kinetics and the insulin and glucose response in healthy volunteers. Pharmacogenetics 12:101–109, 2002a

Kirchheiner J, Brockmoller J, Meineke I, et al: Impact of CYP2C9 amino acid polymorphisms on glyburide kinetics and on the insulin and glucose response in healthy volunteers. Clin Pharmacol Ther 71:286–296, 2002b

Klotz U, Arvela P, Rosenkranz B: Effect of single doses of cimetidine and ranitidine on the steady state plasma levels of midazolam. Clin Pharmacol Ther 38:652–655, 1985

Kobayashi K, Nakajima M, Chiba K, et al: Inhibitory effects of antiarrhythmic drugs on phenacetin O-deethylation catalysed by human CYP1A2. Br J Clin Pharmacol 45:361–368, 1998

Konishi H, Morita K, Minouchi T, et al: Preferential inhibition of CYP1A enzymes in hepatic microsomes by mexiletine. Eur J Drug Metab Pharmacokinet 24:149–153, 1999

Kosoglou T, Salfi M, Lim JM, et al: Evaluation of the pharmacokinetics and electrocardiographic pharmacodynamics of loratadine with concomitant administration of ketoconazole or cimetidine. Br J Clin Pharmacol 50:581–589, 2000

Kosuge K, Nishimoto M, Kimura M, et al: Enhanced effect of triazolam with diltiazem. Br J Clin Pharmacol 43:367–372, 1997

Labbe L: Clinical pharmacokinetics of mexiletine. Clin Pharmacokinet 37:361–384, 1999

Labbe L: Pharmacokinetic and pharmacodynamic interaction between mexiletine and propafenone in human beings. Clin Pharmacol Ther 68:44–57, 2000

Lamberg TS, Kivisto KT, Neuvonen PJ: Effects of verapamil and diltiazem on the pharmacokinetics and pharmacodynamics of buspirone. Clin Pharmacol Ther 63:640–645, 1998

Lee CR, Goldstein JA, Pieper JA: Cytochrome P450 2C9 polymorphisms: a comprehensive review of the in-vitro and human data. Pharmacogenetics 12:251–263, 2002

Lessard E, Yessine MA, Hamelin BA, et al: Diphenhydramine alters the disposition of venlafaxine through inhibition of CYP2D6 activity in humans. J Clin Psychopharmacol 21:175–184, 2001

Lew EA: Review article: pharmacokinetic concerns in the selection of anti-ulcer therapy. Aliment Pharmacol Ther 13 (suppl 5):11–16, 1999

Lilja JJ, Kivisto KT, Neuvonen PJ: Grapefruit juice increases serum concentrations of atorvastatin and has no effect on pravastatin. Clin Pharmacol Ther 66:118–127, 1999

Loi CM, Young M, Randinitis E, et al: Clinical pharmacokinetics of troglitazone. Clin Pharmacokinet 37:91–104, 1999

McClellan K, Jarvis B: Desloratidine. Drugs 61:789–796, 2001

McColl KE, Kennerley P: Proton pump inhibitors—differences emerge in hepatic metabolism. Dig Liver Dis 34:461–467, 2002

Molden E, Asberg A, Christensen H: CYP2D6 is involved in O-demethylation of diltiazem. An in vitro study with transfected human liver cells. Eur J Clin Pharmacol 56:575–579, 2000

Molden E, Johansen PW, Boe GH, et al: Pharmacokinetics of diltiazem and its metabolites in relation to CYP2D6 genotype. Clin Pharmacol Ther 72:333–342, 2002

Monahan BP, Ferguson CL, Killeavy ES, et al: Torsades de pointes occurring in association with terfenadine use. JAMA 264:2788–2790, 1990

Morike KE, Roden DM: Quinidine-enhanced beta-blockade during treatment with propafenone in extensive metabolizer human subjects. Clin Pharmacol Ther 55:28–34, 1994

Mousa O, Brater DC, Sunblad KJ, et al: The interaction of diltiazem with simvastatin. Clin Pharmacol Ther 67:267–274, 2000

Muck W: Rational assessment of the interaction profile of cerivastatin supports its low propensity for drug interactions. Drugs 56 (suppl 1):15–23, 1998

Muck W, Mai I, Fritsche L, et al: Increase in cerivastatin systemic exposure after single and multiple dosing in cyclosporine-treated kidney transplant recipients. Clin Pharmacol Ther 65:251–261, 1999

Mullins ME, Horowitz BZ, Linden DH, et al: Life-threatening interaction of mibefradil and beta-blockers with dihydropyridine calcium channel blockers. JAMA 280:157–158, 1998

Naganuma M, Shiga T, Nishikata K, et al: Role of desethylamiodarone in the anticoagulant effect of concurrent amiodarone and warfarin therapy. J Cardiovasc Pharmacol Ther 6:363–367, 2001

Nakajima M, Kobayashi K, Shimada N, et al: Involvement of CYP1A2 in mexiletine metabolism. Br J Clin Pharmacol 46:55–62, 1998

Negro RD: Pharmacokinetic drug interactions with anti-ulcer drugs. Clin Pharmacokinet 35:135–150, 1998

Neuvonen PJ, Kantola T, Kivisto KT: Simvastatin but not pravastatin is very susceptible to interaction with the CYP3A4 inhibitor itraconazole. Clin Pharmacol Ther 63:332–341, 1998

Niemi M, Cascorbi I, Timm R, et al: Glyburide and glimepiride pharmacokinetics in subjects with different CYP2C9 genotypes. Clin Pharmacol Ther 72:326–332, 2002

Ocran KW, Plauth M, Mai I, et al: Tacrolimus toxicity due to drug interaction with mibefradil in a patient after liver transplantation. Z Gastroenterol 37:1025–1028, 1999

Paoletti R, Corsini A, Bellosta S: Pharmacological interactions of statins. Atheroscler Suppl 3:35–40, 2002

Physicians' Desk Reference, 56th Edition. Montvale, NJ, Medical Economics, 2002

Pieniaszek HJ Jr, Davidson AF, Benedek IH: Effect of moricizine on the pharmacokinetics of single-dose theophylline in healthy subjects. Ther Drug Monit 15:199–203, 1993

Plavix (package insert). New York, Sanofi/Bristol-Myers Squibb Co., 1997

Posicor (package insert). Nutley, NJ, Roche Pharmaceuticals, 1997

Rasmussen BB, Maenpaa J, Pelkonen O, et al: Selective serotonin reuptake inhibitors and theophylline metabolism in human liver microsomes: potent inhibition by fluvoxamine. Br J Clin Pharmacol 39:151–159, 1995

Rasmussen BB, Jeppesen U, Gaist D, et al: Griseofulvin and fluvoxamine interactions with the metabolism of theophylline. Ther Drug Monit 19:56–62, 1997

Renwick AG: The metabolism of antihistamines and drug interactions: the role of cytochrome P450 enzymes. Clin Exp Allergy 29 (suppl 3):116–124, 1999 [This entire supplement of Clinical Experimental Allergy is devoted to antihistamines, with many articles relevant to this topic for psychiatrists.]

Rezulin to be withdrawn from the market. HHS News, US Department of Health and Human Services, March 21, 2000 [www.fda.gov/bbs/topics/NEWS/NEW00721.html]

Robinson M: New-generation proton pump inhibitors: overcoming the limitations of early generation agents. Eur J Gastroenterol Hepatol 13 (suppl 1):S43–S47, 2001

Sanders LD, Whitehead C, Gildersleve CD: Interaction of H_2-receptor antagonists and benzodiazepine sedation: a double-blind placebo-controlled investigation of the effects of cimetidine and ranitidine on recovery after intravenous midazolam. Anaesthesia 48:286–292, 1993

Shum L, Pieniaszek HJ Jr, Robinson CA: Pharmacokinetic interactions of moricizine and diltiazem in healthy volunteers. J Clin Pharmacol 36:1161–1168, 1996

Slater JW, Zechnich AD, Haxby DG: Second generation antihistamines: a comparative review. Drugs 57:31–47, 1999

Spinler SA, Gammaitoni A, Charland SL, et al: Propafenone-theophylline interaction. Pharmacotherapy 13:68–71, 1993

Stedman CA, Barclay ML: Review article: comparison of the pharmacokinetics, acid suppression and efficacy of proton pump inhibitors. Aliment Pharmacol Ther 14:963–978, 2000

Steinijans VW, Huber R, Hartmann M, et al: Lack of pantoprazole drug interactions in man: an updated review. Int J Clin Pharmacol Ther 34:243–262, 1996

Szymanski S, Lieberman JA, Picou D, et al: A case report of cimetidine-induced clozapine toxicity. J Clin Psychiatry 52:21–22, 1991

Tabrizi AR, Zehnbauer BA, Borecki IB, et al: The frequency and effects of cytochrome P450 (CYP) 2C9 polymorphisms in patients receiving warfarin. J Am Coll Surg 194:267–273, 2002

Tanaka M, Ohkubo T, Otani K, et al: Stereoselective pharmacokinetics of pantoprazole, a proton pump inhibitor, in extensive and poor metabolizers of S-mephenytoin. Clin Pharmacol Ther 69:108–113, 2001

Thomas AR, Chan LN, Bauman JL, et al: Prolongation of the QT interval related to cisapride-diltiazem interaction. Pharmacotherapy 18:381–385, 1998

214

Trujillo TC, Nolan PE: Antiarrhythmic agents: drug interactions of clinical significance. Drug Saf 23:509–532, 2000

Tse CS, Akinwande KI, Biallowons K: Phenytoin concentration elevation subsequent to ranitidine administration. Ann Pharmacother 27:1448–1451, 1993

Upton RA: Pharmacokinetic interactions between theophylline and other medication (part I). Clin Pharmacokinet 20:66–80, 1991

Ushiama H, Echizen H, Nachi S, et al: Dose-dependent inhibition of CYP3A activity by clarithromycin during *Helicobacter pylori* eradication therapy assessed by changes in plasma lansoprazole levels and partial cortisol clearance to 6beta-hydroxycortisol. Clin Pharmacol Ther 72:33–43, 2002

van Giersbergen PL, Treiber A, Clozel M, et al: In vivo and in vitro studies exploring the pharmacokinetic interaction between bosentan, a dual endothelin receptor antagonist, and glyburide. Clin Pharmacol Ther 71:253–262, 2002

Van Hecken A, Depre M, Verbesselt R, et al: Effect of montelukast on the pharmacokinetics and pharmacodynamics of warfarin in healthy volunteers. J Clin Pharmacol 39:495–500, 1999

Wang E, Casciano CN, Clement RP, et al: Evaluation of the interaction of loratadine and desloratadine with P-glycoprotein. Drug Metab Dispos 29:1080–1083, 2001

Wei X, Dai R, Zhai S, et al: Inhibition of human liver cytochrome P450 1A2 by the class 1B antiarrhythmics mexiletine, lidocaine, and tocainide. J Pharmacol Exp Ther 289:853–858, 1999

White CM: A review of the pharmacologic and pharmacokinetic aspects of rosuvastatin. J Clin Pharmacol 42:963–970, 2002

Williams D, Feely J: Pharmacokinetic-pharmacodynamic drug interactions with HMG-CoA reductase inhibitors. Clin Pharmacokinet 41:343–370, 2002

Woosley RL: Cardiac actions of antihistamines. Annu Rev Pharmacol Toxicol 36:233–252, 1996

Worz CR, Bottorff M: The role of cytochrome P450-mediated drug-drug interactions in determining the safety of statins. Expert Opin Pharmacother 2:1119–1127, 2001

Yap TG, Camm AJ: The current cardiac safety situation with antihistamines. Clin Exp Allergy 29 (suppl 1):15–24, 1999

Zevin S, Benowitz NL: Drug interactions with tobacco smoking: an update. Clin Pharmacokinet 36:425–438, 1999

14

INFECTIOUS DISEASES

Antimicrobials are the second most commonly prescribed class of medications in the United States. These drugs are associated with many interactions. Antimalarials and antiparasitic drugs are not covered in this book, because they are not regularly encountered in general medical practice in the United States. The antimicrobials with significant drug-interaction activity, as both inducers and inhibitors of enzymes, include macrolide, ketolide, fluoroquinolone, streptogramin, and linezolid antibiotics; imidazole antifungals; antimycobacterials; and antiretrovirals. Each of these antimicrobial classes is dealt with in a separate section below.

> **Reminder:** This chapter is dedicated primarily to metabolic and P-glycoprotein interactions. Interactions due to displaced protein-binding, alterations in absorption or excretion, and pharmacodynamics are not covered.

■ ANTIBIOTICS

Macrolides and Ketolides

General Drug Interactions

Macrolide antibiotics are known for inhibiting the metabolism of drugs dependent on 3A for metabolism—erythromycin and clarithromycin (Biaxin) being the most potent. Azithromycin (Zithromax) appears to be a very mild inhibitor of 3A4, and dirithromycin (Dynabac) does not seem to affect P450 metabolism at all (Watkins et al. 1997).

■ **MACROLIDES AND KETOLIDES**

Drug	Metabolism site(s)	Enzyme(s) inhibited	Enzyme(s) induced
Azithromycin (Zithromax)	3A4	3A4[c]	None known
Clarithromycin (Biaxin)	3A4	**3A4**[a]	None known
Dirithromycin (Dynabac)	3A4	None known	None known
Erythromycin	3A4	**3A4**[a]	None known
Troleandomycin (Tao)	3A4	**3A4**[a]	None known
Telithromycin (Ketek)[1]	3A4, others	**3A4**[a]	None known

[1]Ketolide antibiotic.

[a]Potent (**bold** type).
[b]Moderate.
[c]Mild to not inhibited.

Calcium-channel blockers. Calcium-channel blocker metabolism is inhibited by macrolides (see "Cardiovascular Agents" in Chapter 13 ["Internal Medicine"]), and this inhibition increases the risk of orthostasis, falls, and arrhythmia. One 79-year-old woman who tolerated 480 mg of verapamil a day (the maximum dose approved by the U.S. Food and Drug Administration) without complications developed fatigue and dizziness after administration of erythromycin (2,000 mg/day) for a new-onset productive cough (Goldschmidt et al. 2001). She developed complete atrioventricular heart block and QTc prolongation. Verapamil and erythromycin are both inhibitors of 3A4 and P-glycoprotein.

Cyclosporine. Severe cyclosporine toxicity occurred in a transplant recipient who was concomitantly given clarithromycin (Spicer et al. 1997). (See Chapter 20 ["Transplant Surgery and Rheumatology"] for more on cyclosporine toxicity.)

Ergots. Ausband and Goodman (2001) reported a case of ergotism associated with clarithromycin use. A 41-year-old woman who each day took omeprazole for gastrointestinal upset, a β-blocker for migraine prophylaxis, and an oral caffeine-ergotamine combination for treatment of migraines was prescribed clarithromycin for a nonproductive cough that had lasted 10 days. Shortly after starting clarithromycin therapy, she developed burning leg pain, paresthesias, and edema in both legs, symptoms that progressed to pallor and coolness over 7 days. Ergots are metabolized at 3A4 and their metabolism is inhibited by clarithromycin. Lingual ischemia has also been reported with 2 mg of ergotamine tartrate and clarithromycin (Horowitz et al. 1996).

Hydroxymethylglutaryl–coenzyme A reductase inhibitors ("statins"). The lipid-lowering agents of the hydroxymethylglutaryl–coenzyme A (HMG-CoA) reductase inhibitor class, often called "statins," are greatly affected by P450 inhibition. Erythromycin increases the area under the curve (AUC) and maximal drug concentration (C_{max}) of simvastatin, as evidenced by a randomized, double-blind study involving healthy volunteers. Most statins are metabolized at 3A4, and toxicity leads to muscle pain, fatigue, and potentially rhabdomyolysis (Armstrong et al. 2002). See Chapter 13 ("Internal Medicine") for more details on lipid-lowering agents.

Oral hypoglycemics.   In a randomized, double-blind crossover study, nine healthy volunteers tolerated a single dose of tolbutamide (an oral hypoglycemic of the sulfonylurea class) when given on its own, but when a single dose of clarithromycin was coadministered, seven of the nine volunteers in part one of the study and nine of nine volunteers in part two complained of side effects consistent with hypoglycemia. There was a mean increase in the C_{max} of tolbutamide when the drug was administered with clarithromycin, and the mean bioavailability increased, as did the mean absorption rate constant. Given that the elimination half-life of tolbutamide increased only slightly, it seems that clarithromycin increased the rate of absorption of tolbutamide. Macrolides are known to increase gastric emptying, but clarithromyin may also inhibit P-glycoprotein in the gut (Jayasagar et al. 2000), allowing more tolbutamide into the cells and therefore into the body. (See Chapter 4 ["P-glycoproteins"] for complete a complete review of P-Glycoproteins, and the section on oral hypoglycemics in Chapter 13 ["Internal Medicine"] for further discussion.)

Rifamycin.   Clarithromycin can increase serum levels of rifamycin (rifampin), causing neutropenia and uveitis (Griffith et al. 1995).

Sildenafil.   Sildenafil (Viagra) is metabolized at 3A4. Sildenafil's package insert (Viagra 2000) states that erythromycin increases sildenafil's AUC by 182%. The clinical significance of this increase is unknown. Muirhead et al. (2002) evaluated the effects of multiple doses of erythromycin and azithromycin on sildenafil in a placebo-controlled study. As expected, azithromycin had no effect. Erythromycin caused statistically significant changes in the AUC and C_{max} of sildenafil (increasing both more than twofold in healthy volunteers) and a slight increase in the AUC of sildenafil's primary metabolite.

Psychotropic Interactions

Clozapine.   A single dose of clozapine (Clozaril) given with a single dose of erythromycin did not result in any significant interaction in healthy volunteers (Hagg et al. 1999). Clozapine is known to be metabolized mostly at 1A2 and 2D6, with some 3A4 involvement. An earlier case report implied that clozapine toxicity (somnolence, slurred speech, incoordination, incontinence, and increased serum levels) occurred when erythromycin was added for several days to a stable clozapine regimen (Cohen et al. 1996).

Pimozide.   There have been three reports of sudden death with coadministration of pimozide, an antipsychotic approved for use in patients with Tourette's syndrome (motor and vocal tics), and clarithromycin. Pimozide prolongs QT intervals; therefore, electrocardiographic monitoring is required with pimozide use. Pimozide is a potent inhibitor of 2D6 and a moderate inhibitor of 3A4. The drug is metabolized mainly at 3A4, with some 1A2 contribution (Desta et al. 1998, 1999; Flockhart et al. 2000). We recommend that pimozide not be used with any macrolide antibiotics, and patients must be warned about other moderate to potent 3A4 inhibitors, including grapefruit juice.

Triazolobenzodiazepines.   Prospective, double-blind clinical studies involving small numbers of healthy volunteers have revealed that erythromycin increases the AUCs, decreases oral clearance, and prolongs the elimination half-lives of midazolam and alprazolam (Yasui et al. 1996; Yeates et al. 1997). Most of these formal studies did not reveal significant adverse or prolonged pharmacodynamic effects (oversedation or decreased motor performance), although the duration of saccadic eye movements changed from 15 minutes to 6 hours in one early study (Olkkola et al. 1993). In one controlled, double-blind study, women exhibited a greater extent of interaction with clarithromycin and midazolam than did men (Gorski et al. 1998).

Case reports suggest that some patients may be at risk for prolonged or exaggerated effects when these drugs are combined. Delirium was reported when a patient taking triazolam was given erythromycin (Tokinaga et al. 1996). A healthy male who had been taking flunitrazepam and fluoxetine regularly for depression and sleep apnea developed delirium when clarithromycin was added to his regimen for a respiratory infection (Pollak et al. 1995). The authors of the report thought that the delirium was due to fluoxetine intoxication (which rarely causes delirium), but we believe that the clarithromycin probably increased the effects of the benzodiazepine, which is partially metabolized at 3A4. A child experienced prolonged unconsciousness after minor surgery when administered midazolam while taking prophylactic erythromycin (Hiller et al. 1990). Benzodiazepines that are glucuronidated (and therefore not dependent on phase I metabolism), such as lorazepam, oxazepam, and temazepam, are without these problems.

Azithromycin and dirithromycin mildly inhibit 3A4 and are also without these interactions, as demonstrated in clinical trials and as evidenced by the lack of clinical reports of difficulties (Rapp 1998; Watkins et al. 1997). Rokitamycin needs further clinical study; in vitro human liver enzyme studies indicate that this agent may inhibit 3A4-catalyzed triazolam α-hydroxylation (Zhao et al. 1999). Greenblatt et al. (1998) studied troleandomycin, azithromycin, erythromycin, and clarithromycin in the presence of triazolam (Halcion) in vitro, using human liver microsomes, and then conducted an in vivo study of pharmacodynamic effects of interactions. As expected, troleandomycin, erythromycin, and clarithromycin were potent inhibitors of triazolam metabolism, and erythromycin and clarithromycin enhanced the effects of triazolam. Azithromycin had effects similar to those of placebo.

Buspirone. In a randomized, double-blind study involving healthy volunteers, Kivisto et al. (1997) found that erythromycin increases the AUC of buspirone sixfold, causing psychomotor impairment and an increase in reported buspirone side effects.

Carbamazepine. Carbamazepine toxicity with concomitant use of erythromycin was first reported by Carranco et al. in 1985. Carbamazepine is metabolized at 3A4, which may be inhibited by macrolides and other 3A4 inhibitors (Spina et al. 1996). Yasui et al. (1997) reported on a series of seven psychiatric inpatients receiving 600 mg of carbamazepine a day who then received 400 mg of clarithromycin a day for pneumonia. Four of the seven patients developed carbamazepine toxicity (drowsiness, ataxia) associated with plasma carbamazepine levels that were about twice as high as clarithromycin levels.

Ketolides

Telithromycin (Ketek) is the first of a new subclass of the macrolide-lincosamide-streptogramin group. This class was developed to combat respiratory tract infections that do not respond to macrolides. Telithromycin is a competitive inhibitor of 3A4 but is only partially metabolized there. This new drug has been shown to increase plasma concentrations of drugs dependent on 3A4 for metabolism, including cisapride, simvastatin, and midazolam (Balfour and Figgitt 2001; Bearden et al. 2001).

Summary

The macrolide antibiotics clarithromycin and erythromycin, and potentially the newer ketolide telithromycin, are potent inhibitors of 3A4 and have been shown to increase unwanted side effects and toxicity of medications that are dependent on this enzyme for metabolism. Clarithromycin, erythromycin, and telithromycin should not be administered with any medication that both requires metabolism at 3A4 and has known cardiac or other life-threatening effects (i.e., a narrow therapeutic window). Azithromycin and dirithromycin do not seem prone to these interactions.

Fluoroquinolones

The fluoroquinolones are a large group of antibiotics with a broad spectrum of activity. Between 5% and 8% of patients have difficulty with side effects, gastrointestinal and central nervous system effects being the most common. The latter effects of this class of drugs

■ FLUOROQUINOLONES

Drug	Metabolism	Enzyme(s) inhibited	Enzyme(s) induced
Ciprofloxacin (Cipro)	3A4	1A2,[a] 3A4[a]	None known
Enoxacin (Penetrex)	?	1A2[a]	None known
Gatifloxacin (Tequin)	Renal excretion/?	None known	None known
Levofloxacin (Levaquin)	Renal excretion	None known	None known
Moxifloxacin (Avelox)	Not P450	None known	None known
Norfloxacin (Noroxin)	Renal excretion/?	1A2,[a] 3A4[a]	None known
Ofloxacin (Floxin)	Renal excretion	1A2[c]	None known
Sparfloxacin (Zagam)[1]	3A4, phase II	1A2, 3A4[c]	None known
Trovafloxacin (Trovan)	Phase II	None known	None known

Note.   ? = unknown.
[1]Prolongs the QTc interval and was removed from the United States market.

[a]Potent (**bold** type).
[b]Moderate.
[c]Mild.

include headache, sleep disturbance, irritability, seizures, and psychosis. De Sarro and De Sarro (2001) and Fish (2001) wrote particularly good reviews of the central nervous system–related pharmacodynamic and pharmacokinetic interactions of this class of drugs. Fluoroquinolone antibiotics are also known for being inhibitors of 1A2, with ciprofloxacin (Cipro) and enoxacin (Penetrex) being the most potent. Drugs dependent on 1A2 for more than 50% of their metabolism include theophylline, caffeine, clozapine, amitriptyline, imipramine, cyclobenzaprine (Flexeril), mirtazapine (Remeron), frovatriptan, zolmitriptan (Zomig), and naproxen (Naprosyn) (see Chapter 7 ["1A2"] for full listings). Ciprofloxacin and norfloxacin (Noroxin) potently inhibit both 1A2 and 3A4 and thus may affect many drugs.

General Drug Interactions

Xanthines. Fluoroquinolones affect the metabolism of the xanthine derivatives theophylline, caffeine, and, to some extent, theobromine. These compounds are among the most widely consumed compounds in beverages and pharmaceutical preparations (Robson 1992). Decreased theophylline and caffeine clearance with administration of quinolone antibiotics has been reported since the 1980s (Mizuki et al. 1996). Fish (2001) ranked fluoroquinolones in terms of the potential for interacting with theophylline, as follows (from strongest to weakest potential): enoxacin, ciprofloxacin, norfloxacin, and ofloxacin (Floxin), levofloxacin (Levaquin), trovafloxacin (Trovan), gatifloxacin (Tequin), and moxifloxacin (Avelox). Caffeine metabolism has been found to be decreased by ciprofloxacin and enoxacin, leading to increased side effects (Davis et al. 1996; Fish 2001).

Warfarin. The U.S. Food and Drug Administration reported enhanced warfarin anticoagulation with norfloxacin coadministration, but controlled studies involving healthy volunteers (subjects with no acute illnesses requiring antibiotics) found no such effect. The *R*-enantiomer of warfarin, which is the less potent enantiomer, is metabolized at 1A2. Ravnan and Locke (2001) reported that two patients taking both levofloxacin and warfarin had increased international normalized ratios (INRs). Levofloxacin is the *S*-enantiomer of ofloxacin. Ofloxacin has also been found to increase INRs when administered with warfarin. The enhanced anticoagulation might not be merely a P450-mediated effect; warfarin-drug interactions may be due to displaced protein-binding, altered vitamin K–producing gut flora, or other metabolic drug interactions (Ravnan and Locke 2001). The prothrombin time and INR of warfarin should be monitored when these antibiotics are coadministered.

Psychotropic Interactions

Tricyclic antidepressants. N-Demethylation of doxepin and imipramine occurs at 1A2, as does partial metabolism of other tricyclics (clomipramine and cyclobenzaprine). Despite this knowledge, there are no reports of adverse interactions between tricyclic compounds and fluoroquinolones.

Clozapine. In a case report, Markowitz et al. (1997) suggested that adding ciprofloxacin to the regimen of a patient taking clozapine increased the clozapine levels by 80%. The same authors later reported that ciprofloxacin led to increased plasma concentrations of olanzapine (Markowitz and DeVane 1999). A randomized, double-blind, placebo-controlled study involving schizophrenic patients taking clozapine revealed that ciprofloxacin increased mean serum concentrations of clozapine and its active metabolite, *N*-desmethylclozapine, by about 30% (Raaska and Neuvonen 2000). This study found no clinical signs or symptoms of toxicity, but the patients were not originally taking high-dose clozapine (mean dose, 304 mg/day), only seven patients were studied, and no objective testing of cognitive functioning was performed. We suspect that in the general population, ciprofloxacin would cause significant toxicity, particularly in elderly individuals and chronically medically ill patients (see also Case 3 in the study cases section of Chapter 7 ["1A2"]).

Diazepam. In a controlled, double-blind study in which 12 healthy volunteers were administered ciprofloxacin for 7 days, serum concentrations of diazepam were increased after a single dose of ciprofloxacin (Kamali et al. 1993). This effect was most likely due to inhibition of diazepam metabolism by ciprofloxacin, because diazepam has not been shown to be metabolized by 1A2.

Methadone.   Ciprofloxacin has been found to inhibit metabolism of methadone, leading to profound sedation (reversed by naloxone therapy) (Herrlin et al. 2000). Methadone is metabolized at 3A4 and 2D6. Ciprofloxacin's inhibition of 3A4 leaves the responsibility of metabolism to low-capacity/high-affinity 2D6, which may become overwhelmed, leading to toxicity.

Tacrine.   Hydroxylation of tacrine occurs at 1A2. In an open, randomized crossover study involving 18 healthy volunteers, fluvoxamine was a very potent inhibitor of tacrine metabolism (Larsen et al. 1999). This level of inhibition might enhance tacrine hepatotoxicity. Studies of coadministration of fluoroquinolones and tacrine have not been published to date, but we recommend that this combination not be given until further data are available.

Summary

Most fluoroquinolones are inhibitors of 1A2, and ciprofloxacin and norfloxacin are potent inhibitors of both 1A2 and 3A4. Drugs with significant adverse reactions or toxicity that are dependent on 1A2 for metabolism include clozapine, warfarin, theophylline, caffeine, and the tertiary tricyclic antidepressant (TCA) doxepin. Ciprofloxacin can inhibit metabolism of methadone and the aforementioned drugs. For full lists of drugs dependent on 3A4 and 1A2 for metabolism, please see Chapters 6 ("3A4") and 7 ("1A2").

Streptogramins

The new combination antibiotic quinupristin/dalfopristin (Synercid) is administered intravenously and is used to treat infections caused by resistant gram-positive organisms. Vancomycin was the mainstay for treatment of these infections but is now ineffective in a growing number of patients. Quinupristin/dalfopristin is a potent inhibitor of 3A4 (Allington and Rivey 2001). In in vivo studies involving healthy volunteers, quinupristin/dalfopristin increased the serum levels of cyclosporine, midazolam, and nifedipine ("Quinupristin/Dalfopristin" 1999).

Linezolid

Linezolid (Zyvox) is a member of a new class of antibiotics, the oxazolidinones, which are used against gram-positive bacteria, especially some of the resistant strains. Linezolid is a mild, reversible monoamine oxidase A inhibitor. It may interact with drugs that are adrenergic or serotonergic, leading to serotonin syndrome or hypertensive crisis (Fung et al. 2001). Tyramine-containing foods, meperidine, selective serotonin reuptake inhibitors (SSRIs), TCAs, over-the-counter sympathomimetics such as pseudoephedrine, and other medications may interact pharmacodynamically with linezolid (Fung et al. 2001; Hendershot et al. 2001). In vitro and in vivo studies have found that it is not metabolized by and has no effect on the P450 system.

■ ANTIFUNGALS: AZOLES AND TERBINAFINE

Azoles

Azole antifungals were developed in the 1980s and 1990s as oral systemic antifungal agents and are associated with far fewer side effects and toxicities than are nystatin and amphotericin B. Unfortunately, azoles have their own problems, which include significant P450 interactions and P-glycoprotein activity. Most azole antifungals are inhibitors of 3A4; ketoconazole (Nizoral) is often used as a probe drug to determine indirectly whether a new drug is metabolized at 3A4. Fluconazole (Diflucan) inhibits 3A4 moderately but is a potent inhibitor of 2C9 in vivo and has been identified as an inhibitor of 2C19 in vitro (Venkatakrishnan et al. 2000). Fluconazole therapy has led to increased phenytoin levels, and healthy volunteers receiving fluconazole and warfarin have had increased prothrombin times. Fluconazole may also inhibit the metabolism of nonsteroidal

■ SYSTEMIC ANTIFUNGALS

Drug	Metabolism site(s)	Enzyme(s) inhibited	Enzyme(s) induced
Azoles			
Fluconazole (Diflucan)	3A4	**2C9**,[a] 3A4[b]	None known
Itraconazole (Sporanox)	3A4	**3A4**[a]	None known
Ketoconazole (Nizoral)	3A4	**3A4**[a]	None known
Miconazole	3A4	3A4	
Other antifungals			
Terbinafine (Lamisil)	?	2D6	None known

Note. ? = unknown.

[a]Potent (**bold** type).
[b]Moderate.
[c]Mild.

anti-inflammatory drugs, potentially worsening gastrointestinal side effects. Itraconazole (Sporanox) and ketoconazole inhibit P-glycoprotein function, whereas fluconazole seems to have no activity on P-glycoprotein (Wang et al. 2002). Azole metabolism can be induced at 3A4 (i.e., their plasma concentrations can be reduced) by carbamazepine, phenobarbital, phenytoin, and rifampin, resulting in a reduction in antifungal efficacy.

General Drug Interactions

Cyclosporine.   Ketoconazole has been found to inhibit metabolism of cyclosporine via inhibition of 3A4. Ketoconazole inhibition has been used in an attempt to reduce the amount spent on cyclosporine in transplant recipients, with mixed results. (See Chapter 20 ["Transplant Surgery and Rheumatology"].)

Dexamethasone.   Itraconazole and intravenous and oral dexamethasone were the focus of a randomized, double-blind, placebo-controlled crossover study involving healthy volunteers. Dexamethasone is metabolized at 3A4. The adrenal suppressant effect of dexamethasone was increased in all itraconazole phases (Varis et al. 2000).

HMG-CoA reductase inhibitors ("statins").   Azoles affect the pharmacokinetics of simvastatin and lovastatin (HMG-CoA reductase inhibitors used to decrease low-density lipoprotein levels in hypercholesterolemia). Small doses of itraconazole greatly increase plasma concentrations of lovastatin and simvastatin but not fluvastatin. These increased serum levels of HMG-CoA reductase inhibitors can lead to skeletal muscle toxicity (Kivisto et al. 1998; Maxa et al. 2002; Neuvonen et al. 1998). In the itraconazole manufacturer's package insert, it was reported that rhabdomyolysis occurred in renal transplant recipients given itraconazole and HMG-CoA reductase inhibitors (Sporanox 2000). In two randomized, double-blind crossover studies, in which healthy volunteers were administered fluconazole and fluvastatin (one study) or fluconazole and pravastatin (the other study), fluconazole inhibited the metabolism of fluvastatin, via interaction at 2C9, and did not interact with pravastatin (Kantola et al. 2000). See "Hydroxymethylglutaryl–Coenzyme A Reductase Inhibitors ('Statins')" in Chapter 13 ("Internal Medicine") for further discussion.

Psychotropic Interactions

Buspirone. In a randomized, double-blind crossover study, healthy volunteers received buspirone and either itraconazole or erythromycin (Kivisto et al. 1997). Psychomotor tests were administered, and plasma concentrations, half-lives, and AUCs were determined. All subjects had increased serum buspirone concentrations and significant psychomotor impairments and buspirone-related side effects. In a later study, itraconazole increased serum buspirone levels 14.5-fold and decreased the AUC of buspirone's primary active metabolite by 50% (Kivisto et al. 1999).

Triazolobenzodiazepines. Triazolobenzodiazepines require metabolism at 3A4, and therefore their metabolism may be inhibited by the azoles, resulting in increased drowsiness or sedation and increases in other effects of these medications (Backman et al. 1998).

Terbinafine

Terbinafine (Lamisil) is a topical and systemic antifungal used to treat dermatophytoses. Abdel-Rahman et al. (1999) reported that healthy extensive metabolizers were "converted" to poor metabolizers of dextromethorphan by terbinafine—in vivo evidence that this drug may inhibit 2D6. Concomitant use with other drugs dependent on 2D6 for metabolism (β-blockers, TCAs, codeine) may increase the risk of toxicity of these drugs. Further study is needed.

Summary

The azole antifungal's mechanism of effect is to inhibit P450 fungal enzyme systems. In humans, the antifungals ketoconazole and itraconazole are potent inhibitors of 3A4 and may increase plasma concentrations of cyclosporine, triazolobenzodiazepines, warfarin, vinca alkaloids (antineoplastic agents), felodipine, methylprednisolone, glyburide, phenytoin, rifabutin, ritonavir (Norvir), saquinavir (Invirase), nevirapine (Viramune), tacrolimus, some HMG-CoA reductase inhibitors, and any other drugs dependent on 3A4 for metabolism (Albengres et al. 1998). Fluconazole is the only systemic azole antifungal with mild to moderate inhibition at 3A4 and is thus clinically less problematic at this enzyme. However, fluconazole is a potent inhibitor at 2C9 and may increase the risk of toxicity of phenytoin, warfarin, nonsteroidal anti-inflammatory drugs, and oral hypoglycemics.

■ ANTIMYCOBACTERIALS AND ANTITUBERCULAR AGENTS

Rifamycins

Rifampin (rifampicin) and rifabutin were discovered in 1957 and by 1965 were in wide use for the treatment of tuberculosis. It was quickly learned that the agents *decreased* serum levels of many medications. Where the rifamycins are metabolized has not yet been fully determined, but hepatic and gut wall 3A4 is involved. These drugs are now used in combination therapy for *Mycobacterium avium* complex infection, human immunodeficiency virus (HIV)–related tuberculosis, and community-acquired tuberculosis. The rifamycins induce most P450 enzymes. They also induce the uridine 5'-diphosphate glucuronosyltransferase (UGT) enzyme system (Gallicano et al. 1999) and P-glycoprotein transport systems (Finch et al. 2002).

Rifamycins have been reported to increase (induce) the P450-mediated metabolism of the antiemetics ondansetron and dolasetron (Finch et al. 2002), codeine and methadone (Caraco et al. 1997; Holmes 1990; Kreek et al. 1976), tacrolimus, and cyclosporine (Finch et al. 2002). Rifampin caused SSRI withdrawal syndrome when given with sertraline (Markowitz and DeVane 2000). Coadministration of rifampin and nortriptyline resulted in decreased antidepressant effect (Bebchuk and Stewart 1991; Self et al. 1996). Once rifampin therapy was discontinued, nortriptyline levels in-

■ ANTIMYCOBACTERIALS AND ANTITUBERCULAR AGENTS

Drug	Metabolism site(s)	Enzyme(s) inhibited	Enzyme(s) induced
Isoniazid (INH)	?	2C9, 2E1	2E1
Rifabutin (Mycobutin)	3A4	None known	**3A4**,[a] 1A2, 2C9, 2C19[1]
Rifampin (Rifadin)	3A4	None known	**3A4**,[a] 1A2, 2C9, 2C19[1]
Rifapentine (Priftin)	3A4/?	None known	**3A4**,[a] 2C9

Note.   ? = unknown.

[1] Rifampin and rifabutin induce all enzymes in humans except 2D6 and 2E1.

[a]Potent (**bold** type).
[b]Moderate.
[c]Mild.

creased over a 2-week period to toxic range. The efficacy of buspirone (Kivisto et al. 1999; Lamberg et al. 1998), triazolam (Villikka et al. 1997a), and zolpidem (Villikka et al. 1997b) is considerably reduced via induction by rifampin. Coadministration of rifampin and haloperidol resulted in subtherapeutic haloperidol concentrations and marked clinical ineffectiveness (Kim et al. 1996; Takeda et al. 1986).

> **Reminder:** Induction usually takes a few days and may not wear off for several weeks after discontinuation of the inducing drug. Induction of drugs may lead to ineffectiveness and increase morbidity and mortality. Induction may also result in the production of more toxic metabolites.

Rifamycins are metabolized at 3A4, and their plasma concentrations can be increased by drugs that inhibit 3A4, especially clarithromycin, ketoconazole, and the potent protease inhibitors ritonavir (Norvir) (acutely) and indinavir (Crixivan). Uveitis is one of the toxicities of rifamycins. It is recommended that rifamycin doses be decreased (which may also reduce induction by these medications) when they are administered with potent inhibitors of 3A4 (Strayhorn et al. 1997).

Rifampin induces P-glycoproteins in the duodenum and can decrease levels of digoxin (a P-glycoprotein substrate). Greiner et al. (1999) found that rifampin decreased the AUC and C_{max} of digoxin and reduced digoxin's bioavailability. They noted that intestinal P-glycoprotein levels were 3.5 times greater after rifampin administration. Digoxin may lose its antiarrhythmic effect when taken with rifampin.

Isoniazid

Isoniazid is an old drug (it was developed in the 1950s), and its mechanism of action is still poorly understood. Slow and fast acetylators were first described in reference to this drug. The half-life of isoniazid is influenced by genetic differences in acetyltransferase activity; isoniazid's elimination half-life in rapid acetylators is 50%

that in slow acetylators (Douglas and McLeod 1999). Isoniazid has also been found to inhibit the metabolism of phenytoin, implicating isoniazid as an inhibitor of 2C9 or 2C19 (Kay et al. 1985). Isoniazid may have a biphasic effect at 2E1, greatly affecting acetaminophen metabolism. When first administered with acetaminophen, isoniazid acts as an inhibitor and decreases metabolism to the toxic metabolite *N*-acetyl-*p*-benzoquinone. After 2 weeks, isoniazid becomes an inducer and may increase production of acetaminophen's toxic metabolite and cause hepatotoxicity (Chien et al. 1997; Self et al. 1999). Isoniazid has been found to increase serum haloperidol levels in schizophrenic patients (Takeda et al. 1986), but the mechanism has not been fully elucidated.

Summary

In general, the antitubercular drugs rifampin, rifabutin, and rifapentine induce metabolism at most P450 enzymes and can significantly decrease the efficacy of drugs dependent on active parent drug for effect. In the case of drugs that are metabolized to toxic metabolites, induction may lead to more rapid or severe toxicity. Rifampin is known also to induce phase II UGT metabolism and P-glycoproteins. Isoniazid is a peculiar drug, with many food and drug interactions, and careful monitoring is needed when isoniazid is administered with drugs metabolized at 2C9 and 2E1.

■ ANTIRETROVIRALS

Benjamin Smith, B.S.

HIV-positive patients are frequently administered multiple drugs (typically, the lower the CD4 count, the more medications a patient takes). Polypharmacy places this group at great risk for drug-drug interactions.

The antiretrovirals with P450 considerations are the protease inhibitors and the *non*nucleoside reverse transcriptase inhibitors (NNRTIs) (see the table entitled "Antiretrovirals").

■ ANTIRETROVIRALS

Drug	Metabolism site(s)	Enzyme(s) inhibited	Enzyme(s) induced
Protease inhibitors			
Amprenavir (Agenerase)	3A4	3A4[b]	None known
Indinavir (Crixivan)	3A4	**3A4**[a]	None known
Lopinavir/ritonavir (Kaletra)	3A4	**3A4**,[a] 2D6[1]	3A4, glucuronidation (phase II)
Nelfinavir (Viracept)	3A4, 2C19	3A4,[c] 1A2, 2B6[1]	?2C9
Ritonavir (Norvir)	3A4, 2D6[2]	**3A4, 2D6, 2C9, 2C19**,[a] 2B6[1]	**3A4**,[a] 1A2, 2C9,[b] 2C19
Saquinavir (Invirase)	3A4	3A4[c]	None known
Nonnucleoside reverse transcriptase inhibitors			
Delavirdine (Rescriptor)	3A4, 2D6, 2C9,[2] 2C19[2]	**3A4**,[a] 2C9,[1] 2C19,[1] 2D6[1]	None known
Efavirenz (Sustiva)	3A4, 2B6	**3A4**,[a] 2C9,[1] 2C19,[1] 2B6[1]	3A4,[b] 2B6[c]
Nevirapine (Viramune)	3A4, 2B6	None known	3A4,[b] 2B6[b]

[1]Inhibited in vitro.
[2]Minor pathway.

[a]Potent (**bold** type).
[b]Moderate.
[c]Mild.

The nucleoside reverse transcriptase inhibitors (NRTIs) or nucleoside analogs (which include abacavir [Trizivir], didanosine [Videx], lamivudine [Epivir], stavudine [Zerit], zalcitabine [Hivid], and zidovudine [AZT; Retrovir]) and the new acyclic phosphonate analogs of deoxynucleoside monophosphates (cidofovir [Vistide] and adefovir [Hepsera]) are excreted predominantly by the kidneys and have short half-lives, making P450-mediated drug interactions unlikely. The NRTIs are subject to induction and inhibition of phase II metabolism. The same applies to nucleotide analogs, including the newly introduced tenofovir.

General Drug Interactions

Protease Inhibitors

The class of antiretrovirals known as the protease inhibitors includes powerful drugs with multiple and varied pharmacokinetic and pharmacodynamic interactions. We outline most metabolic interactions here.

Inhibition.   Ritonavir is the most potent acute inhibitor of 3A4 in the protease inhibitor group. In vitro studies have found that, compared with ketoconazole, ritonavir is slightly less inhibitory and amprenavir (Agenerase) is less inhibitory by an order of magnitude (von Moltke et al. 2000). The same warnings apply to the protease inhibitors as to ketoconazole, erythromycin, and clarithromycin. These drugs all potently inhibit 3A4 and can greatly affect drugs with narrow therapeutic indices. Kato et al. (2000) reported that a patient taking carbamazepine developed vomiting, vertigo, and increased liver associated enzyme levels, along with increased serum concentrations of the anticonvulsant, within 12 hours of the first dose of ritonavir. Another patient taking antimigraine medications containing ergotamine began taking ritonavir (Vila et al. 2001). After 5 days of the new therapy, the patient developed ergotism, evidenced by pain, claudication, paresthesia, coldness, and cyanosis of both legs. This is one of six reported cases of serious ergotism associated with ritonavir therapy. Ergots are metabolized at 3A4, which is inhibited by ritonavir. (See Chapter 15 ["Neurology"].)

Other ritonavir interactions may take longer to become apparent. An HIV-positive patient taking ritonavir was administered the glucocorticoid budesonide for radiation colitis. Within 14 days, the patient had developed acute hepatitis, with alanine transaminase levels of 660 (Sagir et al. 2002). Budesonide is used to treat inflammatory bowel disease because the drug's first-pass clearance by 3A4 of more than 90% allows high doses within the lumen of the bowel. When 3A4 metabolism of budesonide was inhibited by ritonavir, a large amount of budesonide accumulated, leading to hepatic parenchymal damage. Patients taking ritonavir have developed Cushing's syndrome after 5 months of inhaled fluticasone because of ritonavir's inhibition of 3A4 metabolism of the corticosteroid (Clevenbergh et al. 2002; Gupta and Dubé 2002). Although inhibition of the substrates at 3A4 was immediate, the pharmacodynamic effects of the higher concentrations of substrate became apparent over time.

Other protease inhibitors, although less potent 3A4 inhibitors than ritonavir, have also demonstrated clinically significant inhibition. In one study, amprenavir so inhibited the metabolism of rifabutin that the combination was not tolerated by many of the patients, who developed flulike symptoms (Polk et al. 2001).

Induction. Ritonavir, a potent inhibitor of 3A4, also *induces* 3A4 metabolism after a few weeks. The balance between induction and inhibition can be quite variable and often unpredictable, ranging from net inhibition to net induction. Thus, close clinical monitoring for several weeks is necessary when ritonavir therapy is begun. Ritonavir has been found to increase or induce the metabolism of meperidine, resulting in increased levels of the neurotoxic metabolite normeperidine, and has been found to reduce the AUC and C_{max} of ethinyl estradiol (Ouellet et al. 1998; Piscitelli et al. 2000b), placing patients at risk for breakthrough bleeding and pregnancy. Ritonavir is also an inducer of 1A2, 2C9, and 2C19. In one case study, a patient taking acenocoumarol (a mixture of *R*- and *S*-warfarin, metabolized at 1A2 and 2C9, respectively) began taking ritonavir (Llibre et al. 2002). The patient's INR decreased dramatically even when the dose of acenocoumarol was tripled. To date, there are no reports of ritonavir inducing metabolism of protease inhibitors that rely on 3A4. In short, ritonavir has been found to be a "pan-*inhibitor*" of P450 enzymes and a specific *inducer* at 3A4, 1A2, 2C9, and 2C19.

The newest protease inhibitor is Kaletra, a combination drug containing ritonavir and lopinavir. Ritonavir, a potent 3A4 inhibitor, increases plasma lopinavir levels, with improved clinical results. Lopinavir induces glucuronidation. This phase II metabolism induction can greatly reduce levels of the NRTIs AZT and abacavir, lowering effectiveness and resulting in viral resistance. Lopinavir has also been found to increase clearance of methadone and ethinyl estradiol. In vitro, lopinavir/ritonavir inhibits 2D6, but clinical studies are pending (Kaletra 2002; C. Koch and R. Hodd, Abbott Laboratories, personal communication, December 19, 2000).

Nonnucleoside Reverse Transcriptase Inhibitors

Inhibition.   NNRTIs also can inhibit P450 enzymes (see the table entitled "Antiretrovirals"). Efavirenz (Sustiva) is a potent inhibitor of 3A4 and, interestingly, also *induces* 3A4 (Sustiva 2002). Delavirdine (Rescriptor) is a potent inhibitor of 3A4, leading to significant effects on the metabolism of clarithromycin and protease inhibitors (Tran et al. 2001). This inhibition has been used in the past to increase concentrations of protease inhibitors to obtain better clinical results.

Induction.   Nevirapine (Viramune) is a 3A4 inducer (Viramune 2002). The drug has been found to reduce the plasma AUC of nelfinavir (Viracept), indinavir, and saquinavir (Invirase). In recent postmarketing surveillance, nevirapine was found to induce methadone metabolism, causing methadone withdrawal in some patients and thus necessitating an increase in methadone (Altice et al. 1999). As noted in the previous paragraph, efavirenz is a potent 3A4 inhibitor but also induces 3A4 (Sustiva 2002). Concomitant use with 3A4 metabolites with narrow therapeutic windows warrants caution.

The doses of drugs such as TCAs, antiarrhythmics, or triazolobenzo-diazepines must immediately be decreased when the drugs are taken with efavirenz, because of efavirenz's inhibition of 3A4. *Induction* may then lead to *decreased* levels of the 3A4-dependent medications, necessitating *increased* doses of them at a later date. In one study, it was demonstrated by an erythromycin breath test that 3A4 induction by efavirenz reached full magnitude on day 10 of administration (Mouly et al. 2002). Efavirenz is often used in combination with protease inhibitors and can induce their metabolism, bringing plasma levels below therapeutic ranges. Efavirenz can decrease amprenavir levels 1–2 weeks after initiation of efavirenz therapy (Duval et al. 2000). Fortunately, this effect can be reversed with the addition of protease inhibitors that inhibit 3A4. Efavirenz induces metabolism of all protease inhibitors except nelfinavir and ritonavir.

Other Drugs

Inhibition and induction.   The metabolism of antiretrovirals can be inhibited as well, leading to greater serum concentrations of drug, as well as potentially intensifying noxious side effects such as nausea, vomiting, and diarrhea. Cimetidine and clarithromycin have increased nevirapine levels, and ketoconazole increased concentrations of delavirdine (Tseng and Foisy 1997). Some centers have reported using inhibition to advantage: plasma levels (and, theoretically, effectiveness) of saquinavir have been increased clinically with the addition of ritonavir, ketoconazole, or grapefruit juice (but concentrations of the latter are inconsistent). One study demonstrated substantial increases in the plasma saquinavir AUC when the drug was given with ketoconazole (69% increase) or erythromycin (99% increase) (Grub et al. 2001).

Antiretrovirals are metabolized at 3A4 and can also be induced by the usual potent inducers: phenytoin, carbamazepine, alcohol, rifamycins, and barbiturates. Rifampin and rifapentine induce protease inhibitors and NNRTIs and can decrease serum concentrations, leading to viral resistance (decreased sensitivity of the virus to the protease inhibitor or NNRTI). St. John's wort was recently found to induce 3A4, decreasing mean plasma indinavir concentrations by 57% and trough levels by 81% (Piscitelli et al. 2000a). Garlic supplements were found to decrease plasma saquinavir levels by approximately 50% (Piscitelli et al. 2002).

Psychotropic Interactions

Triazolobenzodiazepines

A 32-year-old man with HIV infection tolerated midazolam for bronchoscopy while taking AZT and lamivudine. Saquinavir was added without problems. However, when he needed another bronchoscopy, the same dose of midazolam necessitated the addition of flumazenil for prolonged sedation, and the patient remained impaired for more than 5 hours (Merry et al. 1997). Midazolam's metabolism was inhibited by the protease inhibitor, prolonging midazolam's sedating effects.

Ritonavir's interaction with alprazolam and triazolam has proven to be more complex. Short-term use of ritonavir has been shown to potently inhibit metabolism of these drugs, resulting in enhanced sedation and impairment (Greenblatt et al. 2000). However, after ritonavir has been used for more than a few days, clearance of the benzodiazepines increases, even to the point of there being a slight net 3A4 induction by ritonavir.

Tricyclic Antidepressants

TCAs may be affected by ritonavir, because all metabolic routes may be inhibited, leading to toxicity.

SSRIs

Patients taking fluoxetine and ritonavir may develop serotonin syndrome (a constellation of symptoms including mental status changes, diarrhea, and myoclonus) 1–2 weeks after initiation of ritonavir therapy (DeSilva et al. 2001). SSRIs are mostly metabolized at

2D6 and 3A4, which are both inhibited by ritonavir. To date, no cases have been reported of SSRI withdrawal syndrome due to 3A4 induction with prolonged ritonavir or efavirenz use.

Antipsychotics

Clozapine metabolism may be inhibited by ritonavir. For treatment of psychosis in a patient who must take ritonavir, olanzapine may be used because this drug is metabolized by several P450 enzymes and by phase II enzymes. A better choice may be ziprasidone, since olanzapine is 30%–40% metabolized at 1A2 as well.

Methadone and Buprenorphine

In vitro studies involving human microsomes revealed that protease inhibitors inhibit methadone N-demethylation and buprenorphine N-dealkylation, which could lead to respiratory compromise secondary to opiate toxicity (Iribarne et al. 1998). In one case study, however, a patient taking methadone experienced withdrawal symptoms within 7 days of initiation of ritonavir therapy and was noted to have decreased plasma methadone levels (Geletko and Erickson 2000). This effect may have been due to a net 3A4 induction by ritonavir.

In a study involving 11 patients receiving methadone, a decrease in methadone AUC of more than 50% occurred after only 24 hours of efavirenz administration (Clarke et al. 2001). This led to nine patients complaining of withdrawal symptoms, beginning on day 8 of efavirenz treatment.

Summary

Ritonavir is a very potent pan-inhibitor, with activity at most P450 enzymes. Whenever a patient is administered ritonavir, caution must be taken with all additional drugs that have narrow therapeutic windows. All protease inhibitors are metabolized at 3A4, and all exhibit some inhibition at 3A4. The NNRTIs efavirenz and delavirdine are potent inhibitors of 3A4, and nevirapine, ritonavir, and efavirenz are inducers of 3A4. Lopinavir/ritonavir carries all of the warnings for ritonavir and may also induce metabolism of methadone, oral contraceptives, and NRTIs via induction of glucuronidation. Metabolism of all protease inhibitors and NNRTIs may be induced by antitubercular drugs such as rifampin, leading to ineffectiveness and viral resistance.

■ REFERENCES

Abdel-Rahman SM, Gotschall RR, Kauffman RE, et al: Investigation of terbinafine as a CYP2D6 inhibitor in vivo. Clin Pharmacol Ther 65:465–472, 1999

Albengres E, LeLouet H, Tillement JP: Systemic antifungal agents: drug interactions of clinical significance. Drug Saf 18:83–97, 1998

Allington DR, Rivey MP: Quinupristin/Dalfopristin: a therapeutic review. Clin Ther 23:24–44, 2001

Altice FL, Friedland GH, Cooney EL: Nevirapine induced opiate withdrawal among injection drug users with HIV infection receiving methadone. AIDS 13:957–962, 1999

Armstrong SC, Cozza KL, Oesterheld JR: Med-psych drug-drug interactions update. Psychosomatics 43:79–81, 2002

Ausband SC, Goodman PE: An unusual case of clarithromycin associated ergotism. J Emerg Med 21:411–413, 2001

Backman JT, Kivisto KT, Olkkola KT, et al: The area under the plasma concentration-time curve for oral midazolam is 400-fold larger during treatment with itraconazole than with rifampicin. Eur J Clin Pharmacol 54:53–58, 1998

Balfour JA, Figgitt DP: Telithromycin. Drugs 61:815–829, 2001

Balfour JA, Wiseman LR: Moxifloxacin. Drugs 57:363–373, 1999

Bearden DT, Neuhauser MM, Garey KW: Telithromycin: an oral ketolide for respiratory infections. Pharmacotherapy 21:1204–1222, 2001

Bebchuk JM, Stewart DE: Drug interaction between rifampin and nortriptyline: a case report. Int J Psychiatry Med 21:183–187, 1991

Caraco Y, Sheller J, Wood AJ: Pharmacogenetic determinants of codeine induction by rifampin: the impact on codeine's respiratory, psychomotor and miotic effects. J Pharmacol Exp Ther 281:330–336, 1997

Carranco E, Kareus J, Co S, et al: Carbamazepine toxicity induced by concurrent erythromycin therapy. Arch Neurol 42:187–188, 1985

Chien JY, Peter RM, Nolan CM, et al: Influence of polymorphic *N*-acetyl-transferase phenotype on the inhibition and induction of acetaminophen bioactivation with long-term isoniazid. Clin Pharmacol Ther 61:24–34, 1997

Clarke SM, Mulcahy FM, Tjia J, et al: The pharmacokinetics of methadone in HIV-positive patients receiving the non-nucleoside reverse transcriptase inhibitor efavirenz. Br J Clin Pharmacol 51:213–217, 2001

Clevenbergh P, Corcostegui M, Gerard D, et al: Iatrogenic Cushing's syndrome in an HIV-infected patient with inhaled corticosteroids (fluticasone propionate) and low dose ritonavir enhanced PI containing regimen. J Infect 44:194–195, 2002

Cohen LG, Chesley S, Eugenio L, et al: Erythromycin-induced clozapine toxic reaction. Arch Intern Med 156:675–677, 1996

Davis R, Markham A, Balfour JA: Ciprofloxacin: an updated review of its pharmacology, therapeutic efficacy and tolerability. Drugs 51:1019–1074, 1996

De Sarro A, De Sarro G: Adverse reactions to fluoroquinolones: an overview on mechanistic aspects. Curr Med Chem 8:371–384, 2001

DeSilva KE, Le Flore DB, Marston BJ, et al: Serotonin syndrome in HIV-infected individuals receiving antiretroviral therapy and fluoxetine. AIDS 15:1281–1285, 2001

Desta Z, Kerbusch T, Soukhova N, et al: Identification and characterization of human cytochrome P450 isoforms interacting with pimozide. J Pharmacol Exp Ther 285:428–437, 1998

Desta Z, Kerbusch T, Flockhart DA: Effect of clarithromycin on the pharmacokinetics and pharmacodynamics of pimozide in healthy poor and extensive metabolizers of cytochrome P450 2D6 (CYP2D6). Clin Pharmacol Ther 65:10–20, 1999

Douglas JG, McLeod M: Pharmacokinetic factors in modern drug treatment of tuberculosis. Clin Pharmacokinet 37:127–146, 1999

Duval X, Le Moing V, Longuet C, et al: Efavirenz-induced decrease in plasma amprenavir levels in human immunodeficiency virus-infected patients and correction by ritonavir (letter). Antimicrob Agents Chemother 44:2593, 2000

Eagling VA, Back DJ, Barry MG: Differential inhibition of cytochrome P450 isoforms by the protease inhibitors, ritonavir, saquinavir and indinavir. Br J Clin Pharmacol 44:190–194, 1997

Efthymiopoulos C: Pharmacokinetics of grepafloxacin. J Antimicrob Chemother 40 (suppl A):35–43, 1997

Finch CK, Chrisman CR, Baciewicz AM, et al: Rifampin and rifabutin drug interactions. Arch Intern Med 162:985–992, 2002

Fish DN: Fluoroquinolone adverse effects and drug interactions. Pharmacotherapy 21:253S–272S, 2001

Flockhart DA, Drici M, Kerbusch T, et al: Studies on the mechanism of a fatal clarithromycin-pimozide interaction in a patient with Tourette syndrome. J Clin Psychopharmacol 20:317–324, 2000

Fung HB, Kirschenbaum HL, Ojofeitimi BO: Linezolid: an oxazolidinone antimicrobial agent. Clin Ther 23:356–391, 2001

Gallicano KD, Sahai J, Shukla VK, et al: Induction of zidovudine glucuronidation and amination pathways by rifampicin in HIV-infected patients. Br J Clin Pharmacol 48:168–179, 1999

Geletko SM, Erickson AD: Decreased methadone effect after ritonavir initiation. Pharmacotherapy 20:93–94, 2000

Gorski JC, Jones DR, Haehner-Daniels BD, et al: The contribution of intestinal and hepatic CYP3A to the interaction between midazolam and clarithromycin. Clin Pharmacol Ther 64:133–143, 1998

Greenblatt DJ, von Moltke LL, Harmatz JS, et al: Inhibition of triazolam clearance by macrolide antimicrobial agents: in vitro correlates and dynamic consequences. Clin Pharmacol Ther 64:278–285, 1998

Greenblatt DJ, von Moltke LL, Harmatz JS, et al: Alprazolam-ritonavir interaction: implications for product labeling. Clin Pharmacol Ther 67: 335–341, 2000

Greiner B, Eichelbaum M, Fritz P, et al: The role of intestinal P-glycoprotein in the interaction of digoxin and rifampin. J Clin Invest 104:147–153, 1999

Griffith DE, Brown BA, Girard WM, et al: Adverse events associated with high-dose rifabutin in macrolide-containing regimens for the treatment of *Mycobacterium avium* complex lung disease. Clin Infect Dis 21:594–598, 1995

Grub S, Bryson H, Goggin T, et al: The interaction of saquinavir (soft gelatin capsule) with ketoconazole, erythromycin and rifampicin: comparison of the effect in healthy volunteers and in HIV-infected patients. Eur J Clin Pharmacol 57:115–121, 2001

Gupta SK, Dubé MP: Exogenous Cushing syndrome mimicking human immunodeficiency virus lipodystrophy. Clin Infect Dis 35:E69–E71, 2002

Hagg S, Spigset O, Mjorndal T, et al: Absence of interaction between erythromycin and a single dose of clozapine. Eur J Clin Pharmacol 55:221–226, 1999

Hendershot PE, Antal EJ, Welshman IR, et al: Linezolid: pharmacokinetic and pharmacodynamic evaluation of coadministration with pseudo-ephedrine HCl, phenylpropanolamine HCl, and dextromethorphan HBr. J Clin Pharmacol 41:563–572, 2001

Herrlin K, Segerdahl M, Gustafsson LL, et al: Methadone, ciprofloxacin, and adverse drug reactions. Lancet 356:2069–2070, 2000

Hesse LM, von Moltke LL, Shader RI, et al: Ritonavir, efavirenz, and nelfinavir inhibit CYP2B6 activity in vitro: potential drug interactions with bupropion. Drug Metab Dispos 29:100–102, 2001

Hiller A, Olkkola KT, Isohanni P, et al: Unconsciousness associated with midazolam and erythromycin. Br J Anaesth 65:826–828, 1990

Holmes VF: Rifampin-induced methadone withdrawal in AIDS (letter). J Clin Psychopharmacol 10:443–444, 1990

Horowitz RS, Dart RC, Gomez HF: Clinical ergotism with lingual ischemia induced by clarithromycin-ergotamine interaction. Arch Intern Med 156: 456–458, 1996

Iatsimirskaia E, Tulebaev S, Storozhuk E, et al: Metabolism of rifabutin in human enterocyte and liver microsomes: kinetic parameters, identification of enzyme systems, and drug interactions with macrolides and antifungal agents. Clin Pharmacol Ther 61:554–562, 1997

Iribarne C, Berthou F, Carlhant D, et al: Inhibition of methadone and buprenorphine N-dealkylations by three HIV-1 protease inhibitors. Drug Metab Dispos 26:257–260, 1998

Jayasagar G, Dixit AA, Kishan V, et al: Effect of clarithromycin on the pharmacokinetics of tolbutamide. Drug Metabol Drug Interact 16:207–215, 2000

Kaletra (package insert). Abbott Park, IL, Abbott Laboratories, 2002

Kamali F, Thomas SHL, Edwards C: The influence of steady-state ciprofloxacin on the pharmacokinetics and pharmacodynamics of a single dose of diazepam in healthy volunteers. Eur J Clin Pharmacol 44:365–367, 1993

Kantola T, Kivisto KT, Neuvonen PJ: Erythromycin and verapamil considerably increase serum simvastatin and simvastatin acid concentrations. Clin Pharmacol Ther 64:177–182, 1998

Kantola T, Backman JT, Niemi M, et al: Effect of fluconazole on plasma fluvastatin and pravastatin. Eur J Clin Pharmacol 56:225–229, 2000

Kato Y, Fujii T, Mizoguchi N, et al: Potential interaction between ritonavir and carbamazepine. Pharmacotherapy 20:851–854, 2000

Kay L, Kampmann JP, Svendsen T, et al: Influence of rifampicin and isoniazid on the kinetics of phenytoin. Br J Clin Pharmacol 20:323–326, 1985

Kim YH, Cha IJ, Shim JC, et al: Effect of rifampin on the plasma concentration and the clinical effect of haloperidol concomitantly administered to schizophrenic patients. J Clin Psychopharmacol 16:247–252, 1996

Kinzig-Schippers M, Fuhr U, Cesana M, et al: Absence of effect of rufloxacin on theophylline pharmacokinetics in steady state. Antimicrob Agents Chemother 42:2359–2364, 1998

Kinzig-Schippers M, Fuhr U, Zaigler M, et al: Interaction of pefloxacin and enoxacin with the human cytochrome P450 enzyme CYP1A2. Clin Pharmacol Ther 65:262–274, 1999

Kivisto KT, Lamberg TS, Kantola T, et al: Plasma buspirone concentrations are greatly increased by erythromycin and itraconazole. Clin Pharmacol Ther 62:348–354, 1997

Kivisto KT, Kantola T, Neuvonen PJ: Different effects of itraconazole on the pharmacokinetics of fluvastatin and lovastatin. Br J Clin Pharmacol 46:49–53, 1998

Kivisto KT, Lamberg TS, Neuvonen PJ: Interactions of buspirone with itraconazole and rifampicin: effects on the pharmacokinetics of the active 1-(2-pyrimidinyl)-piperazine metabolite of buspirone. Pharmacol Toxicol 84:94–97, 1999

Kreek MJ, Garfield JW, Gutjahr CL, et al: Rifampin induced methadone withdrawal. N Engl J Med 294:1104–1106, 1976

Lamberg TS, Kivisto KT, Neuvonen PJ: Concentrations and effects of buspirone are considerably reduced by rifampin. Br J Clin Pharmacol 45:381–385, 1998

Larsen JT, Hansen LL, Spigset O, et al: Fluvoxamine is a potent inhibitor of tacrine metabolism in vivo. Eur J Clin Pharmacol 55:375–382, 1999

Lazar JD, Wilner KD: Drug interactions with fluconazole. Rev Infect Dis 12 (suppl 3):S327–S333, 1990

Llibre JM, Romeu J, Lopez E, et al: Severe interaction between ritonavir and acenocoumarol. Ann Pharmacother 36:621–623, 2002

Lomaestro BM, Piatek MA: Update on drug interactions with azole antifungal agents. Ann Pharmacother 32:915–928, 1998

Luurila H, Olkkola KT, Neuvonen PJ: Interaction between erythromycin and the benzodiazepines diazepam and flunitrazepam. Pharmacol Toxicol 78:117–122, 1996

Mandell GL, Bennett JE, Dolin R (eds): Principles and Practice of Infectious Diseases. Philadelphia, PA, Churchill Livingstone, 2000, pp 404–422

Markowitz JS, DeVane CL: Suspected ciprofloxacin inhibition of olanzapine resulting in increased plasma concentration. J Clin Psychopharmacol 19:289–291, 1999

Markowitz JS, DeVane CL: Rifampin-induced selective serotonin reuptake inhibitor withdrawal syndrome in a patient treated with sertraline (letter). J Clin Psychopharmacol 20:109–110, 2000

Markowitz JS, Gill HS, DeVane CL, et al: Fluoroquinolone inhibition of clozapine metabolism (letter). Am J Psychiatry 154:881, 1997

Maxa JL, Melton LB, Ogu CC, et al: Rhabdomyolysis after concomitant use of cyclosporine, simvastatin, gemfibrozil, and itraconazole. Ann Pharmacother 36:820–823, 2002

Merry C, Mulcahy F, Barry M, et al: Saquinavir interaction with midazolam: pharmacokinetic considerations when prescribing protease inhibitors for patients with HIV disease. AIDS 11:268–269, 1997

Mizuki Y, Fujiwara I, Yamaguchi T: Pharmacokinetic interactions related to the chemical structures of fluoroquinolones. J Antimicrob Chemother 37 (suppl A):41–55, 1996

Mouly S, Lown KS, Kornhauser D, et al: Hepatic but not intestinal CYP3A4 displays dose-dependent induction by efavirenz in humans. Clin Pharmacol Ther 72:1–9, 2002

Muirhead GJ, Faulkner S, Harness JA, et al: The effects of steady-state erythromycin and azithromycin on the pharmacokinetics of sildenafil in healthy volunteers. Br J Clin Pharmacol 53 (suppl 1):375–435, 2002

Neuvonen PJ, Kantola T, Kivisto KT: Simvastatin but not pravastatin is very susceptible to interaction with the CYP3A4 inhibitor itraconazole. Clin Pharmacol Ther 63:332–341, 1998

Olkkola KT, Aranko K, Luurila H, et al: A potentially hazardous interaction between erythromycin and midazolam. Clin Pharmacol Ther 53:298–305, 1993

Ouellet D, Hsu A, Qian J, et al: Effect of ritonavir on the pharmacokinetics of ethinyl oestradiol in healthy female volunteers. Br J Clin Pharmacol 46:111–116, 1998

Piscitelli SC, Burstein AH, Chaitt D, et al: Indinavir concentrations and St John's wort. Lancet 355:547–548, 2000a

Piscitelli SC, Kress DR, Bertz RJ, et al: The effect of ritonavir on the pharmacokinetics of meperidine and normeperidine. Pharmacotherapy 20:549–553, 2000b

Piscitelli SC, Burstein AH, Welden N, et al: The effect of garlic supplements on the pharmacokinetics of saquinavir. Clin Infect Dis 34:234–238, 2002

Polk RE, Brophy DF, Israel DS, et al: Pharmacokinetic interaction between amprenavir and rifabutin or rifampin in healthy males. Antimicrob Agents Chemother 45:502–508, 2001

Pollak PT, Sketris IS, MacKenzie SL, et al: Delirium probably induced by clarithromycin in a patient receiving fluoxetine. Ann Pharmacother 29: 486–488, 1995

Quinupristin/dalfopristin. Med Lett Drugs Ther 41:109–110, 1999

Raaska K, Neuvonen PJ: Ciprofloxacin increases serum clozapine and N-desmethylclozapine: a study in patients with schizophrenia. Eur J Clin Pharmacol 56:585–589, 2000

Rapp RP: Pharmacokinetics and pharmacodynamics of intravenous and oral azithromycin: enhanced tissue activity and minimal drug interactions. Ann Pharmacother 32:785–793, 1998

Ravnan SL, Locke C: Levofloxacin and warfarin interaction. Pharmacotherapy 21:884–885, 2001

Robson RA: The effects of quinolones on xanthine pharmacokinetics. Am J Med 92:22S–25S, 1992

Rubenstein E, Prokocimer P, Talbot GH: Safety and tolerability of quinupristin/dalfopristin: administration guidelines. J Antimicrob Chemother 44 (suppl A):37–46, 1999

Sagir A, Wettstein M, Oette M, et al: Budesonide-induced acute hepatitis in an HIV-positive patient with ritonavir as a co-medication. AIDS 16: 1191–1192, 2002

Self T[H], Corley CR, Nabhan S, et al: Case report: interaction of rifampin and nortriptyline. Am J Med Sci 311:80–81, 1996

Self TH, Chrisman CR, Baciewicz AM, et al: Isoniazid drug and food interactions. Am J Med Sci 317:304–311, 1999

Smith PF, DiCenzo R, Morse GD: Clinical pharmacokinetics of non-nucleoside reverse transcriptase inhibitors. Clin Pharmacokinet 40:893–905, 2001

Sovner R, Fogelman S: Ketoconazole therapy for atypical depression. J Clin Psychiatry 57:227–228, 1996

Spicer ST, Liddle C, Chapman JR, et al: The mechanism of cyclosporine toxicity induced by clarithromycin. Br J Clin Pharmacol 43:194–196, 1997

Spina E, Pisani F, Perucca E: Clinically significant pharmacokinetic drug interactions with carbamazepine: an update. Clin Pharmacokinet 31: 198–214, 1996

Sporanox (package insert). Titusville, NJ, Janssen Pharmaceutica Products, LP, 2000

Staas H, Kubitza D: Profile of moxifloxacin drug interactions. Clin Infect Dis 32 (suppl 1):S47–S50, 2001

Strayhorn VA, Baciewicz AM, Self TH: Update on rifampin drug interactions, III. Arch Intern Med 157:2453–2458, 1997

Sustiva (package insert). Wilmington, DE, DuPont Pharmaceuticals, 2002

Takeda M, Nishinuma K, Yamashita S, et al: Serum haloperidol levels of schizophrenics receiving treatment for tuberculosis. Clin Neuropharmacol 9:386–397, 1986

Temple ME, Nahata MC: Rifapentine: its role in the treatment of tuberculosis. Ann Pharmacother 33:1203–1210, 1999

Tokinaga N, Kondo T, Kaneko S, et al: Hallucinations after a therapeutic dose of benzodiazepine hypnotics with co-administration of erythromycin. Psychiatry Clin Neurosci 50:337–339, 1996

Tran JQ, Gerber JG, Kerr BM: Delavirdine: clinical pharmacokinetics and drug interactions. Clin Pharmacokinet 40:207–226, 2001

Tseng AL, Foisy MM: Management of drug interactions in patients with HIV. Ann Pharmacother 31:1040–1058, 1997

Varis T, Kivisto KT, Backman JT, et al: The cytochrome P450 3A4 inhibitor itraconazole markedly increases the plasma concentrations of dexamethasone and enhances its adrenal-suppressant effect. Clin Pharmacol Ther 68:487–494, 2000

Venkatakrishnan K, von Moltke LL, Greenblatt DJ: Effects of the antifungal agents on oxidative drug metabolism: clinical relevance. Clin Pharmacokinet 38:111–180, 2000

Viagra (package insert). New York, Pfizer Inc., 2000

Vila A, Mykietiuk A, Bonvehì P, et al: Clinical ergotism induced by ritonavir. Scand J Infect Dis 33:788–789, 2001

Villikka K, Kivisto KT, Backman JT, et al: Triazolam is ineffective in patients taking rifampin. Clin Pharmacol Ther 61:8–14, 1997a

Villikka K, Kivisto KT, Luurila H, et al: Rifampin reduces plasma concentrations and effects of zolpidem. Clin Pharmacol Ther 62:629–634, 1997b

Villikka K, Kivisto KT, Neuvonen PJ: The effect of rifampin on the pharmacokinetics of oral and intravenous ondansetron. Clin Pharmacol Ther 65:377–381, 1999

Viramune (package insert). Ridgefield, CT, Boehringer Ingelheim Pharmaceuticals, Inc., and Roxane Laboratories, 2002

von Moltke LL, Durol AL, Duan SX, et al: Potent mechanism-based inhibition of human CYP3A in vitro by amprenavir and ritonavir: comparison with ketoconazole. Eur J Clin Pharmacol 56:259–261, 2000

Voorman RL, Payne NA, Wienkers LC, et al: Interaction of delavirdine with human liver microsomal cytochrome P450: inhibition of CYP2C9, CYP2C19, and CYP2D6. Drug Metab Dispos 29:41–47, 2001

Wang EJ, Lew K, Casciano CN, et al: Interaction of common azole antifungals with P-glycoprotein. Antimicrob Agents Chemother 46:160–165, 2002

Watkins JS, Polk RE, Stotka JL: Drug interactions of macrolides: emphasis on dirithromycin. Ann Pharmacother 31:349–356, 1997

Yasui N, Otani K, Kaneko S, et al: A kinetic and dynamic study of oral alprazolam with and without erythromycin in humans: in vivo evidence for the involvement of CYP3A4 in alprazolam metabolism. Clin Pharmacol Ther 59:514–519, 1996

Yasui N, Otani K, Kaneko S, et al: Carbamazepine toxicity induced by clarithromycin coadministration in psychiatric patients. Int Clin Psychopharmacol 12:225–229, 1997

Yeates RA, Laufen H, Zimmermann T, et al: Pharmacokinetic and pharmacodynamic interaction study between midazolam and the macrolide antibiotics, erythromycin, clarithromycin, and the azalide azithromycin. Int J Clin Pharmacol Ther 35(12):577–599, 1997

Zhao XJ, Koyama E, Ishizaki T: An in vitro study on the metabolism and possible drug interactions of rokitamycin, a macrolide antibiotic, using human liver microsomes. Drug Metab Dispos 27:776–785, 1999

15

NEUROLOGY

Neurology and psychiatry share many pharmacological treatments and oftentimes patients. The use of tricyclic antidepressants (TCAs) and selective serotonin reuptake inhibitors for poststroke depression, TCAs for migraine prophylaxis, and cholinesterase inhibitors for dementia, and the overlapping psychiatric and neurological uses of antiepileptic drugs are just a few examples. The antiepileptics have significant potential for phase I and phase II drug-drug interactions. These agents are substrates of phase I and phase II enzymes, but they also interact to both induce and inhibit these enzymes as well. In this chapter, we cover antiepileptic agents, antiparkinsonian drugs, cholinesterase inhibitors for dementia, and triptans and ergots for migraine headaches.

> **Reminder:** This chapter is dedicated primarily to metabolic and P-glycoprotein interactions. Interactions due to displaced protein-binding, alterations in absorption or excretion, and pharmacodynamics are not covered.

■ ANTIEPILEPTIC DRUGS

Phenobarbital was noted to be efficacious for seizure control in 1912, phenytoin (Dilantin) was marketed in 1938, and valproic acid (VPA; Depakote) was marketed in 1968. The metabolism of these three drugs was and in some ways remains a mystery. Drugs developed after the late 1980s have undergone human liver microsome studies and some in vivo testing with probes. Unfortunately, many older drugs, being off patent, have not been reevaluated with this

■ ANTIEPILEPTIC DRUGS

Drug	Metabolism	Enzyme(s) inhibited	Enzyme(s) induced
Carbamazepine (Tegretol)	3A4, 2C8, 2C9, 1A2, phase II	None known	**3A4,**[a] 1A2, 2C19
Ethosuximide (Zarontin)	3A4, phase II	None known	?Pan-inducer
Felbamate (Felbatol)	3A4, 2E1	2C19	3A4
Gabapentin (Neurontin)	Excreted in urine unchanged	None known	None known
Lamotrigine (Lamictal)	UGTs; excreted in urine unchanged	None known	UGTs (mild, autoinduction)
Levetiracetam (Keppra)	Non-P450 phase I hydrolysis	None known	None known
Methsuximide (Celontin)	3A4, phase II	None known	?Pan-inducer
Oxcarbazepine (Trileptal)	3A4	2C19	3A4[b]
Phenobarbital	2C9, 2C19, 2E1; 25% excreted in urine unchanged	3A4, ?phase II	UGTs, 3A4, 2C9, 2C19, 1A2, ?others
Phenytoin (Dilantin)	2C9, 2C19, 2E1, phase II	None known	3A4, 2C9, 2C19, phase II
Primidone (Mysoline)	2C9, 2C19, 2E1; 25% excreted in urine unchanged	3A4, ?phase II	UGTs, 3A4, 2C9, 2C19, 1A2, ?others
Tiagabine (Gabitril)	3A4, UGTs	2D6	None known
Topiramate (Topamax)	70% excreted in urine unchanged; phase I, phase II	2C19[b]	None known; decreases ethinyl estradiol levels

■ ANTIEPILEPTIC DRUGS (continued)

Drug	Metabolism	Enzyme(s) inhibited	Enzyme(s) induced
Valproic acid (Depakote/ Depakene)	Complex: 2C9, 2C19, 2A6, phase II	**2D6, 2C9**, UGTs, epoxide hydroxylase	None known; indirect evidence of 2C9, 2C19, and phase II
Vigabatrin (Sabril)	Primarily excreted in urine unchanged	None known	Decreases phenytoin levels by unknown mechanism
Zonisamide (Zonegran)	Acetylation, sulfonation, 3A4	None known	None known

Note. UGT = uridine 5'-diphosphate glucuronosyltransferase.

[a]Potent (**bold** type).
[b]Moderate.
[c]Mild.

new technology. The hepatic enzymes involved in the metabolism of phenobarbital and VPA have been deduced from their in vivo drug interactions, and the older literature is sometimes confusing. Phenytoin has been studied more extensively, having become a probe drug for 2C9 and 2C19. In this section, we briefly discuss the numerous antiepileptic drugs and their P450 and phase II profiles.

General Drug Interactions

Barbiturates

Twenty-five percent of primidone (Mysoline) is metabolized to phenobarbital; primidone is also metabolized to phenylethyl-malonamide (a weak anticonvulsant). Therefore, primidone's pharmacokinetic effects on other drugs may be similar to those of phenobarbital.

Phenobarbital is metabolized at 2C9, 2C19, and 2E1 (Tanaka 1999). 2C9 is the drug's major enzyme of metabolism. Interestingly, 25% of phenobarbital is excreted unchanged in the urine, and this percentage increases as the alkalinity of the urine is increased. Metabolism of phenobarbital may be inhibited by potent inhibitors of these enzymes, including other anticonvulsants such as felbamate (Felbatol) (Reidenberg et al. 1995) and VPA (Bernus et al. 1994). It would be expected that potent 2C9 and 2C19 inhibitors such as fluvoxamine and the "pan-inhibitor" ritonavir would also inhibit the metabolism of phenobarbital and other barbiturates; however, we are not aware of any published case reports.

Barbiturates have been known for decades to be metabolic inducers. All barbiturates induce enzyme metabolism and are "pan-inducers," meaning that they affect all inducible metabolic enzymes. In a 1993 prospective study involving neonates in the intensive care setting, Yoshida et al. found that when phenobarbital was given to patients with therapeutic phenytoin levels, their phenytoin levels decreased significantly shortly after phenobarbital was added. Phenobarbital induces the metabolism of oral contraceptives as well (see Chapter 12 ["Gynecology"]).

Psychotropics are greatly affected by phenobarbital. von Bahr et al. (1998) administered nortriptyline to six healthy volunteers for 4 weeks, adding phenobarbital on days 8–21. Nortriptyline levels decreased after 2 days of phenobarbital administration, and clearance of nortriptyline increased twofold. Induction of 3A4, and perhaps 2D6, is the probable mechanism of this interaction. Spina et al. (1996a) compared desipramine metabolism in eight epileptic patients and eight control subjects who were all extensive metabolizers at 2D6. The epileptic patients were undergoing steady-state phenobarbital therapy. A single dose of desipramine was administered to all, and the area under the curve (AUC) and maximal drug concentration (C_{max}) were lower and the elimination half-life was shorter among the epileptic patients. This study suggests that 2D6 can be induced. Clozapine's metabolism was shown to be induced by phenobarbital in a study comparing schizophrenic patients and healthy control subjects (Facciola et al. 1998).

Carbamazepine

Carbamazepine (Tegretol) is a commonly used antiepileptic with several off-label uses. The drug induces its own metabolism. The half-life decreases from 35.6 to 20.9 hours after multiple doses, with the steady-state concentration reducing 50% after 3 weeks. Carbamazepine also induces the metabolism of other drugs, particularly those dependent on 3A4 for metabolism; however, it has been found to induce 1A2 as well, affecting the metabolism of caffeine (Parker et al. 1998). Carbamazepine has been shown to reduce the half-life and increase oral clearance of ethosuximide (Zarontin) (Giaccone et al. 1996), an agent that depends in part on 3A4 for clearance. More potent inducers of 3A4, such as rifampin or phenobarbital, may decrease serum carbamazepine levels.

Epoxidation of carbamazepine occurs via 3A4, its major metabolic pathway, 2C9 and 1A2 being minor pathways (Spina et al. 1996b). Therefore, potent inhibitors of 3A4 (ketoconazole, ritonavir, erythromycin, and clarithromycin) may increase carbamazepine levels beyond the therapeutic window (Spina et al. 1997). Flucona-zole, a modest inhibitor of 3A4 but a potent inhibitor of 2C9, has been noted in a few case reports to increase carbamazepine concentrations (Nair and Morris 1999).

Oxcarbazepine

Oxcarbazepine (Trileptal) was developed in part to sidestep the aforementioned problems associated with carbamazepine. Oxcarbazepine is supposed to have a low level of hepatic induction. When carbamazepine is replaced by oxcarbazepine in the treatment of patients taking other P450-dependent antiepileptic drugs, the other antiepileptic drugs may reach toxic levels after 2–4 weeks of oxcarbazepine. These increased drug levels occur after the carbamazepine-induced enzymes return to normal functioning (Tecoma 1999).

Oxcarbazepine is metabolized quickly to a 10-monohydroxy metabolite, which is thought to be the active compound. Most of the 10-monohydroxy metabolite is conjugated by various phase II enzymes, with about 5% metabolized by 3A4 oxidation (Hachad et al. 2002). The metabolite does not induce its own metabolism. Oxcarbazepine seems not to be affected itself by potent inhibitors of P450 enzymes such as erythromycin and cimetidine. Tecoma (1999) suggested that oxcarbazepine dosing may need to be increased if the agent is administered with potent P450-inducing drugs.

Oxcarbazepine does seem to induce P450 metabolism of ethinyl estradiol (EE) and levonorgestrel, probably at 3A4. Fattore et al. (1999) studied 16 healthy women over two menstrual cycles in a randomized, double-blind crossover study. AUCs, peak plasma concentrations, and half-lives of EE and levonorgestrel were decreased with oxcarbazepine coadministration. Breakthrough bleeding occurred with these combinations, but the authors found no surge in progesterone levels (ovulation).

Oxcarbazepine may also inhibit 2C19; there have been reports of increases in levels of phenytoin (which is primarily dependent on 2C9 and 2C19) of up to 40% (Trileptal 2001).

Oxcarbazepine may have better side-effect, autoinduction, and toxicity profiles than carbamazepine, but its P450 induction and inhibition profile may be comparable to those of other common antiepileptic drugs—carbamazepine, phenytoin, and the barbiturates (Armstrong and Cozza 2000).

Felbamate

Because of its potential for hepatotoxicity and for producing aplastic anemia, felbamate (Felbatol) is reserved for treatment of refractory seizures (Felbatol 2000). The drug is metabolized by 3A4 and 2E1, and its metabolism has been induced by carbamazepine, phenytoin, and phenobarbital. The manufacturer recommends a 33% reduction in phenytoin dose when felbamate is added to a regimen. The presumed mechanism is 2C19 inhibition by felbamate. Felbamate also induces 3A4, reducing stable carbamazepine levels (Glue et al. 1997) and concentrations of oral contraceptives (Wilbur and Ensom 2000).

Gabapentin

Gabapentin (Neurontin) is distributed throughout the body, largely unbound with proteins (less than 3%), and is excreted unchanged in the urine (Neurontin 1998). In clinical studies, there were no significant interactions with phenytoin, carbamazepine, valproic acid, phenobarbital, cimetidine, or oral contraceptives.

Lamotrigine

Lamotrigine (Lamictal) is mostly metabolized by glucuronic acid conjugation but is also affected by enzyme-inducing and enzyme-inhibiting drugs, the mechanisms of which have not been fully evaluated. Valproic acid increases lamotrigine's half-life and appears to decrease clearance of lamotrigine, necessitating a reduction in lamotrigine dose when the two drugs are coadministered. The mechanism for this interaction seems to be inhibition of phase II glucuronidation (Anderson et al. 1996). Carbamazepine, phenytoin, phenobarbital, and primidone all decrease lamotrigine's half-life and increase its oral clearance (Bottiger et al. 1999; Matsuo 1999). In healthy subjects, lamotrigine induces its own metabolism (Lamictal 2001). Nevertheless, lamotrigine itself seems to cause no clinically significant changes with regard to other antiepileptics when it is added to regimens of patients in whom drug concentrations have achieved a steady state. Lamotrigine is associated with multiorgan failure (rarely) and with severe skin rashes, so careful dosing in patients receiving valproic acid or other inhibiting drugs is prudent.

Levetiracetam

Levetiracetam (Keppra) was developed in the late 1990s as an agent for add-on therapy in patients with refractory complex partial seizures. The agent has a limited metabolism in humans, with 66% of the dose excreted in the urine unchanged (Keppra 2001). Twenty-four percent is metabolized through enzymatic hydrolysis by the acetamide group, resulting in a carboxylic acid metabolite. Levetiracetam is not metabolized by P450 enzymes, nor does the drug inhibit or induce these enzymes. Studies by the manufacturer indicated no significant interactions with phenytoin, carbamazepine, valproic acid, phenobarbital, lamotrigine, gabapentin, primidone, oral contraceptives, digoxin, or warfarin.

Phenytoin

The study of phenytoin (Dilantin) has been complicated. Phenytoin is highly protein bound and can displace or be displaced by many other drugs. In addition, because phenytoin is metabolized at 2C9 and 2C19, genetic polymorphisms affect the metabolism of this drug: this was not known to early investigators, to whom the reasons for such varying individual responses were a mystery. Drugs that inhibit 2C9 and 2C19 (see tables in Chapters 8 ["2C9"] and 9 ["2C19"]) will "convert" extensive metabolizers to poor metabolizers and increase phenytoin levels in those individuals while not apparently slowing the metabolism in persons who are already poor metabolizers. Potent 2C9 inhibitors include fluvoxamine (Luvox) and fluconazole (Diflucan); fluoxetine (Prozac) and modafinil (Provigil) are moderate inhibitors. Potent inhibitors of 2C19 include fluvoxamine, ticlopidine (Ticlid), and omeprazole (Prilosec); again, fluoxetine is a moderate inhibitor. Rifamycins induce phenytoin metabolism.

Phenytoin itself is a potent inducer of 3A4, phase II enzymes, and possibly 2C9 and 2C19. When phenytoin is added to stable 3A4-dependent drug regimens, it may decrease serum levels of these drugs after the first few weeks, necessitating dose adjustment.

Tiagabine

Tiagabine (Gabitril) is metabolized at 3A4, and its metabolism is susceptible to induction by other antiepileptic drugs that induce this enzyme (Gabitril 2000); use with carbamazepine, phenytoin, and phenobarbital caused a 60% increase in the clearance of tiagabine. Tiagabine administration in patients taking VPA has been associated with a mild decrease in VPA levels (10%), the mechanism of which is unclear (Brodie 1995; Gustavson et al. 1998); in general, however, tiagabine is not considered a P450 inhibitor or inducer (Kalviainen 1998).

Topiramate

Seventy percent of topiramate (Topamax) is excreted unchanged in the urine, with six other metabolites making up the rest of the clearance through various enzymes of phase I and phase II (Topamax 2000). Nevertheless, topiramate's metabolism appears to be inducible, and topiramate concentrations seem to be decreased by 40%–48% when the drug is used with phenytoin or carbamazepine. Topiramate modestly inhibits 2C19 (Anderson 1998; Sachdeo et al. 2002). It is unclear whether topiramate induces any enzymes; however, when it was used with oral contraceptives containing EE, the mean total exposure to EE decreased by 18%, 21%, and 30% at daily doses of 200, 400, and 800 mg of topiramate. Therefore, efficacy of oral contraceptives may be compromised by topiramate through an unknown mechanism.

Valproic Acid

Valproic acid (Depakene, Depakote)—also called valproate, valprote, VPA (we use VPA here)—is highly protein bound and is involved in many interactions because of protein-binding displacement. The agent also is extensively metabolized in the liver to 50 or more metabolites (Pisani 1992). VPA metabolism is induced by carbamazepine, phenobarbital, primidone, and phenytoin, resulting in an increase in total valproate clearance of 30%–85%. When VPA is induced, the production of a toxic metabolite, 4-ene-valproic acid, is increased. Levels of this toxic metabolite are not measured in routine valproic acid laboratory tests. The metabolite 4-ene-valproic acid is a suspect in the hepatotoxicity of VPA. The risk factors for valproic acid–induced hepatotoxicity are male gender, age less than 2 years, neurological disease (other than seizures), and treatment with a P450-inducing medication in conjunction with VPA therapy. Sadeque et al. (1997) studied 4-ene-valproic acid reactions in vitro. These researchers' findings suggest that 3A4 is not responsible for the increase in toxic metabolite production but that 2C9 and 2A6 catalyze terminal desaturation of VPA.

VPA is a mild to moderate inhibitor of 2D6 and an inhibitor of 2C9 (Anderson 1998; Wen et al. 2001), UGTs, and epoxide hydroxylase (Anderson 1998). It is unclear whether VPA induces any enzymes, but deductive reasoning indicates it may (see "Zonisamide," later in this chapter).

Vigabatrin

Vigabatrin (Sabril) is excreted almost entirely unchanged in the urine, so pharmacokinetic drug-drug interactions are not expected. However, through an unknown mechanism, vigabatrin decreases phenytoin levels by 20% (Richens 1995).

Zonisamide

Zonisamide (Zonegran) undergoes acetylation to form *N*-acetyl-zonisamide and reduction to form the open-ring metabolite 2-sulfamoylacetylphenol (SMAP). Of the excreted dose, 35% was recovered as zonisamide, 15% as *N*-acetylzonisamide, and 50% as the glucuronide of SMAP. Reduction of zonisamide to SMAP is mediated by 3A4. Zonisamide does not induce its own metabolism (Zonegran 2000). Zonisamide has a long half-life (63 hours), but because of induction (probably of 3A4), its half-life is significantly shorter when the drug is used with phenytoin (27 hours), phenobarbital (38 hours), or valproic acid (46 hours).

Psychotropic Drug Interactions

Induction

Carbamazepine, phenytoin, phenobarbital, and felbamate may all decrease drug levels by induction, especially if the other drug is metabolized primarily by 3A4. Therefore, TCAs, clozapine, and the triazolobenzodiazepines may need dosage adjustments when administered along with these 3A4 inducers (Facciola et al. 1998). Olanzapine (Zyprexa) is induced by carbamazepine, even though olanzapine is not dependent on 3A4 for metabolism. Carbamazepine has been shown to induce 1A2 in vitro and in vivo (Lucas et al. 1998).

In a controlled clinical trial, Hesslinger et al. (1999) studied the effects of carbamazepine and VPA on the pharmacokinetics of haloperidol (Haldol). Subjects with schizophrenia or schizoaffective disorder received haloperidol alone, haloperidol and carbamazepine, or haloperidol and VPA. The haloperidol dose remained stable, and the antiepileptic agents were adjusted to therapeutic levels. Carbamazepine significantly decreased plasma haloperidol levels, producing worsened clinical symptoms compared with symptoms in patients taking haloperidol only. VPA had no effect on haloperidol levels or clinical outcome. The authors suggested that haloperidol taken with carbamazepine may result in treatment failure if haloperidol doses are not increased. Patients are at risk for haloperidol toxicity if they discontinue carbamazepine—a process that may take 1–2 weeks to develop by uninduction (see Chapter 2 ["Definitions and Phase I Metabolism"]).

Inhibition

Fluvoxamine and fluoxetine are inhibitors of 2C9 and 2C19, and phenytoin levels have increased with the addition of fluoxetine. Shad and Preskorn (1999) reported a decrease in phenytoin levels and effect when fluoxetine was discontinued.

VPA is a moderate inhibitor. In an open-label, sequential, two-period study involving healthy volunteers, valproic acid increased amitriptyline serum levels by 31% and increased combined TCA levels 19% (Wong et al. 1996).

Summary

Antiepileptic drugs are generally inducers of P450 enzymes and can therefore reduce the efficacy of coadministered drugs, particularly oral contraceptives (Guberman 1999) and drugs in combination antiepileptics. Carbamazepine and many other agents are metabolized at 3A4 and may reach toxic levels when administered with potent inhibitors such as erythromycin, ritonavir, or grapefruit juice. Phenytoin is metabolized at 2C9 and 2C19, so administration with drugs such as fluvoxamine and ticlopidine may lead to phenytoin toxicity. VPA is a drug with a complicated metabolism and the potential for hepatotoxicity; therefore, serum levels of all coadministered medications with the potential for toxicity should be carefully monitored, as should levels of liver-associated enzymes.

■ ANTIPARKINSONIAN DRUGS

Bromocriptine

Bromocriptine (Parlodel), an ergot alkaloid, was first released in the United States in 1978 for the treatment of amenorrhea and galactorrhea secondary to hyperprolactinemia. In 1982, the agent was approved for use in patients with Parkinson's disease. Because it is an older drug, little known is about its metabolism or its potential to inhibit or induce liver enzymes. There is evidence that some of bromocriptine's metabolism is through 3A4 (Peyronneau et al. 1994) and that the drug inhibits 3A4 (Wynalda and Wienkers 1997).

■ ANTIPARKINSONIAN DRUGS

Drug	Metabolism	Enzyme(s) inhibited	Enzyme(s) induced
COMT inhibitors			
Entacapone (Comtan)	UGTs	P450[c]	None known
Tolcapone (Tasmar)	UGTs, COMT, 3A4, 2A6	2C9[c]	None known
Dopamine agonists			
Bromocriptine (Parlodel)	3A4, ?others	3A4[b]	None known
Carbidopa-levodopa (Sinemet)	Carbidopa: excreted unchanged; Levodopa: aromatic amino acid decarboxylase	None known	None known
Pergolide (Permax)	Phase II, 3A4	3A4	None known
Pramipexole (Mirapex)	Excreted in urine unchanged	None known	None known
Ropinirole (Requip)	1A2, 3A4	1A2[c]	None known
Monoamine oxidase B inhibitors			
Selegiline (Eldepryl)	2D6 and 3A4 or 2B6 and 2C19	2C19[1]	None known

Note. COMT=catechol *O*-methyltransferase; UGT=uridine 5′-diphosphate glucuronosyltransferase.
[1]Significance unknown.

[a]Potent (**bold** type).
[b]Moderate.
[c]Mild.

Carbidopa-Levodopa

Carbidopa-levodopa (Sinemet) is the mainstay for treatment of symptoms of Parkinson's disease and has been available in the United States since 1982. Levodopa is easily metabolized to dopamine in the central nervous system (CNS) and peripherally, and carbidopa is added to inhibit peripheral destruction of the levodopa so that more levodopa can enter the CNS. Carbidopa does not cross the blood-brain barrier and is not appreciably metabolized but is excreted unchanged (Sinemet 1999). Although pharmacokinetic drug-drug interactions are not a problem with carbidopa-levodopa, significant pharmacodynamic drug-drug interactions do occur. Carbidopa-levodopa should not be administered with monoamine oxidase inhibitors (MAOIs), and problems are associated with concomitant use of carbidopa-levodopa and antipsychotics.

Entacapone

Entacapone (Comtan) is a reversible catecholamine O-methyltransferase (COMT) inhibitor used as an adjunct in the treatment of Parkinson's disease. It is metabolized primarily through glucuronidation. However, the glucuronidated metabolite is primarily (90%) excreted through the biliary system, so caution should be used in patients with the potential for biliary obstruction (Comtan 2000). Although in vitro studies by the manufacturer revealed that entacapone is a very mild inhibitor of nearly all P450 enzymes, this inhibition is considered clinically insignificant, and there are no reports to date of significant drug-drug interactions involving entacapone. However, because most of entacapone's excretion is through the biliary system, as noted above, caution should be exercised when entacapone is administered with drugs known to interfere with biliary excretion or glucuronidation. These drugs include probenecid, cholestyramine, and some antibiotics (e.g., erythromycin, rifampicin, ampicillin, and chloramphenicol).

Pergolide

In 1988, pergolide (Permax), an ergot alkaloid, received approval in the United States for use in patients with Parkinson's disease. Pergolide and bromocriptine work in a similar way, but pergolide is much more potent. This drug is metabolized through multiple mechanisms and has 10 known metabolites, both oxidative metabolites and conjugates from various phase II enzymes (Permax 2000). It appears to inhibit 3A4 (Wynalda and Wienkers 1997), but no case reports exist to elucidate the clinical significance of this inhibition.

Pramipexole

When pramipexole (Mirapex) was released in the United States in 1997, it represented the first new agent for the treatment of Parkinson's disease in nearly 10 years. Although it is not an ergot like bromocriptine and pergolide, it is a dopamine agonist. Because of its chemical structure, it is classified as an aminobenzothiazole (Hubble 2000). It is excreted unchanged in the urine, and there are no known metabolites (Mirapex 1999). Drug-drug interactions involving this drug have not been reported.

Ropinirole

Ropinirole (Requip) was released in the United States soon after pramipexole, in late 1997. This nonergot dopamine agonist is primarily metabolized by 1A2 (Kaye and Nicholls 2000; Requip 2001), with a contribution by 3A4. There are no known active metabolites. Most of the 1A2 metabolite is excreted unchanged, with a smaller amount glucuronidated before excretion.

Because 1A2 represents the major means of clearance for ropinirole, clinicians must remember, when using ropinirole, that 1A2 can be induced (most commonly by smoking, omeprazole, and esomeprazole [Nexium]) or inhibited (particularly by ciprofloxacin and fluvoxamine). A search for reports of drug-drug interactions involving ropinirole and the aforementioned drugs revealed no cases or studies. However, the manufacturer stated that when ropinirole was used with ciprofloxacin (a potent inhibitor of 1A2), ropinirole's AUC increased by 84% and its C_{max} by 60% (Requip 2001). The AUC and C_{max} of theophylline, a drug that is dependent on 1A2 for clearance and has a narrow therapeutic or safety window, did not change significantly when the agent was used with ropinirole, which indicates that ropinirole probably has minimal 1A2 inhibition (Thalamas et al. 1999).

Tolcapone

Tolcapone (Tasmar), like entacapone, is a reversible COMT inhibitor, but tolcapone is relegated as a second-line agent for the treatment of Parkinson's disease because of its potential for liver toxicity (Tasmar 2002). Tolcapone is primarily metabolized through glucuronidation, but it is also metabolized by COMT, 3A4, and 2A6. Premarketing in vitro studies by the manufacturer revealed that tolcapone may inhibit 2C9 (Tasmar 2002), but when tolbutamide (which is metabolized by 2C9) was used with tolcapone in an in vivo study, the pharmacokinetics of tolbutamide remained unchanged.

Selegiline

Selegiline (Eldepryl) is an irreversible monoamine oxidase B (MAO B) inhibitor. Because of its selectivity, it is presumed to have less potential for side effects and pharmacodynamic interactions (e.g., hypertensive crisis) associated with other MAOIs. Selegiline is used in treatment for Parkinson's disease because MAO B is responsible for most of dopamine's metabolism in the brain, and inhibition of MAO B thus increases dopamine levels but has no effect on CNS serotonin or epinephrine levels. Early in vitro studies indicated that it was metabolized oxidatively primarily by 2D6 to N-desmethyldeprenyl (Grace et al. 1994). N-Desmethyldeprenyl has some mild MAO B inhibition (Eldepryl 1998). A secondary metabolite, levomethamphetamine, is formed from 3A4 (Taavitsainen et al. 2000). There is controversy, however, about selegiline's metabolism. Hidestrand et al. (2001) showed that when in vitro cultures of multiple human cytochromes were used, *N*-desmethyl-deprenyl and levomethamphetamine were produced by 2B6 and 2C19, respectively. No definitive in vivo studies of selegiline metabolism have been conducted. It appears that selegiline moderately inhibits 2C19, but no case reports have yet indicated that this effect is clinically relevant.

■ CHOLINESTERASE INHIBITORS

Cholinesterase inhibitors have become popular medications in the last 10 years because they are the only drugs approved for use in the treatment and management of Alzheimer's dementia in the United States. Because they are prescribed to elderly patients, who are often taking multiple drugs, the potential for pharmacokinetic drug-drug interactions is high.

Tacrine

Tacrine (Cognex) was the first cholinesterase inhibitor to be released; it was made available in 1993. Tacrine is rarely used now, primarily because of its association with liver toxicity. In addition, the agent must be taken four times a day, which makes it the least convenient of the four available cholinesterase inhibitors (the others can be prescribed for once or twice a day). Use of tacrine all but ceased after donepezil (Aricept) became available in 1997.

Tacrine is metabolized by 1A2 and, to a smaller extent, 2D6 (Cognex 2000). Tacrine also inhibits 1A2. Because theophylline's metabolism is highly dependent on 1A2, theophylline levels are increased twofold when that drug is used with tacrine. Concentrations of caffeine and pentoxifylline, which are also dependent on 1A2 for metabolic clearance, would be expected to be increased with tacrine coadministration. Tacrine levels increase significantly when tacrine is administered with cimetidine (Tagamet), a pan-inhibitor of the P450 enzymes. Also, 40 mg of fluvoxamine (a 1A2

■ CHOLINESTERASE INHIBITORS

Drug	Metabolism	Enzyme(s) inhibited	Enzyme(s) induced
Donepezil (Aricept)	2D6, 3A4, UGTs	None known	None known
Galantamine (Reminyl)	2D6, 3A4, UGTs; 50% excreted in urine unchanged	None known	None known
Rivastigmine (Exelon)	Local cholinesterases; excreted in urine	None known	None known
Tacrine (Cognex)	1A2,[1] 2D6[2]	1A2	None known

Note. UGT = uridine 5'-diphosphate glucuronosyltransferase.
[1]Major metabolizer.
[2]Minor metabolizer.

inhibitor) increased the AUC and C_{max} of tacrine five- to eightfold in 13 healthy men.

Interestingly, levels of tacrine are twice as high in females, possibly because 1A2 activity is less in females. Finally, smoking decreases tacrine levels by one-third, because tobacco smoke induces 1A2. Clinicians should expect tacrine levels to increase in patients who quit smoking.

Donepezil

Donepezil (Aricept) was introduced in 1997. It is metabolized by 2D6 and 3A4 (Aricept 2000). Any potential for pharmacokinetic drug-drug interactions appears to be minor because donepezil does not have a narrow margin of safety. In addition, unlike tacrine, donepezil does not inhibit or induce any metabolic enzymes that could affect clearance of other drugs. Induction of 3A4 by phenobarbital, carbamazepine, oxcarbazepine, rifampins, phenytoin, or St. John's wort may decrease levels of donepezil. Ketoconazole and quinidine—known inhibitors of 3A4 and 2D6, respectively—have been shown to increase donepezil levels in vitro. This result may lead to enhancement of donepezil's side effects, particularly nausea and diarrhea.

Rivastigmine

Rivastigmine (Exelon) was introduced in the United States in 2000. It has a unique metabolic profile compared with other cholinesterase inhibitors. Rivastigmine is metabolized at its site of action—the cholinesterases—and this product is then cleared almost entirely by the kidneys (Exelon 2001). Grossberg et al. (2000) found few clinically significant pharmacokinetic and pharmacodynamic drug-drug interactions between rivastigmine and 22 classes of medications.

Galantamine

Galantamine (Reminyl) is the newest cholinesterase inhibitor on the United States market, introduced in 2001. The manufacturer studied many facets of potential pharmacokinetic drug-drug interactions before releasing galantamine (Reminyl 2001). Fifty-percent of galantamine is metabolized by 2D6, 3A4, and UGTs; the other 50% is excreted in the urine unchanged. The C_{max} in poor metabolizers at 2D6 (7% of Caucasians) is similar to that in normal metabolizers at 2D6. Galantamine does not inhibit or induce any metabolic enzymes. Because no single metabolic or clearance pathway predominates, galantamine is less likely to interact with drugs that inhibit or induce metabolic enzymes. Known inhibitors of 2D6 (fluoxetine, paroxetine, quinidine, and cimetidine) and 3A4 (erythromycin and ketoconazole) increase AUCs by 10%–40%, but the clinical significance of this effect appears to be small.

■ TRIPTANS

Triptans are potent serotonin$_{1B/1D}$ (5-HT$_{1B/1D}$) receptor agonists used to abort and treat migraine headaches. They are believed to cause vasoconstriction of cranial blood vessels at arteriovenous anastomoses (sites of many 5-HT$_{1B/1D}$ receptors, whereas serotonin$_2$ receptors are found in peripheral arteries) and reduce inflammation. Sumatriptan (Imitrex) is a first-generation triptan but has many limitations, including poor oral bioavailability, a short half-life, and an inability to cross the blood-brain barrier. Newer and better-tolerated triptans have been developed. All triptans have very similar pharmacodynamic (receptor) characteristics but differ pharmacokinetically (for further discussion, see the review by Deleu and Hanssens [2000]).

All triptans go through phase I (oxidative) metabolism. Unlike most drug classes, however, triptans undergo oxidative metabolism through both the P450 system and monoamine oxidase (MAO). MAO exists to metabolize endogenous biogenic amines. The two MAO enzymes are MAO A and MAO B. A particular triptan may be metabolized by the P450 system, MAO, or both. None of the triptans appear to actively inhibit or induce P450 metabolism themselves.

■ TRIPTANS

Drug	Metabolism	Enzyme(s) inhibited	Enzyme(s) induced
Almotriptan (Axert)	MAO A, 3A4, 2D6	None known	None known
Eletriptan (Relpax)	3A4	None known	None known
Frovatriptan (Frova)	1A2	None known	None known
Naratriptan (Amerge)	P450, MAO A, excreted in urine	None known	None known
Rizatriptan (Maxalt)	MAO A	None known	None known
Sumatriptan (Imitrex)	MAO A	None known	None known
Zolmitriptan (Zomig)	1A2, MAO A	None known	None known

Note. MAO A=monoamine oxidase A.

Triptan metabolism may be affected by competing drugs that use, inhibit, or induce the P450 system, particularly if the triptan in question is dependent on a specific P450 enzyme for its metabolism or is administered with drugs that inhibit MAO activity. Triptan toxicities and side effects include dizziness, chest or neck tightness, palpitations, shortness of breath, and acute anxiety. Myocardial ischemia has been reported with triptan use, especially in patients with coronary artery disease (Jhee et al. 2001). MAOIs—particularly MAO A inhibitors such as moclobemide—are contraindicated with triptans whose metabolism is solely dependent on MAO (rizatriptan [Maxalt] and sumatriptan). Gardner and Lynd (1998) found no reports of adverse events with simultaneous administration of sumatriptan and MAOIs, but the manufacturer has listed this combination as absolutely contraindicated (Imitrex 2001). Propranolol may be an inhibitor of MAO A and has been found to increase plasma concentrations of rizatriptan, so dose reduction of MAO A–dependent triptans is recommended with concomitant use of propranolol. The other β-blockers do not seem to be associated with the same interaction (Goldberg et al. 2001).

P450 interactions with triptans are predictable, based as they are on the P450 enzymes on which triptans are dependent. Eletriptan (Relpax) and almotriptan (Axert) are primarily metabolized at 3A4. One would predict that potent inhibitors of 3A4 such as nefazodone (Serzone), clarithromycin (Biaxin), erythromycin, ketoconazole, itraconazole (Sporanox), ritonavir (Norvir), ciprofloxacin (Cipro), and grapefruit juice might increase plasma levels of the triptans and worsen side effects or toxicity. In healthy volunteers, verapamil (a moderate inhibitor of 3A4) and fluoxetine (a moderate inhibitor of both 3A4 and 2D6) caused a moderate increase in the C_{max} and AUC of almotriptan, which is metabolized by MAO, 3A4, and 2D6 (Fleishaker et al. 2000, 2001). In both of these studies, no significant clinical events occurred, and the authors suggested that no dose adjustment is necessary. These modest findings reflect almotriptan's multiple avenues of metabolism, which allow the drug to be biotransformed despite roadblocks at some of its metabolic sites. At the time of writing, there were no reports on the use of triptans with potent 3A4 inhibitors. However, caution is advised, particularly with eletriptan, which is predominantly metabolized at 3A4.

Triptans dependent on 1A2 (frovatriptan [Frova] and zolmitriptan [Zomig]) may become toxic when administered with potent 1A2 inhibitors such as fluvoxamine and ciprofloxacin (Millson et al. 2000). Buchan et al. (2002) reviewed results of in vitro studies, healthy-volunteer studies, and a retrospective analysis of phase I clinical data concerning triptans and drugs commonly coadministered with frovatriptan. In addition to noting inhibition by the aforementioned potent 1A2 inhibitors, they found the AUC and C_{max} of frovatriptan to be lower in tobacco smokers (tobacco smoke is a potent inducer of 1A2). Eletriptan requires higher dosing than other second-generation triptans because of an active P-glycoprotein efflux system at the blood-brain barrier (Millson et al. 2000).

■ ERGOTAMINES

Ergot derivatives are used as vasodilators in migraine treatment and, more recently, in the treatment of dementia. Ergotamines are metabolized at 3A4 and are mild to moderate inhibitors of 3A4 as well. Potent 3A4 inhibitors, particularly the macrolide antibiotics, have caused frank ergotism in patients. Horowitz et al. (1996) reported that a patient receiving clarithromycin therapy developed lingual ischemia after taking 2 mg of ergotamine tartrate. Nicergoline, an ergot not yet available in the United States, has been used for the treatment of dementia in Europe. This agent seems to be metabolized by 2D6, as determined in studies involving healthy volunteers (Bottiger et al. 1996). Studies of this drug in combination with potent 2D6 inhibitors have not yet been conducted.

■ REFERENCES

Anderson GD: A mechanistic approach to antiepileptic drug interactions. Ann Pharmacother 32:554–563, 1998

Anderson GD, Yua MK, Gidal BE, et al: Bidirectional interaction of valproate and lamotrigine in healthy subjects. Clin Pharmacol Ther 60: 145–156, 1996

Aricept (package insert). Teaneck, NJ, Eisai Inc., 2000

Armstrong SC, Cozza KL: Consultation-liaison psychiatry drug-drug interactions update. Psychosomatics 41:541–543, 2000

Bernus I, Dickinson RG, Hooper WD, et al: Inhibition of phenobarbitone N-glucosidation by valproate. Br J Clin Pharmacol 38:411–416, 1994

Bottiger Y, Dostert P, Benedetti MS, et al: Involvement of CYP2D6 but not CYP2C19 in nicergoline metabolism in humans. Br J Clin Pharmacol 42:707–711, 1996

Bottiger Y, Svensson JO, Stahle L: Lamotrigine drug interactions in a TDM material. Ther Drug Monit 21:171–174, 1999

Brodie JM: Tiagabine pharmacology in profile. Epilepsia 36 (suppl 6):S7–S9, 1995

Buchan P, Wade A, Ward C, et al: Frovatriptan: a review of drug-drug interactions. Headache 42 (suppl 2):63–73, 2002

Carrier L: Donepezil and paroxetine: possible drug interaction (letter). J Am Geriatr Soc 47:1037, 1999

Cognex (package insert). Morris Plains, NJ, Parke Davis Pharmaceuticals, Ltd., 2000

Comtan (package insert). East Hanover, NJ, Novartis Pharmaceuticals Corp., 2000

Deleu D, Hanssens Y: Current and emerging second-generation triptans in acute migraine therapy: a comparative review. J Clin Pharmacol 40: 687–700, 2000

Donahue S, Flockhart DA, Abernethy DR: Ticlopidine inhibits phenytoin clearance. Clin Pharmacol Ther 66:563–568, 1999

Eldepryl (package insert). Tampa, FL, Somerset Pharmaceuticals, Inc., 1998

Exelon (package insert). East Hanover, NJ, Novartis Pharmaceuticals Corp., 2001

Facciola G, Avenoso A, Spina E, et al: Inducing effect of phenobarbital on clozapine metabolism in patients with chronic schizophrenia. Ther Drug Monit 20:628–630, 1998

Fattore C, Cipolla G, Gatti G, et al: Induction of ethinylestradiol and levonorgestrel metabolism by oxcarbazepine in healthy women. Epilepsia 40:783–787, 1999

Felbatol (package insert). Cranbury, NJ, Wallace Laboratories, 2000

Fleishaker JC, Sisson TA, Carel BJ, et al: Pharmacokinetic interaction between verapamil and almotriptan in healthy volunteers. Clin Pharmacol Ther 67:498–503, 2000

Fleishaker JC, Ryan KK, Carel BJ, et al: Evaluation of the potential pharmacokinetic interaction between almotriptan and fluoxetine in healthy volunteers. J Clin Pharmacol 41:217–223, 2001

Forgue ST, Reece PA, Sedman AJ, et al: Inhibition of tacrine metabolism by cimetidine. Clin Pharmacol Ther 59:444–449, 1996

Gabitril (package insert). West Chester, PA, Cephalon Inc., 2000

Gardner DM, Lynd LD: Sumatriptan contraindications and the serotonin syndrome. Ann Pharmacother 32:33–38, 1998

Giaccone M, Bartoli A, Gatti G, et al: Effect of enzyme inducing anticonvulsants on ethosuximide pharmacokinetics in epileptic patients. Br J Clin Pharmacol 41:575–579, 1996

Glue P, Banfield CR, Perhach JL, et al: Pharmacokinetic interactions with felbamate: in vitro–in vivo correlation. Clin Pharmacokinet 33:214–224, 1997

Goldberg MR, Sciberras D, De Smet M, et al: Influence of beta-adrenoceptor antagonists on the pharmacokinetics of rizatriptan, a 5-HT1B/1D agonist: differential effects of propranolol, nadolol and metoprolol. Br J Clin Pharmacol 52:69–76, 2001

Grace JM, Kinter MT, Macdonald TL: Atypical metabolism of deprenyl and its enantiomer, *(S)*-(+)-*N*,alpha-dimethyl-*N*-propynylphenethylamine, by cytochrome P450 2D6. Chem Res Toxicol 7:286–290, 1994

Grossberg GT, Stahelin HB, Messina JC, et al: Lack of adverse pharmacodynamic drug interactions with rivastigmine and twenty-two classes of medications. Int J Geriatr Psychiatry 15:242–247, 2000

Guberman A: Hormonal contraception with epilepsy. Neurology 53:S38–S40, 1999

Gustavson LE, Sommerville KW, Boellner SW, et al: Lack of a clinically significant pharmacokinetic drug interaction between tiagabine and valproate. Am J Ther 5:73–79, 1998

Hachad H, Ragueneau-Majlessi I, Levy RH: New antiepileptic drugs: review on drug interactions. Ther Drug Monit 24:91–103, 2002

Hesslinger B, Normann C, Langosch JM, et al: Effects of carbamazepine and valproate on haloperidol plasma levels and on psychopathologic outcome in schizophrenic patients. J Clin Psychopharmacol 19:310–315, 1999

276

Hidestrand M, Oscarson M, Salonen JS, et al: CYP2B6 and CYP2C19 as the major enzymes responsible for the metabolism of selegiline, a drug used in the treatment of Parkinson's disease, as revealed from experiments with recombinant enzymes. Drug Metab Dispos 29:1480–1484, 2001

Horowitz RS, Dart RC, Gomez HF: Clinical ergotism with lingual ischemia induced by clarithromycin-ergotamine interaction. Arch Intern Med 156: 456–458, 1996

Hubble JP: Pre-clinical studies of pramipexole: clinical significance. Eur J Neurol 7 (suppl 1):15–20, 2000

Imitrex (package insert). Research Triangle Park, NC, GlaxoSmithKline, 2001

Jhee SS, Shiovitz T, Crawford AW, et al: Pharmacokinetics and pharmacodynamics of the triptan antimigraine agents. Clin Pharmacokinet 40: 189–205, 2001

Kalviainen R: Tiagabine: a new therapeutic option for people with intellectual disability and partial epilepsy. J Intellect Disabil Res 42 (suppl 1):63–67, 1998

Kaye CM, Nicholls B: Clinical pharmacokinetics of ropinirole. Clin Pharmacokinet 39:243–254, 2000

Keppra (package insert). Smyrna, GA, UCB Pharmaceuticals, Inc., 2001

Laine K, Palovaara S, Tapanainen P, et al: Plasma tacrine concentrations are significantly increased by concomitant hormone replacement therapy. Clin Pharmacol Ther 66:602–628, 1999

Lamictal (package insert). Research Triangle Park, NC, GlaxoSmithKline, 2001

Larsen JT, Hansen LL, Spigset O, et al: Fluvoxamine is a potent inhibitor of tacrine metabolism in vivo. Eur J Clin Pharmacol 55:375–382, 1999

Lucas RA, Gilfillan DJ, Bergstrom RF: A pharmacokinetic interaction between carbamazepine and olanzapine: observations on possible mechanism. Eur J Clin Pharmacol 54:639–643, 1998

Madden S, Spaldin V, Park BK: Clinical pharmacokinetics of tacrine. Clin Pharmacokinet 28:449–457, 1995

Matsuo F: Lamotrigine. Epilepsia 40 (suppl 5):S30–S36, 1999

Millson DS, Tepper SJ, Rapoport AM: Migraine pharmacotherapy with oral triptans: a rational approach to clinical management. Expert Opin Pharmacother 1:391–404, 2000

Mirapex (package insert). Kalamazoo, MI, Pharmacia & Upjohn, Inc., 1999

Nair DR, Morris HH: Potential fluconazole-induced carbamazepine toxicity. Ann Pharmacother 33:790–792, 1999

Neurontin (package insert). Morris Plains, NJ, Parke-Davis, 1998

Nordberg A, Svensson AL: Cholinesterase inhibitors in the treatment of Alzheimer's disease: a comparison of tolerability and pharmacology. Drug Saf 19:465–480, 1998

Parker AC, Pritchard P, Preston T, et al: Induction of CYP1A2 activity by carbamazepine in children using the caffeine breath test. Br J Clin Pharmacol 45:176–178, 1998

Permax (package insert). South San Francisco, CA, Elan Pharmaceuticals, Inc, 2000

Peyronneau MA, Delaforge M, Riviere R, et al: High affinity of ergopeptides for cytochromes P450 3A. Importance of their peptide moiety for P450 recognition and hydroxylation of bromocriptine. Eur J Biochem 223:947–956, 1994

Pisani F: Influence of co-medication on the metabolism of valproate. Pharma Weekbl Sci 14:108–113, 1992

Reidenberg P, Glue P, Banfield CR, et al: Effects of felbamate on the pharmacokinetics of phenobarbital. Clin Pharmacol Ther 58:279–287, 1995

Reminyl (package insert). Titusville, NJ, Janssen Pharmaceutica Products, LP, 2001

Requip (package insert). Research Triangle Park, NC, GlaxoSmithKline, 2001

Richens A: Pharmacokinetic and pharmacodynamic drug interactions during treatment with vigabatrin. Acta Neurol Scand Suppl 162:43–46, 1995

Sachdeo RC, Sachdeo SK, Levy RH, et al: Topiramate and phenytoin pharmacokinetics during repetitive monotherapy and combination therapy to epileptic patients. Epilepsia 43:691–696, 2002

Sadeque AJM, Fisher MB, Korzekwa KR, et al: Human CYP2C9 and CYP2A6 mediate formation of the hepatotoxin 4-ene-valproic acid. J Pharmacol Exp Ther 283:698–703, 1997

Schmider J, Greenblatt DJ, von Moltke LL, et al: Inhibition of CYP2C9 by selective serotonin reuptake inhibitors in vitro: studies of phenytoin p-hydroxylation. Br J Clin Pharmacol 44:495–498, 1997

Shad MU, Preskorn SH: Drug-drug interaction in reverse: possible loss of phenytoin efficacy as a result of fluoxetine discontinuation. J Clin Psychopharmacol 19:471–472, 1999

Sinemet (package insert). Wilmington, DE, DuPont Pharmaceuticals, 1999

Spina E, Avenoso A, Campo GM, et al: Phenobarbital induces the 2-hydroxylation of desipramine. Ther Drug Monit 18:60–64, 1996a

Spina E, Pisani F, Perucca E: Clinically significant pharmacokinetic drug interactions with carbamazepine. Clin Pharmacokinet 31:198–214, 1996b

Spina E, Arena D, Scordo MG, et al: Elevation of plasma carbamazepine concentrations by ketoconazole in patients with epilepsy. Ther Drug Monit 19:535–538, 1997

Taavitsainen P, Antilla M, Nyman L, et al: Selegiline metabolism and cytochrome P450 enzymes: in vitro study in human liver microsomes. Pharmacol Toxicol 86:215–221, 2000

Tanaka E: Clinically significant pharmacokinetic drug interactions between antiepileptic drugs. J Clin Pharm Ther 24:87–92, 1999

Tasmar (package insert). Montvale, NJ, Roche Laboratories Inc., 2002

Tecoma ES: Oxcarbazepine. Epilepsia 40 (suppl 5):S37–S46, 1999

Thalamas C, Taylor A, Brefel-Courbon C, et al: Lack of pharmacokinetic interaction between ropinirole and theophylline in patients with Parkinson's disease. Eur J Pharmacol 55:299–303, 1999

Tiseo PJ, Perdomo CA, Friedhoff LT: Concurrent administration of donepezil HCl and cimetidine: assessment of pharmacokinetic changes following single and multiple doses. Br J Clin Pharmacol 46 (suppl 1):25–29, 1998

Topamax (package insert). Raritan NJ, Ortho-McNeil Pharmaceutical, Inc., 2000

Trileptal (package insert). Huningue, France, Novartis Pharma S.A., 2001

von Bahr C, Steiner E, Koike Y, et al: Time course of enzyme induction in humans: effect of pentobarbital on nortriptyline metabolism. Clin Pharmacol Ther 64:18–26, 1998

Wen X, Wang JS, Kivisto KT, et al: In vitro evaluation of valproic acid as an inhibitor of human cytochrome P450 isoforms: preferential inhibition of cytochrome P450 2C9 (CYP2C9). Br J Clin Pharmacol 52:547–553, 2001

Wilbur K, Ensom MH: Pharmacokinetic drug interactions between oral contraceptives and second-generation anticonvulsants. Clin Pharmacokinet 38:355–365, 2000

Wong SL, Cavanaugh J, Shi H, et al: Effects of divalproex sodium on amitriptyline and nortriptyline pharmacokinetics. Clin Pharmacol Ther 60:48–53, 1996

Wynalda MA, Wienkers LC: Assessment of potential interactions between dopamine receptor agonists and various human cytochrome P450 enzymes using a simple in vitro inhibition screen. Drug Metab Dispos 25:1211–1214, 1997

Yoshida N, Oda Y, Nishi S, et al: Effect of barbiturate therapy on phenytoin pharmacokinetics. Crit Care Med 21:1514–1522, 1993

Zonegran (package insert). South San Francisco, CA, Elan Pharmaceuticals, Inc., 2000

16

ONCOLOGY

Gary H. Wynn, M.D.
Michael A. Cole, M.D.

The pharmacology of oncology is exceptionally complex. Accelerated approval of uses of new agents by the U.S. Food and Drug Administration means that medications are hitting the market nearly continuously. Polypharmacy is the norm, so attention needs to be paid to the interactions between drugs. The P450 effects of oncology drugs are in varying stages of investigation.

The elucidation of oncology drug interactions is hampered for several reasons. Many of the medications used are old and have not been studied comprehensively. The toxicity of these medications makes in vivo pharmacokinetic studies both difficult for and unattractive to primary investigators. Also, many oncology agents are used together, making identification of some interactions and effects difficult. Additionally, many cancer patients receive a wide variety of medications for disease- and pain-related complications; these complications range from mucositis to cytopenias to depression. Given these issues, much of the knowledge of oncology drug metabolism comes from in vitro cell studies, tissue culture studies, and even animal models.

In pediatric patients, isoforms of enzymes are known to develop at different rates, with some enzymes not being present at all and others not present in amounts equivalent to amounts in adults. For example, fetal liver microsomes have approximately 1% of adult activity levels, and these levels increase to an average of 70% by day 7 of extrauterine life. The majority of the data in this chapter can be extrapolated to apply to children older than 10–12 years, but a more thorough review of developmental pharmacokinetics in the pediatric subpopulation is warranted. A good review can be found in a report by Leeder and Kearns (1997).

This chapter is arranged by major classes of agents, and drugs in each class are discussed individually. These drugs are then evaluated in light of current available research, with attention accorded to in vivo studies primarily, in vitro studies secondarily, and animal studies lastly. We also provide an overview of the classes and drugs routinely used in clinical oncology practice—including, but in less detail, new and investigational agents.

> **Reminder:** This chapter is dedicated primarily to metabolic and P-glycoprotein interactions. Interactions due to displaced protein-binding, alterations in absorption or excretion, and pharmacodynamics are not covered.

■ ANTINEOPLASTIC DRUGS

Alkylating Agents

Alkylating agents are some of the more frequently used drugs in chemotherapy. The main effect of these drugs is the cross-linking of strands of DNA, resulting in breakage and cell death. Although the cross-linking of DNA strands works most effectively in cells that are rapidly proliferating, alkylating agents can damage cells during any phase of the cell cycle.

Busulfan

The primary site of metabolism of busulfan (Myleran) is 3A4. Buggia and colleagues (1996) studied the effects of itraconazole (Sporanox) and fluconazole (Diflucan) on busulfan levels. Itraconazole and fluconazole are known to be potent inhibitors of 3A4 and 2C9, respectively. The subjects who received coadministered itraconazole had a roughly 20% decrease in busulfan clearance compared with those receiving fluconazole and busulfan, which implies that busulfan metabolism occurs at 3A4. An additional study showed increased clearance of busulfan with coadministration of phenytoin (Dilantin) (a known 3A4 inducer), which further indicates 3A4 metabolism of busulfan (Hassan et al. 1993).

Cyclophosphamide, Ifosfamide, and Trofosfamide

Cyclophosphamide (Cytoxan), ifosfamide (Ifex), and trofosfamide (Ixoten) are alkylating pro-drugs that require metabolism by P450 enzymes for antitumor activity. The primary mechanism of bioactivation of cyclophosphamide and ifosfamide is via 4-hydroxylation at 2B6 and 3A4 (Brain et al. 1998; Huang et al. 2000b). Inactivation of these metabolites occurs via N-dechloroethylation to a potent neurotoxin, chloroacetaldehyde. Chloroacetaldehyde's neurotoxic effect is commonly known as "ifosfamide encephalopathy," which may present with cerebellar ataxia, confusion, complex visual hallucinations, extrapyramidal signs, mutism, and seizures (Primavera et al. 2002). Cyclophosphamide is N-dechloroethylated—or inactivated—at 3A4. Ifosfamide is N-dechloroethylated (and also inactivated) through 3A4 and 2B6. Since they have somewhat different inactivation sites, the production of the potent neurotoxin chloroacetaldehyde may vary under different circumstances. Ifosfamide-treated patients with increased metabolism at 2B6 because of genetic predisposition or induction of 2B6 by other factors may have an increased ability to form chloroacetaldehyde, resulting in increased levels of chloroacetaldehyde; in ifosfamide-treated patients who have lower capacity at 2B6 and 3A4, or who are not taking inducing comedications, this risk is less. According to Huang et al. (2001a), there may be clinical benefit to medically inhibiting 2B6 in patients known to have higher capacity at 2B6, given the risk of neurotoxic metabolite formation.

Schmidt et al. (2001) showed that in female hepatic microsomes treated with ifosfamide, more chloroacetaldehyde was produced than in male-counterpart microsomes. Further research is needed on the possible clinical relevance of gender difference in chloroacetaldehyde formation.

Clinical anecdotes suggest that cyclophosphamide may induce its own metabolism. These anecdotes are supported by an in vitro study using human liver microsomes that showed that administration of either cyclophosphamide or ifosfamide results in increased production of several P450 enzymes, including 3A4 and 2C9 (T. K. Chang et al. 1997). In a study by Baumhakel et al. (2001), human liver microsomes of 3A4 were given a stable substrate of dihydropyridine denitronifedipine with cyclophosphamide and ifosfamide. Both ifosfamide and cyclophosphamide significantly inhibited oxidation of dihydropyridine denitronifedipine, indicating that treatment with either drug may have clinical implications, given the drugs' effective inhibition of 3A4. Because of conflicting evidence on the activity of these medications, and the lack of in vivo studies confirming their activity, further research into the autoinduction of cyclophosphamide and inhibition at 3A4 is needed.

Trofosfamide is a newer alkylating agent that also requires metabolism for activation. Trofosfamide is bioactivated by being metabolized to ifosfamide and cyclophosphamide (Hempel et al. 1997) through 3A4 and 2B6 (May-Manke et al. 1999). Brinker et al. (2002) found low levels of ifosfamide and cyclophosphamide present during treatment, which would suggest there is a component of direct 4-hydroxylation. Given that trofosfamide has several pathways of metabolism to include metabolism to cyclophosphamide and ifosfamide as well as direct 4-hydroxylation, the findings by May-Manke et al. (1999) demonstrating minimal induction or inhibition are likely due to the minimal available inhibiting metabolites. The amount of available neurotoxic metabolite from the conversion of cyclophosphamide and ifosfamide is also lowered because of the variety of pathways of metabolism.

Carmustine and Lomustine

Delineating the metabolism of carmustine (BCNU) and lomustine (belustine) has proven difficult. In 1975, Hill et al. demonstrated that carmustine is metabolized by mice via microsomal enzymes in the liver and lungs. In 1979, Levin et al. showed that pretreatment with phenobarbital (in a rat model) increases the clearance of carmustine and lomustine, whereas pretreatment with phenytoin or dexamethasone, both inducers of 3A4, does not affect clearance rates. Weber and Waxman (1993) demonstrated that phenytoin and dexamethasone induce metabolism of carmustine and lomustine when the glutathione-*S*-transferase system is inhibited. Both the P450 system (only 2%–3% of overall metabolism) and the glutathione-*S*-transferase system play a role in the metabolism of these drugs, because of the need for both denitrosation and nicotinamide adenine dinucleotide phosphate (reduced form) (NADPH)–dependent P450 metabolism. More research, including studies beyond animal models, needs to be done to determine the clinical implications of this complicated system of metabolism.

Streptozocin

P. Chang et al. (1976) reported decreased clearance of doxorubicin (Adriamycin) in patients who were also receiving streptozocin (Zanosar). The increased severity of side effects of doxorubicin in that study suggests hepatic dysfunction due to streptozocin, but no specific mention was made of P450 involvement.

Thiotepa

Thiotepa (Testamine) is an alkylating agent that requires metabolism to its pharmacologically active metabolite, TEPA. Jacobson et al. (2002) showed that thiotepa's metabolism is primarily by 3A4, with a minor portion performed by 2B6. Huitema et al. (2001) and Rae et al. (2002) showed reversible inhibition of 2B6 by thiotepa through increased levels of cyclophosphamide when coadministered with thiotepa. These studies suggest that clinicians using chemotherapeutic regimens including thiotepa should be aware of its inhibitory effects on drugs metabolized by 2B6.

Antimetabolites

Antimetabolites come in many forms, with multiple mechanisms of action. These drugs exert their cytotoxicity by acting as false substrates in multiple biochemical pathways. Nucleoside analogs are incorporated into newly formed DNA and result in termination of DNA growth. Other antimetabolite agents include enzyme inhibitors such as methotrexate, and all antimetabolites ultimately result in faulty DNA synthesis.

Methotrexate

Methotrexate is metabolized by oxidation but not via P450 enzymes (Chladek et al. 1997). Subsequent studies have reconfirmed that the P450 system plays no role in methotrexate metabolism (Baumhakel et al. 2001; Rozman 2002). A study using human liver microsomes showed that ethanol and acetaminophen, both inducers of 2E1, also increase levels of tumor necrosis factor-α, interleukin (IL)-6, and IL-8 (Neuman et al. 1999). These increases led to reduced mitochondrial and cytosolic glutathione levels and an increase in the oxidative stress on cell cultures. These same cells were then exposed to methotrexate and showed increased methotrexate-induced cytotoxicity and an increased rate of programmed cell death (apoptosis). This phenomenon is not specifically related to P450 enzymes, but it is important to consider, given the known effects of cytokines on P450 activity. (See "Immunomodulators" later in this chapter.)

Fluorouracil

van Meerten et al. (1995) reviewed the then-available literature on drug-drug interactions and antineoplastic agents. They noted that both cimetidine and metronidazole (Flagyl) inhibit metabolism of fluorouracil, which suggests metabolism by P450 enzymes (3A4, 2D6). Interferon-α appears to decrease clearance of fluorouracil (Efudex), a finding that is consistent with findings of studies showing interferon's effect on the downregulation of some P450 enzymes.

Taxanes

The taxanes are a group of compounds isolated from plants, specifically yews. Taxanes are antineoplastic because of their ability to stabilize cellular microtubules, which are necessary during mitosis, and prevent their disassembly.

Docetaxel and Paclitaxel

Both docetaxel (Taxotere) and paclitaxel (Taxol) are metabolized to their inactive metabolites by liver microsomal enzymes and are further eliminated through the biliary system. Taxanes are also affected by the P-glycoprotein system. (See Chapter 4 ["P-Glycoproteins"] for more on P-glycoproteins.)

Cresteil et al. (2002) showed that docetaxel is metabolized by 3A4 oxidation of the *tert*-butyl group on the lateral chain to its inactive form before removal through the biliary system. Royer et al. (1996) demonstrated that ketoconazole and erythromycin (known 3A4 inhibitors) significantly inhibit oxidation of docetaxel. Malingre et al. (2001) determined that coadministration of cyclosporine (Neoral) (a known 3A4 and P-glycoprotein inhibitor) and docetaxel increases the bioavailability of docetaxel. Given the presence of P-glycoprotein in the intestine, as well as first-pass P450 metabolism by 3A4, coadministration should increase levels of docetaxel.

Cresteil et al. (2002) showed that paclitaxel is metabolized by 2C8 6-hydroxylation of the taxane ring before further removal. Dai et al. (2001) demonstrated that metabolism of paclitaxel by 2C8 is affected by the allele coding the 2C8 enzyme. *2C8* alleles vary according to the coding allele, and these alleles are present in various amounts in different ethnic groups. In patients homozygous for the allele that shows decreased ability to metabolize paclitaxel, the ability to metabolize the drug is significantly decreased, and thus the incidence of toxicity is higher.

Britten et al. (2000) studied the effect of oral paclitaxel and cyclosporine coadministration. Use of oral paclitaxel typically does not result in therapeutic levels of the agent, but with coadministration of cyclosporine, effective blood concentrations of paclitaxel can be achieved. Given that cyclosporine is a potent 3A4 and P-glycoprotein inhibitor, this result is likely due to cyclosporine's effect on the P-glycoprotein system.

It is well established that paclitaxel and docetaxel are metabolized by the P450 system, and the P-glycoprotein system seems to have a significant effect on these drugs as well. Data indicate that inhibition of P-glycoprotein activity in normal tissues by effective modulators, and the physiological and pharmacological consequences of this treatment, cannot be predicted only by monitoring plasma drug levels. More research is needed on the effect of P-glycoproteins on docetaxel and paclitaxel.

Vinca Alkaloids

Vinca alkaloids are another group of plant-derived drugs. Like the taxanes, vinca alkaloids disrupt cells in mitosis. These agents' mechanism of action is slightly different in that vinca alkaloids inhibit microtubule assembly by binding to tubulin.

Vincristine

Chan (1998) conducted a thorough review of case reports on and clinical studies of vinca alkaloids and their pharmacokinetics. All inhibitors of 3A4 reduce the metabolism of vincristine in vitro, and several case reports have indicated increased vincristine toxicity with concomitant use of 3A4 inhibitors such as itraconazole and cyclosporine.

Drugs such as carbamazepine (Tegretol) and phenytoin (Dilantin), known inducers of 3A4, have been shown to increase the metabolism of vincristine (used in combination with lomustine and procarbazine) in human volunteer subjects (Villikka et al. 1999). No studies have evaluated efficacy during concomitant administration.

Vinorelbine

Kajita et al. (2000) used human liver microsome preparations to demonstrate that 3A4 is the main P450 enzyme responsible for metabolism of vinorelbine. The same investigators showed that high concentrations (100 µM) also inhibit 3A4 activity without inhibiting other P450 enzymes, but that this level is likely higher than that found in human plasma concentrations.

Topoisomerase Inhibitors

Replication of DNA is a complex process that is mediated by several enzymes. Tension is created in the DNA molecule during normal replication. Topoisomerase enzymes are crucial to making the DNA molecule flexible during replication. If topoisomerase enzymes are inhibited, this tension is not relieved, and DNA replication and cell production cannot take place.

Etoposide and Teniposide

Etoposide (Toposar) and teniposide (Vumon) are metabolized mainly by 3A4 and partially by 1A2 and 2E1 (Kawashiro et al. 1998; McLeod 1998; Relling et al. 1994). Cyclosporine's ability to decrease clearance of etoposide both in vitro and clinically has been noted in several reports, as has the need to decrease the dose of etoposide when the two agents are used concomitantly. Although both drugs are metabolized by 3A4, the need to decrease the dose is not due to a P450-mediated effect. Cyclosporine is a known inhibitor of P-glycoprotein, and this inhibition causes cells to retain etoposide longer.

Bagniewski et al. (1996) showed that glucocorticoids and anticonvulsants increase clearance of etoposide, a finding that is explained by etoposide's 3A4-mediated metabolism and the known P450 induction of 3A4 by glucocorticoids and anticonvulsants.

Irinotecan

Irinotecan (Camptosar) is a topoisomerase inhibitor used in treating patients with lung or colon cancer (Berkery et al. 1997). Santos et al. (2000) used human liver microsome preparations to demonstrate that irinotecan is metabolized predominantly at 3A4 and to a varying degree at 3A5. More recent studies have shown that irinotecan metabolism is vulnerable to both inhibition (by potent 3A4 inhibitors such as ketoconazole) and induction (by 3A4-inducing antiepileptics) (Kehrer et al. 2002). Additionally, the decrease in irinotecan concentrations that occurs with phenytoin coadministration is likely mediated by uridine 5′-diphosphate glucuronosyltransferase (UGT) 1A1. Given the multiple avenues of irinotecan metabolism—3A4, 3A5, and UGT1A1, and a likely P-glycoprotein effect—there is a need for further study of irinotecan and its effects on these systems.

Antitumor Antibiotics

Often referred to as anthracyclines, antitumor antibiotics are cytotoxic by a variety of mechanisms, but the underlying mechanism of these drugs is DNA damage. Some antitumor antibiotics lead to creation of free radicals that make double- and single-strand breaks in the DNA, whereas others in this group of agents cross-link the DNA strands and prevent replication.

Doxorubicin

Balis (1986) showed that P450 enzymes are involved in anthracycline metabolism, although no specific enzymes were delineated. Use of either phenytoin or phenobarbital induces metabolism of doxorubicin (Adriamycin). These data suggest that doxorubicin is partially metabolized at 3A4. Baumhakel et al. (2001) showed that doxorubicin has an inhibitory effect on 3A4 in vitro. There are multiple reports of in vitro studies of doxorubicin's effects on taxane metabolism, but no in vivo data could be found to demonstrate clinical relevance of this possible interaction.

Antiandrogens and Antiestrogens

The enzyme responsible for conversion of androgens to estrogens in many human tissues is P450 aromatase, an important member of the P450 family that is also found in adipose, neural, and skin tissues. Because androgens (e.g., testosterone) and estrogens have such dramatic effects on some carcinomas (e.g., breast and prostate cancer), modulation of aromatase activity is a useful therapeutic modality.

Aminoglutethimide

Aminoglutethimide (Cytadren) is a potent P450 aromatase inhibitor that is used in the treatment of metastatic breast cancer. Santner et al. (1984) studied preparations of human placental microsomes with inhibitors of aromatase and noted that coadministration of two aromatase inhibitors, aminoglutethimide and testolactone, produces an additive effect, evidenced by a decrease in aromatase activity greater than that seen with either agent alone. These investigators suggested that a reduction in aminoglutethimide dose might be possible with coadministration of aminoglutethimide and testolactone. This reduction would decrease possible side effects such as sedation, rash, and orthostatic hypotension.

Anastrozole

Anastrozole (Arimidex) is a third-generation aromatase inhibitor used in the treatment of breast cancer (usually advanced-stage disease in postmenopausal women). It is a potent inhibitor of P450 aromatase and decreases the pro-growth effect of estrogen on breast tissue—specifically, cancerous breast tissue. Grimm and Dyroff (1997) used in vitro studies to show that anastrozole inhibits 1A2, 2C9, and 3A4. No clinical or in vivo studies have been performed, but if the usual dose of anastrozole were administered in vivo, inhibition of P450 enzymes in vivo would be minimal (given the findings of Grimm and Dyroff [1997] in their in vitro study) and likely not clinically relevant. There are currently no case reports of clinically relevant drug-drug interactions due to P450 inhibition by anastrozole. Discussion of the genetics and expression of aromatase can be found in a report by Simpson et al. (1997).

Flutamide

Flutamide (Eulexin) is an androgen receptor antagonist that is often used in the treatment of prostate cancer. Using human liver microsome preparations, Shet and colleagues (1997) demonstrated that flutamide is metabolized to its primary metabolite by 1A2. A minor metabolite was formed by 3A4. The primary metabolite of fluta- mide, 2-hydroxyflutamide, is a more potent androgen receptor antagonist and can inhibit 1A2. No in vivo studies were found that focused on this phenomenon, and the clinical implications of 1A2 inhibition by 2-hydroxyflutamide cannot be estimated adequately from these data.

Tamoxifen

Tamoxifen (Nolvadex) is an older chemotherapy drug that works as an antiestrogen. Tamoxifen is metabolized through both N-demeth- ylation and 4-hydroxylation. Tamoxifen's 4-hydroxylation metabo- lite is intrinsically 100 times more potent and is predominantly created by 2D6 metabolism of tamoxifen (Crewe et al. 1997). Human liver microsome studies showed that N-demethylation of tamoxifen by 3A4 produces a less potent antiestrogen (Dehal and Kupfer 1997). Christians et al. (1996) determined that several drugs, includ- ing tamoxifen, may inhibit P450 metabolism of tacrolimus, a known 3A4 substrate. This finding strongly suggests that tamoxifen inhib- its 3A4.

A study of the interaction between rifampin and tamoxifen found a marked reduction in the serum levels of tamoxifen in pa- tients also taking rifampin, a potent inducer of 3A4 (Kivisto et al. 1998).

Toremifene

In a study involving healthy male volunteers, plasma concentra- tions of toremifene (Fareston) were decreased when the drug was given in concert with rifampin, a known 3A4 and 1A inducer (Kivisto et al. 1998). This finding suggests that toremifene is me- tabolized at 3A4 and 1A. In vitro studies using human liver micro- some preparations with known inhibitors showed that the majority (but not all) of the metabolites of the drug are created by these two isoforms (Berthou et al. 1994).

Miscellaneous Agents

Cisplatin and Other Platinum Agents

Platinum agents are the only heavy metal compounds used for anti-neoplastic chemotherapy. Administration of these drugs results in covalent cross-linking strands of DNA, leading to an inability to replicate the DNA strands.

There are numerous reports that the use of cisplatin may decrease serum levels of anticonvulsants, although none of these reports include comments on a specific mechanism. Although platinum agents are predominantly cleared renally, there is a need for further explanation of their P450-mediated effects.

Ando and colleagues (1998) reported that JM216, an oral platinum agent, inhibited several P450 enzymes, including 3A4, 2C9, 1A1, 1A2, 2A6, 2E1, and 2D6. These authors provided no in vivo data and suggested that further studies need to be done.

Dacarbazine

Dacarbazine (DTIC), a pro-drug like cyclophosphamide, was recently found to be metabolized to active forms by 1A1, 1A2, and 2E1 (Patterson and Murray 2002). Inhibitors of these enzymes significantly decreased N-demethylation of dacarbazine in vitro (Reid et al. 1999).

Retinoids

Retinoic acid, a vitamin A derivative, plays an important role in maintaining normal cell growth and structure but has been shown to induce cell differentiation and development in both healthy cells and cancer cells, leading to early cell death. Retinoic acid was initially administered only in cases of acute promyelocytic leukemia, but the drug is now used in patients with other tumors. Early trials examined retinoic acid's effect on prostate cancers. More recent studies also evaluated its effect on breast carcinoma. Han and Choi (1996) found that retinoic acid is metabolized to 4- and 18-hydroxy metabolites. Retinoic acid induces its own metabolism, but human liver microsome assays of known inhibitors and inducers revealed no P450-mediated interactions.

All-*trans*-retinoic acid (ATRA) also induces its own metabolism. In a Phase II study of ATRA in prostate cancer patients, subjects who underwent 14 days of ATRA therapy had an 83% increase in activity of 2E1 as well as of phase II *N*-acetyltransferase (Adedoyin et al. 1998). Subjects showed no appreciable differences in 1A2, 2C19, 2D6, or 3A4 activity. Krekels et al. (1997) performed in vitro assays with breast cancer cells and found that autoinduction of ATRA metabolism is dose dependent.

An in vitro study of several head and neck cancer cell lines showed that the oxidative catabolism of retinoids is inhibited by fluconazole (suggesting 3A4 or 2C9 catabolism) and induced by 13-*cis*-retinoic acid, 9-*cis*-retinoic acid, and retinal but not retinol (Kim et al. 1998). These findings corroborated those of Schwartz and colleagues (1995) from a prospective study involving patients with acute promyelocytic leukemia. However, Lee et al. (1995) found no differences in the area under the curve of ATRA with or without ketoconazole coadministration. 3A4 may or may not be involved in ATRA metabolism, but extrapolation of the data from these studies suggests that ATRA is metabolized by 2C9 to a much greater extent than by 3A4.

CYP26 is a P450 enzyme that has not been extensively characterized. Sonneveld et al. (1998) reviewed retinoid metabolism and its probable hydroxylation by CYP26, which is induced by ATRA. CYP26 was specific for the hydroxylation of ATRA only, not other isomers of retinoic acid. Although CYP26 is not a prominent P450 enzyme, its effect on retinoids is notable.

Steroids

Glucocorticoids are a common addition to many chemotherapeutic regimens. Many studies, including those by Christian et al. (1996), Liddle et al. (1998), and El-Sankary et al. (2002), show both metabolism and induction of 3A4. Given the frequency of use of glucocorticoids, care must be taken when these drugs are used with either pro-drugs whose active metabolites of induced 3A4 may cause toxic side effects, or drugs requiring 3A4 for deactivation.

■ IMMUNOMODULATORS

Much of the communication between cells, both healthy and diseased, is accomplished chemically. Cytokines are intercellular mediators that are released by cells in response to antigens or disease states in an effort to communicate with other cells, the immune system, or the body in general. Cytokines include chemical signals by interleukins, interferons, and other nonantibody proteins.

There has been a rapid increase in the number of drugs and synthetic antibodies routinely used in oncology as well as other areas of medicine. Many of these compounds are not metabolized by P450 enzymes but can have significant effects on the regulation of the activity level of these enzymes. Additionally, P450 activity has been noted to fluctuate in many disease states, a concept supported by several in vitro human liver microsome studies showing changes in enzyme activity due to the effects of cytokines.

Interferon-α

Dorr (1993) reviewed available literature on the effects of interferon-α (Intron-A) in multiple disease states and cited evidence that P450 enzymes, along with general cellular protein synthesis, are inhibited by interferon-α. Both Leeder and Kearns (1997) and Dorr (1993) noted increased clearance of theophylline in inflammatory states, suggesting possible 1A2 induction, although no reference was made to specific enzymes.

Cytokines and Interleukins

Gorski et al. (2000) briefly reviewed the decreases in P450 function observed with IL-6, tumor necrosis factor-α, and IL-1β therapy. In a study of IL-10 in healthy human volunteers, these investigators demonstrated a decrease in 3A4 activity without any effect on 1A2, 2C9, or 2D6. Observations in more clinical settings suggest that theophylline clearance is decreased during serologically confirmed upper respiratory tract infections (Leeder and Kearns 1997).

Elkahwaji et al. (1999) found that in patients with metastatic disease in the liver, high doses of IL-2 decreased the total P450 and monooxygenase activity—specifically, the activity of 1A2, 2C, 2E1, and 3A4.

Oncostatin M is a cytokine in the IL-6 receptor family. Although oncostatin M is not used in clinical oncology, this cytokine's presence in disease states makes it notable. Guillen et al. (1998) compared the effects of oncostatin M with those of interferon-γ and IL-6. The activity of 1A2 was noted to be significantly reduced by all three cytokines but most strongly by oncostatin M. Similar reductions in activity of 2A6, 2B6, and 3A4 were noted with exposure to oncostatin M.

■ SUMMARY

There are many classes and subclasses of chemotherapeutic agents. Many of these drugs are too old or too new to be well understood pharmacokinetically. Oncology patients are routinely on polypharmacy to address the many side effects of these agents. The in vitro data for these agents are burgeoning, and more in vivo study of metabolic and P-glycoprotein interaction is needed to improve outcome and avoid toxicities.

■ REFERENCES

Adedoyin A, Stiff DD, Smith DC, et al: All-*trans*-retinoic acid modulation of drug-metabolizing enzyme activities: investigation with selective metabolic drug probes. Cancer Chemother Pharmacol 41:133–139, 1998

Ando Y, Shimizu T, Nakamure K, et al: Potent and non-specific inhibition of cytochrome P450 by JM216, a new oral platinum agent. Br J Cancer 18:1170–1174, 1998

Bagniewski PG, Reid JM, Ames MM, et al: Increased etoposide clearance in patients with glioma may be associated with concurrent glucocorticoid or anticonvulsant treatment (abstract). Proceedings of the Annual Meeting of the American Association for Cancer Research 37:A1224, 1996

Balis FM: Pharmacokinetic drug interactions of commonly used anticancer drugs. Clin Pharmacokinet 11:223–235, 1986

Baumhakel M, Kasel D, Rao-Schymanski RA, et al: Screening for inhibitory effects of antineoplastic agents on CYP3A4 in human liver microsomes. Int J Clin Pharmacol Ther 39:517–528, 2001

Berkery R, Cleri LB, Skarin AT: Oncology: Pocket Guide to Chemotherapy. St. Louis, MO, Mosby Year–Book, 1997

Berthou F, Dreano Y, Belloc C, et al: Involvement of cytochrome P450 3A family in the major metabolic pathways of toremifene in human liver microsomes. Biochem Pharmacol 47:1883–1895, 1994

Bohnenstengel F, Hofmann U, Eichelbaum M, et al: Characterization of the cytochrome P450 involved in side-chain oxidation of cyclophosphamide in humans. Eur J Clin Pharmacol 51:297–301, 1996

Brain EG, Yu LJ, Gustafsson K, et al: Modulation of P450 dependent ifosfamide pharmacokinetics: a better understanding of drug activation in vivo. Br J Cancer 77:1768–1776, 1998

Brinker A, Kisro J, Letsch C, et al: New insights into the clinical pharmacokinetics of trofosfamide. Int J Clin Pharmacol Ther 40:376–381, 2002

Britten CD, Baker SD, Denis LJ, et al: Oral paclitaxel and concurrent cyclosporin A: targeting clinically relevant systemic exposure to paclitaxel. Clin Cancer Res 6:3459–3468, 2000

Buggia I, Zecca M, Alessandrino EP, et al: Itraconazole can increase systemic exposure to busulfan in patients given bone marrow transplantation. GITMO (Gruppo Italiano Trapianto di Midollo Osseo). Anticancer Res 16:2083–2088, 1996

Chan JD: Pharmacokinetic drug interactions of vinca alkaloids: summary of case reports. Pharmacotherapy 18:1304–1307, 1998

Chang P, Riggs CE Jr, Scheerer MT, et al: Combination chemotherapy with Adriamycin and streptozotocin, II: clinicopharmacologic correlation of augmented Adriamycin toxicity caused by streptozotocin. Clin Pharmacol Ther 20:611–616, 1976

Chang TK, Yu L, Maurel P, et al: Enhanced cyclophosphamide and ifosfamide activation in primary human hepatocyte cultures: response to cytochrome P-450 inducers and autoinduction by oxazaphosphorines. Cancer Res 57:1946–1954, 1997

Chen L, Yu LJ, Waxman DJ: Potentiation of cytochrome P450/cyclophos-phamide-based cancer gene therapy by coexpression of the P450 reductase gene. Cancer Res 57:4830–4837, 1997

Chladek J, Martinkova J, Sispera L: An in vitro study on methotrexate hydroxylation in rat and human liver. Physiol Res 46:371–379, 1997

Christians U, Schmidt G, Bader A, et al: Identification of drugs inhibiting the in-vitro metabolism of tacrolimus by human liver microsomes. Br J Clin Pharmacol 41:187–190, 1996

Clarke SJ, Rivory LP: Clinical pharmacokinetics of docetaxel. Clin Pharmacokinet 36:99–114, 1999

Cresteil T, Monsarrat B, Dubois J, et al: Regioselective metabolism of taxoids by human CYP3A4 and 2C8: structure-activity relationship. Drug Metab Dispos 30:438–445, 2002

Crewe HK, Ellis SW, Lennard MS, et al: Variable contribution of cytochromes P450 2D6, 2C8 and 3A4 to the 4-hydroxylation of tamoxifen by human liver microsomes. Biochem Pharmacol 53:171–178, 1997

Dai D, Zeldin D, Blaisdell JA, et al: Polymorphisms in human CYP2C8 decrease metabolism of the anticancer drug paclitaxel and arachidonic acid. Pharmacogenetics 11:597–607, 2001

Debruyne FJ, Murray R, Fradet Y, et al: Liarozole—a novel treatment approach for advanced prostate cancer: results of a large randomized trial versus cyproterone acetate. Liarozole Study Group. Urology 52:72–81, 1998

Dehal SS, Kupfer D: CYP2D6 catalyzes tamoxifen 4-hydroxylation in human liver. Cancer Res 57:3402–3406, 1997

Desai PB, Duan JZ, Zhu YW, et al: Human liver microsomal metabolism of paclitaxel and drug interactions. Eur J Drug Metab Pharmacokinet 23:417–424, 1998

Dorr RT: Interferon-alpha in malignant and viral diseases: a review. Drugs 45:177–211, 1993

Elkahwaji J, Robin MA, Berson A, et al: Decrease in hepatic cytochrome P450 after interleukin-2 immunotherapy. Biochem Pharmacol 57:951–954, 1999

El-Sankary W, Bombail V, Gibson GG, et al: Glucocorticoid mediated induction of CYP3A4 is decreased by disruption of a protein: DNA interaction distinct from the pregnane X receptor response element. Drug Metab Dispos 30(9):1029–1034, 2002

Gorski JC, Hall SD, Becker P, et al: In vivo effects of interleukin-10 on human cytochrome P450 activity. Clin Pharmacol Ther 67:32–43, 2000

Goss PE: Pre-clinical and clinical review of vorozole, a new third generation aromatase inhibitor. Breast Cancer Res Treat 49 (suppl 1):S59–S65, 1998

Goss PE, Oza A, Blackstein M, et al: A Phase II study of liarozole fumarate in postmenopausal women with metastatic breast cancer (abstract). Proceedings of the Annual Meeting of the American Society of Clinical Oncology 15:A156, 1996

Grimm SW, Dyroff MC: Inhibition of human drug metabolizing cytochromes P450 by anastrozole, a potent and selective inhibitor of aromatase. Drug Metab Dispos 25:598–601, 1997

Guillen MI, Donato MT, Jover R, et al: Oncostatin M down-regulates basal and induced cytochromes P450 in human hepatocytes. J Pharmacol Exp Ther 285:127–134, 1998

Han IS, Choi JH: Highly specific cytochrome P450-like enzymes for all-*trans*-retinoic acid in T47D human breast cancer cells. J Clin Endocrinol Metab 81:2069–2075, 1996

Harris JW, Rahman A, Kim BR, et al: Metabolism of taxol by human hepatic microsomes and liver slices: participation of P450 3A4 and an unknown P450 enzyme. Cancer Res 54:4026–4035, 1994

Hassan M, Oberg G, Bjorkholm M, et al: Influence of prophylactic anticonvulsant therapy on high-dose busulfan kinetics. Cancer Chemother Pharmacol 33:181–186, 1993

Hempel G, Krumpelman S, May-Manke A, et al: Pharmacokinetics of trofosfamide and its dechloroethylated metabolites. Cancer Chemother Pharmacol 40:45–50, 1997

Hill DL, Kirk MC, Struck RF: Microsomal metabolism of nitrosoureas. Cancer Res 35:296–301, 1975

Huang Z, Raychowdhurry MK, Waxman DJ: Impact of liver P450 reductase suppression on cyclophosphamide activation, pharmacokinetics and antitumoral activity in a cytochrome p450 based cancer gene therapy model. Cancer Gene Ther 7:1034–1042, 2000a

Huang Z, Roy P, Waxman DJ: Role of human liver microsomal CYP 3A4 and CYP 2B6 in catalyzing N-dechloroethylation of cyclophosphamide and ifosfamide. Biochem Pharmacol 59:961–972, 2000b

Huitema AD, Mathot RA, Tibben MM, et al: A mechanism based model for the cytochrome P450 drug-drug interaction between cyclophosphamide and thioTEPA and the autoinduction of cyclophosphamide. J Pharmacokinet Pharmacodyn 28:211–230, 2001

Jamis-Dow CA, Pearl ML, Watkins PB, et al: Predicting drug interactions in-vivo from experiments in-vitro: human studies with paclitaxel and ketoconazole. Am J Clin Oncol 20:592–599, 1997

Jacobson PA, Green K, Birnbaum A, et al: Cytochrome P450 isozymes 3A4 and 2B6 are involved in the in vitro human metabolism of thiotepa to TEPA. Cancer Chemother Pharmacol 49:461–467, 2002

Kajita J, Kuwabara T, Kobayashi H, et al: CYP3A4 is mainly responsible for the metabolism of a new vinca alkaloid, vinorelbine, in human liver microsomes. Drug Metab Dispos 28:1121–1127, 2000

Kawashiro T, Yamashita K, Zhao XJ, et al: A study on the metabolism of etoposide and possible interactions with antitumor or supporting agents by human liver microsomes. J Pharmacol Exp Ther 286:1294–1300, 1998

Kehrer DF, Mathijssen RH, Verweij J, et al: Modulation of irinotecan metabolism by ketoconazole. J Clin Oncol 20:3122–3129, 2002

Kerbusch T, Jansen RL, Mathot RA, et al: Modulation of the cytochrome P450-mediated metabolism of ifosfamide by ketoconazole and rifampin. Clin Pharmacol Ther 70:132–141, 2001

Kim SY, Han IS, Yu HK, et al: The induction of P450-mediated oxidation of all-*trans* retinoic acid by retinoids in head and neck squamous cell carcinoma cell lines. Metabolism 47:955–958, 1998

Kivisto KT, Villikka K, Nyman L, et al: Tamoxifen and toremifene concentrations in plasma are greatly decreased by rifampin. Clin Pharmacol Ther 64:648–654, 1998

Krekels MD, Verhoeven A, van Dun J, et al: Induction of the oxidative catabolism of retinoid acid in MCF-7 cells. Br J Cancer 75:1098–1104, 1997

Kusuhara H, Suzuki H, Sugiyama Y: The role of P-glycoprotein in the liver. Nippon Rinsho 55:1069–1076, 1997

Lee JS, Newman RA, Lippman SM, et al: Phase I evaluation of all-*trans* retinoic acid with and without ketoconazole in adults with solid tumors. J Clin Oncol 13:1501–1508, 1995

Leeder JS, Kearns GL: Pharmacogenetics in pediatrics. Implications for practice. Pediatr Clin North Am 44:55–77, 1997

Levin VA, Stearns J, Byrd A, et al: The effect of phenobarbital pretreatment on the antitumor activity of 1,3-bis(2-chloroethyl)-1-nitrosourea (BCNU), 1-(2-chloroethyl)-3-cyclohexyl-1-nitrosourea (CCNU) and 1-(2-chloroethyl)-3-(2,6-dioxo-3-piperidyl)-1-nitrosourea (PCNU), and on the plasma pharmacokinetics and biotransformation of BCNU. J Pharmacol Exp Ther 208:1–6, 1979

Liddle C, Goodwin BJ, George J, et al: Separate and interactive regulation of cytochrome P450 3A4 by triiodothyronine, dexamethasone, and growth hormone in cultured hepatocytes. J Clin Endocrinol Metab 83:2411–2416, 1998

Malingre MM, Ten Bokkel Huinink WW, Mackay M, et al: Pharmacokinetics of oral cyclosporin A when co-administered to enhance the absorption of orally administered docetaxel. Eur J Clin Pharmacol 57:305–307, 2001

May-Manke A, Kroemer H, Hempel G, et al: Investigation of the major human hepatic cytochrome P450 involved in 4-hydroxylation and N-dechloroethylation of trofosfamide. Cancer Chemother Pharmacol 44:327–334, 1999

McLeod HL: Clinically significant drug-drug interactions in oncology. Br J Clin Pharmacol 45:539–544, 1998

Monsarrat B, Chatelut E, Alvinerie P, et al: Modification of paclitaxel metabolism by drug induction of cytochrome P450A4 in a cancer patient (abstract). Proceedings of the Annual Meeting of the American Association for Cancer Research 38:A31, 1997

Neuman MG, Cameron RG, Haber JA, et al: Inducers of cytochrome P450 2E1 enhance methotrexate-induced hepatotoxicity. Clin Biochem 32:519–536, 1999

Patterson LH, Murray GI: Tumour cytochrome P450 and drug activation. Curr Pharm Des 8:1335–1347, 2002

Philip PA, Ali-Sadat S, Doehmer J, et al: Use of V79 cells with stably transfected cytochrome P450 cDNAs in studying the metabolism and effects of cytotoxic drugs. Cancer Chemother Pharmacol 43:59–67, 1999

Primavera A, Audenino D, Cocito L: Ifosfamide encephalopathy and nonconvulsive status epilepticus. Can J Neurol Sci 29:180–183, 2002

Rahman A, Korzekwa KR, Grogan J, et al: Selective biotransformation of taxol to 6-alpha-hydroxytaxol by human cytochrome P450 2C8. Cancer Res 54:5543–5546, 1994

Rae JM, Soukhova NV, Flockhart DA: Triethylenethiophosphamide is a specific inhibitor of cytochrome P450 2B6: implications for cyclophosphamide metabolism. Drug Metab Dispos 30:525–530, 2002

Reid JM, Kuffel MJ, Miller JK, et al: Metabolic activation of dacarbazine by human cytochromes P450: the role of CYP1A1, CYP1A2, and CYP2E1. Clin Cancer Res 5:2192–2197, 1999

Relling MV, Nemec J, Schuetz EG, et al: O-Demethylation of epipodophyllotoxins is catalyzed by human cytochrome P450 3A4. Mol Pharmacol 45:352–358, 1994

Rochat B, Morsman JM, Murray GI, et al: Human CYP1B1 and anticancer agent metabolism: mechanism for tumor-specific drug inactivation? J Pharmacol Exp Ther 296:537–541, 2001

Royer I, Monsarrat B, Sonnier M, et al: Metabolism of docetaxel by human cytochromes P450: interactions with paclitaxel and other antineoplastic drugs. Cancer Res 56:58–65, 1996

Rozman B: Clinical pharmacokinetics of leflunomide. Clin Pharmacokinet 41:421–430, 2002

Santner SJ, Rosen H, Osawa Y, et al: Additive effects of aminoglutethimide, testololactone, and 4-hydroxyandrostenedione as inhibitors of aromatase. J Steroid Biochem 20:1239–1242, 1984

Santos A, Zanetta S, Cresteil T, et al: Metabolism of irinotecan (CPT-11) by CYP3A4 and CYP3A5 in humans. Clin Cancer Res 6:2012–2020, 2000

Schmidt R, Baumann F, Hanschmann H, et al: Gender differences in ifosfamide metabolism by human liver microsomes. Eur J Drug Metab Pharmacokinet 26:193–200, 2001

Schwartz EL, Hallam S, Gallagher RE, et al: Inhibition of all-*trans*-retinoic acid metabolism by fluconazole in-vitro and in patients with acute promyelocytic leukemia. Biochem Pharmacol 50:923–928, 1995

Seidmon EJ, Trump DL, Kreis W, et al: Phase I/II dose-escalation study of liarozole in patients with stage D, hormone-refractory carcinoma. Ann Surg Oncol 2:550–556, 1995

Shet MS, McPhaul M, Fisher CW, et al: Metabolism of the antiandrogenic drug (flutamide) by human CYP1A2. Drug Metab Dispos 25:1298–1303, 1997

Shou M, Martinet M, Korzekwa KR, et al: Role of human cytochrome P450 3A4 and 3A5 in the metabolism of Taxotere and its derivatives: enzyme specificity, interindividual distribution and metabolic contribution in human liver. Pharmacogenetics 8:391–401, 1998

Simpson ER, Zhao Y, Agarwal VR, et al: Aromatase expression in health and disease. Recent Prog Horm Res 52:185–214, 1997

Sonneveld E, van den Brink CE, van der Leede BM, et al: Human retinoic acid (RA) 4-hydroxylase (CYP26) is highly specific for all-*trans*-RA and can be induced through RA receptors in human breast and colon carcinoma cells. Cell Growth Differ 9:629–637, 1998

van Meerten E, Verweij J, Schellens JH: Antineoplastic agents: drug interactions of clinical significance. Drug Saf 12:168–182, 1995

Villikka K, Kivisto KT, Maenpaa H, et al: Cytochrome P450-inducing antiepileptics increase the clearance of vincristine in patients with brain tumors. Clin Pharmacol Ther 66:589–593, 1999

Weber GF, Waxman DJ: Denitrosation of the anti-cancer drug 1,3-bis(2-chloroethyl)-1-nitrosourea catalyzed by microsomal glutathione S-transferase and cytochrome P450 monooxygenases. Arch Biochem Biophys 307:369–378, 1993

■ CHEMOTHERAPEUTIC AGENTS METABOLIZED AT P450 ENZYMES

3A4	2B6	2C9	2C19	1A2	1A1, 2E1
Busulfan	Cyclophosphamide	Carmustine	Cyclophosphamide	Dacarbazine	Dacarbazine
Cyclophosphamide[1]	Ifosfamide	Paclitaxel	Ifosfamide	Flutamide	
Daunorubicin	Thiotepa	Tamoxifen			
Dexamethasone	Trofosfamide				
Docetaxel					
Doxorubicin					
Etoposide					
Ifosfamide					
Ondansetron					
Paclitaxel					
Tamoxifen					
Teniposide					
Thiotepa					
Toremifene					
Trofosfamide					
Vinblastine					
Vincristine					
Vindesine					
Vinorelbine					

[1]N-Dealkylation to a neurotoxic agent, chloroacetaldehyde.

■ CHEMOTHERAPEUTIC AGENTS THAT ARE INHIBITORS OF P450 ENZYMES

3A4	1A2	2C9	2B6
Anastrozole	Anastrozole	Anastrozole	Thiotepa
?Doxorubicin	Flutamide[1]		
?Paclitaxel			
Tamoxifen			

[1]Flutamide's primary metabolite is a **potent** 1A2 inhibitor.

■ CHEMOTHERAPEUTIC AGENTS THAT ARE INDUCERS OF P450 ENZYMES

3A4	2C9	2E1
Cisplatin	Cyclophosphamide	Retinoids
Cyclophosphamide	Ifosfamide	
Ifosfamide		

17

PAIN MANAGEMENT I:
NONNARCOTIC ANALGESICS

The nonnarcotic analgesics discussed in this chapter include a wide array of medications: "coxib" cyclooxygenase-2 (COX-2) inhibitors, noncoxib COX-2 inhibitors, aspirin, aspirin-like products, acetaminophen (Tylenol), and nonsteroidal anti-inflammatory drugs (NSAIDs). Generally, little has been written about pharmacokinetic drug interactions involving these medications, for two reasons:

1. Nonnarcotic analgesics have broad safety margins, and any drug interactions that do occur rarely have dire consequences. Indeed, many of these drugs are available over the counter in the United States.
2. What is known about the metabolism of nonnarcotic analgesics is sketchy at times. Many nonnarcotic analgesics are older medications that have gone off patent, and drug companies and researchers have been less interested in profiling their metabolisms. In addition, determining exactly how these drugs are metabolized can be difficult because many are metabolized by the uridine 5′-diphosphate glucuronosyltransferase (UGT) system, which has only recently been characterized (see Chapter 3 ["Metabolism in Depth: Phase II"]) and is not as well delineated as the P450 system.

There are five overriding themes that are important to know regarding potential pharmacokinetic drug-drug interactions of nonnarcotic analgesics:

1. Some nonnarcotic analgesics (aspirin, salsalate [Disalcid], nabumetone [Relafen]) are pro-drugs. Such drugs require an oxidative reaction to achieve their pharmacological effects. They must be "activated." If that process is inhibited, the drugs' effectiveness may be decreased.

2. Many nonnarcotic analgesics are oxidatively metabolized by 2C9, and so, theoretically, levels and side effects of the drugs could be increased in poor metabolizers (PMs) at 2C9 or with the addition of a 2C9 inhibitor (such as fluvoxamine [Luvox] or fluconazole [Diflucan]). This result is rarely, if ever, reported, since many nonnarcotic analgesics that are 2C9 substrates also progress directly to UGT conjugation even if they are not oxidatively changed by 2C9. In addition, nonnarcotic analgesics have wide safety margins, so inhibition of metabolism may have only modest consequences, except perhaps for pro-drug nonnarcotic analgesics.

3. Some nonnarcotic analgesics are inhibitors of UGT enzymes. Many traditional NSAIDs inhibit UGT2B7. In particular, some have been shown to inhibit conjugation of zidovudine (AZT) and oxazepam by this mechanism. However, there is scant clinical evidence that these interactions are clinically relevant.

4. Most nonnarcotic analgesics that are conjugated go through a process of recirculation in the hepatic system and are deconjugated and become active again. This could be important if an inhibitor of conjugation is added, but, again, little to no information exists on this potential drug-drug interaction.

5. Nonnarcotic analgesics are not known to induce any metabolic enzymes.

Reminder: This chapter is dedicated primarily to metabolic and P-glycoprotein interactions. Interactions due to displaced protein-binding, alterations in absorption or excretion, and pharmacodynamics are not covered. In addition, the two most common and potentially serious side effects secondary to most nonnarcotic analgesic use—gastrointestinal bleeding and liver toxicity—are not covered in this chapter.

■ CYCLOOXYGENASE-2 INHIBITORS

"Coxibs"

Celecoxib

Celecoxib (Celebrex) is a commonly used coxib for chronic pain due to osteoarthritis. It is metabolized chiefly through hydroxylation by 2C9 (Celebrex 2002) and by one or more unspecified UGT enzymes to form a 1-*O*-glucuronide (Paulson et al. 2000). Because 2C9 is considered the major enzyme for clearance of celecoxib, there has been some concern that celecoxib's effectiveness may be altered in PMs at 2C9 or by inhibitors or inducers of 2C9 (see Chapter 8 ["2C9"]). C. Tang et al. (2001) demonstrated that celecoxib's area under the curve (AUC) was increased 2.2-fold in three volunteers who were PMs at 2C9 and who received a single 200-mg dose. Werner et al. (2002) obtained a similar finding in one PM, with the AUC doubling compared with the AUCs in extensive metabolizers at 2C9, although the half-life of the drug was unchanged. We are not aware of any pharmacokinetic studies examining celecoxib use with 2C9 inhibitors such as fluvoxamine or fluconazole. In addition, there are no studies of celecoxib's analgesic efficacy or untoward side effects (from higher AUCs) in PMs or with coadministration of 2C9 inhibitors. Nevertheless, the manufacturer has recommended caution when the drug is used in known or suspected PMs at 2C9 (Celebrex 2002)—and we would add, with potent 2C9 inhibitors. Finally, there is some evidence that celecoxib may inhibit 2D6 (Garnett 2001), but no further evidence has been reported.

Rofecoxib

The metabolism of rofecoxib (Vioxx) differs from the metabolisms of the other two coxibs. Rofecoxib is not metabolized appreciably by P450 enzymes (Garnett 2001; Vioxx 2002). It is reduced and not conjugated. The enzymes responsible for this reduction are non-P450 cytosolic enzymes. "Pan-inducers" of hepatic enzymes, such as rifampin or phenobarbital, may decrease serum rofecoxib levels.

■ CYCLOOXYGENASE-2 (COX-2) INHIBITORS

Drug	P450 enzyme(s) drug is metabolized by	UGT(s) drug is metabolized by	Other metabolism	Enzyme(s) inhibited	Pro-drug?[1]
"Coxibs"					
Celecoxib (Celebrex)	2C9	Unspecified UGT(s)	None	2D6	No
Rofecoxib (Vioxx)	None	None	Non-P450 reduction	None	No
Valdecoxib (Bextra)	3A4, 2C9	Unspecified UGTs	None	2C19	No[2]
Other COX-2 inhibitors					
Diclofenac (Voltaren)	2C9, 2C8, 2C18, 2C19, 3A4	UGT2B7, others	Sulfation	UGT2B7, ?SULTs	No
Etodolac (Tedolan)	Unspecified P450 enzymes	Unspecified UGTs	None	None	No
Meloxicam (Mobic)	2C9, 3A4	None	None	None	No
Nabumetone (Relafen)	Unspecified phase I enzyme	Unspecified UGTs	None	None	Yes[3]

Note. SULT=sulfotransferase; UGT=uridine 5′-diphosphate glucuronosyltransferase.
[1]Drug is metabolized to an active analgesic metabolite.
[2]Parenteral parecoxib is rapidly metabolized to valdecoxib.
[3]Metabolized by phase I enzymes to the active analgesic 6-methoxy-2-naphthylacetic acid (6-MNA).

The manufacturer reported that rofecoxib levels decreased 50% when the drug was given with 600 mg of rifampin a day (Vioxx 2002).

Valdecoxib

Valdecoxib (Bextra) is the third COX-2 inhibitor available in the United States. It is rapidly absorbed and is highly protein bound. Valdecoxib is metabolized by 3A4 and 2C9 (Bextra 2002). A parenteral version of the drug, parecoxib, is hydrolyzed to valdecoxib within minutes. Further metabolism of the P450 products occurs with conjugation by UGTs (Bextra 2002; Yuan et al. 2002). Because of the drug's reliance on 3A4 and 2C9 for oxidative metabolism, the manufacturer has warned that use with 3A4 or 2C9 inhibitors or inducers may alter valdecoxib's efficacy (Bextra 2002). In addition, valdecoxib is a moderate inhibitor of 2C19 (6 μg/mL inhibits 50%) and a very mild inhibitor of 3A4 and 2C9. Ketoconazole (Nizoral) and fluconazole (both inhibitors of 3A4) have been shown to increase valdecoxib's AUC by 40%–60%. The potential for pharmacokinetic drug-drug interactions involving valdecoxib has been researched in only two other studies: in one, midazolam (a 3A4 substrate) was coadministered (Ibrahim et al. 2002a), and in the other, propofol (a 2C9 substrate) was the second drug (Ibrahim et al. 2002b). The pharmacokinetics of midazolam (Versed) and propofol were not altered.

Other Cyclooxygenase-2 Inhibitors

Diclofenac

Diclofenac (Voltaren) is metabolized by both oxidative and conjugation processes. Oxidative clearance is considered a minor role, and most of the oxidative products are conjugated. 2C9 appears to be the main enzyme involved in creating the 4-hydroxylation metabolite of diclofenac (Bort et al. 1999; W. Tang et al. 1999). This reaction has often been considered specific for 2C9, and researchers have used this reaction as a probe for 2C9 activity. However, a recent in vivo study with PMs at 2C9 indicated that other 2Cs (2C8, 2C18, and 2C19) or 3A4 may be involved in 4-hydroxylation of diclofenac (Yasar et al. 2001). Diclofenac's hydroxylation has been the subject of much research: it has been proposed that diclofenac may increase liver associated enzymes without (or rarely) causing hepatotoxicity. It seems possible that the hydroxylation of diclofenac—and changes by PMs, inhibitors, or inducers—is in part responsible for the altered liver enzymes. Other reports appear to cast doubt on this theory (Aithal et al. 2000; Yasar et al. 2001).

Most of diclofenac—either the parent compound or hydroxylated diclofenac—is cleared by glucuronidation and sulfation (Voltaren 2000). UGT2B7 seems to be the major glucuronidation enzyme involved (King et al. 2001). It appears that diclofenac may inhibit UGT2B7; metabolism of morphine by UGT2B7 (which activates morphine to a potent morphine-6-glucuronide) was reduced by diclofenac (Voltaren 2000).

Etodolac

Etodolac (Tedolan) is oxidatively metabolized to at least four metabolites (Humber et al. 1988). P450 enzymes are presumed to be involved in some of these reactions, but the exact enzymes have not been described. In addition, acyl glucuronidation occurs, yielding 1-*O*-glucuronides (Berendes and Blaschke 1996), but the exact UGT enzymes have also not been reported. These findings have been confirmed by renal elimination studies, which showed that glucuronides and various hydroxylated etodolac compounds are found in the urine (Strickmann and Blaschke 2001).

Meloxicam

The major metabolites of meloxicam (Mobic) are produced by 2C9 and 3A4 (Chesne et al. 1998). 2C9 appears to be the major enzyme involved, with 3A4 playing a lesser role. The two metabolites, 5-hydroxymethylmeloxicam and 5-carboxymeloxicam, are the primary forms found in urine and feces (Mobic 2000), indicating that phase II has little involvement in the metabolism of meloxicam. It is not known whether the efficacy of meloxicam is altered in PMs at 2C9 or by inhibitors or inducers of 2C9.

Nabumetone

Nabumetone (Relafen) is a pro-drug that is metabolized to 6-methoxy-2-naphthylacetic acid (6-MNA), the active compound that has inhibitory effects on COX-2 (Davies and McLachlan 2000). This transformation is very rapid, and little parent compound is found in the serum after ingestion of the drug (Relafen 2001). The advantage of this rapid transformation is that nabumetone is inactive as it enters the gastrointestinal tract, and so, unlike other NSAIDs, it is less likely to cause gastrointestinal distress and bleeding. It has other metabolites, including inactive oxidative metabolites and glucuronides. Liver failure may decrease the rate of 6-MNA formation. Unfortunately, the enzyme responsible for 6-MNA formation has not been determined, so drug interactions relating to inhibition of the enzyme or relating to PMs at the enzyme cannot be predicted. Nabumetone is highly protein bound, and thus most drug interactions that have been described have been presumed to be connected with this mechanism.

■ ASPIRIN AND ACETAMINOPHEN

Aspirin

Aspirin (acetylsalicylic acid) is metabolized through oxidative demethylation to salicylic acid (Salacid and many others) by non-P450 carboxylesterases (Miners 1989). Salicylic acid interacts with other drugs because it is extensively protein bound. There is no evidence that salicylic acid can induce any metabolic enzymes. Salicylic acid is metabolized extensively by phase II enzymes to salicyluric acid (glycine conjugation) and to at least three glucuronides (*Goodman and Gilman's The Pharmacological Basis of Therapeutics* 2001, pp. 467, 1534). One of the UGTs involved appears to be UGT2B7 (de Wildt et al. 1999). Because salicylic acid is so extensively metabolized, it is not surprising that it may com-

■ ASPIRIN AND ACETAMINOPHEN

Drug	P450 enzyme(s) drug is metabolized by	UGT(s) drug is metabolized by	Other metabolism	Enzyme(s) inhibited	Pro-drug?[1]
Acetaminophen (Tylenol)	2E1, others	UGT1A1, UGT1A6, UGT1A9	Sulfation by SULT1A1	None	No
Aspirin	None	None	Metabolized to salicylic acid by carboxylesterases	None	Yes
Salicylic acid (Salacid)	None	UGT2B7, others	Glycine conjugation	UGT2B7, ?other UGTs, SULTs	No
Salsalate (Disalcid)	None	UGT2B7, others	Split by esterases into two salicylic acids	UGT2B7, ?other UGTs, SULTs	Yes

Note. SULT = sulfotransferase; UGT = uridine 5'-diphosphate glucuronosyltransferase.
[1] Drug is metabolized to an active analgesic metabolite.

petitively inhibit other drugs that rely on the same phase II enzymes for clearance. It is suspected that levels of valproic acid, which relies in part on UGT2B7 for clearance, are increased because of salicylic acid's competitive inhibition at UGT2B7. AZT levels have been increased with acetylsalicylic acid use—more evidence that UGT2B7 may be inhibited (Sim et al. 1991). There is also evidence that salicylic acid may inhibit sulfation conjugation (Vietri et al. 2000a), which could increase acetaminophen levels. Finally, salicylic acid levels may be reduced when it is used with phase II inducers, such as some oral contraceptives, corticosteroids, or rifampin (Miners 1989).

Salsalate (Disalcid), a related compound, is inactive as an analgesic. However, it is metabolized by esterases in the liver and elsewhere to two moieties of salicylic acid.

Acetaminophen

Acetaminophen (Tylenol) is metabolized through glucuronidation (50%; via UGT1A1, UGT1A6, and UGT1A9 [Court et al. 2001]), sulfation conjugation (30%–40%; via sulfotransferase [SULT] 1A1 [Dooley 1998]), and oxidative metabolism (via 2E1 and, to a lesser extent, 3A4 and 1A2 [Manyike et al. 2000]). 2E1 is typically a minor pathway, but it does create a metabolite that is toxic to the liver. If acetaminophen is taken in overdose or if 2E1 is induced, there is risk of hepatic injury. For more details, see Chapter 10 ("2E1").

■ NONSTEROIDAL ANTI-INFLAMMATORY DRUGS

Diflunisal

Diflunisal (Dolobid) is metabolized chiefly through glucuronidation, with two soluble glucuronides in the urine accounting for 90% of the administered dose (Dolobid 1998). UGT1A3 and UGT1A9 seem to be the predominant enzymes in this process (Ritter 2000; Sallustio et al. 2000). There appears to be no metabolism by P450 enzymes. Diflunisal may inhibit UGT1A9 (Vietri et al. 2000a) and sulfation enzymes (Vietri et al. 2000b).

■ NONSTEROIDAL ANTI-INFLAMMATORY DRUGS

Drug	P450 enzyme(s) drug is metabolized by	UGT(s) drug is metabolized by	Other metabolism	Enzyme(s) inhibited
Diflunisal (Dolobid)	None	UGT1A3, UGT1A9	None	UGT1A9, SULTs
Fenoprofen (Fepron)	None	UGT1A3, UGT2B7	None	UGT2B7
Flurbiprofen (Ansaid)	2C9	Unspecified UGTs	None	None
Ibuprofen (Advil)	2C9	UGT1A3, UGT2B7	None	UGT2B7
Indomethacin (Indocin)	2C9, 2C19	Unspecified UGTs	None	UGT2B7
Ketoprofen (Orudis)	?2C9	UGT1A3, UGT1A6, UGT2B7	None	?2C9, UGT2B7
Ketorolac (Toradol)	Unspecified P450 enzyme	Unspecified UGT	60% excreted in urine unchanged	None
Meclofenamate (Meclomen)	2C9	UGT1A9, others	None	SULTs
Mefenamic acid (Ponstel)	2C9	UGT1A9, others	None	SULTs
Naproxen (Naprosyn)	2C9, 2C8, 1A2	UGT1A3, UGT1A6, UGT1A9, UGT2B7	None	UGT2B7
Oxaprozin (Daypro)	Unspecified P450 enzymes	Unspecified UGTs	None	None
Piroxicam (Feldene)	2C9, ?others	None	None	None
Sulindac (Clinoril)[1]	None known	Unspecified UGTs	Activated by FMO₃	None
Tolmetin (Tolmene)	Unspecified P450 enzymes	Unspecified UGTs	None	None

Note. FMO₃=flavin-containing monooxygenase 3; SULT=sulfotransferase; UGT=uridine 5'-diphosphate glucuronosyltransferase.
[1]Sulindac is a pro-drug activated by enzymatic activity of FMO₃.

Fenoprofen

Fenoprofen (Nalfon) is metabolized by UGT1A3 (Green et al. 1998) and UGT2B7 (Patel et al. 1995). There is some evidence that fenoprofen inhibits UGT2B7; when administered with oxazepam (Serax), fenoprofen decreased glucuronidation of oxazepam (which is conjugated by UGT2B7) (Patel et al. 1995). However, other NSAIDs decreased glucuronidation of that drug to a greater extent.

Flurbiprofen

Flurbiprofen (Ansaid) is 4-hydroxylated by 2C9 (Tracy et al. 1996). This reaction appears to be specific for 2C9 and no other P450 enzyme, indicating that flurbiprofen's hydroxylation could be a probe for 2C9 activity. Much of the parent compound and the hydroxylated compound is also conjugated by UGT enzymes (Ansaid 2002), but the specific UGTs have not been determined.

Ibuprofen

Ibuprofen (Advil, Motrin) is 2- and 3-hydroxylated by 2C9 (Klose et al. 1998). As with other NSAIDs, the hydroxylated compounds and the parent compound are conjugated by UGT1A3 (Green et al. 1998) and UGT2B7 (de Wildt et al. 1999). Kirchheiner et al. (2002) found that in 2C9 PMs who took ibuprofen, there was more pharmacological activity (from thromboxane B_2 formation, which reflects COX-1 inhibition), but the clinical significance of this is not clear. Ibuprofen also appears to inhibit UGT2B7, as demonstrated by its inhibition of oxazepam glucuronidation (Patel et al. 1995).

Indomethacin

Indomethacin (Indocin) is metabolized through O-demethylation by 2C9 (Nakajima et al. 1998), although 2C19 also plays a minor role in production of the metabolite. O-Demethylation by 2C9 appears to be the major metabolic pathway for indomethacin. Urine recovery after drug ingestion indicates that most of the drug is eliminated as the parent compound or the oxidative metabolite, with a small portion of glucuronide metabolites (Indocin 1999). The UGTs that metabolize indomethacin have not been elucidated. Indomethacin may inhibit UGT2B7; there is evidence of indomethacin's increasing AZT concentrations (Sim et al. 1991).

Ketoprofen

Sabolovic et al. (2000) indicated that UGT1A3, UGT1A6, and UGT2B7 conjugate ketoprofen (Orudis). According to the package insert, the acyl glucuronide formed by UGTs is unstable (Orudis 1997). This implies that the glucuronide creates a reservoir for the parent compound, with metabolite going back to parent compound. Indeed, much of the parent compound is found unchanged in the urine along with the acyl glucuronide. Many secondary sources indicate that ketoprofen may have an oxidative metabolite and be a 2C9 substrate and inhibitor. However, we could not substantiate that with primary source bench research data. There is some evidence that ketoprofen may inhibit UGT2B7; the drug was found to increase levels of oxazepam (Grancharov et al. 2001) and AZT (Patel et al. 1995).

Ketorolac

The liver only modestly metabolizes ketorolac (Toradol). The drug is hydroxylated by an unknown P450 enzyme and glucuronidated by an unknown UGT enzyme. After ingestion, 60% is found unchanged in the urine, with 28% as glucuronides and 12% as *p*-hydroxyketorolac (Mroszczak et al. 1990). Pharmacokinetic drug interactions have not been well established, but the agent is highly protein bound, so displacement of other compounds is the most likely interaction (Toradol 1997).

Mefenamic Acid

Mefenamic acid (Ponstel) (and meclofenamate [Meclomen]) has long been known to be primarily metabolized via oxidation at 2C9 (Leemann et al. 1993). Mefenamic acid is metabolized by 2C9 to two metabolites: 3-hydroxymethyl mefenamic acid and 3-carboxy-mefenamic acid (Ponstel 2000). The drug and its 2C9 metabolites also undergo glucuronidation, with three separate glucuronides identified in humans (McGurk et al. 1996), one of them UGT1A9 (Ritter 2000). Vietri et al. (2001) demonstrated that mefenamic acid inhibits phenol SULTs. Like diclofenac, mefenamic acid has been known to produce an idiosyncratic reaction with rare hepatotoxicity. However, there is no evidence that the risk of this side effect is increased in 2C9 PMs or by inhibitors or inducers of 2C9.

Naproxen

Naproxen (Naprosyn, Aleve) is oxidatively metabolized through 6-O-demethylation primarily by 2C9, but 2C8 and 1A2 also contribute (Tracy et al. 1997). Naproxen and its oxidative metabolite are further metabolized by several UGTs, including UGT1A3, UGT1A6, UGT1A9, and UGT2B7 (Ritter 2000; Sabolovic et al. 2000). The manufacturer has claimed that both the parent compound and the 6-O-demethylation metabolite do not induce any enzymes (Naprosyn 2001). However, naproxen has been shown to inhibit UGT2B7—specifically, to inhibit the metabolism of AZT (Grancharov et al. 2001; Veal and Back 1995) and oxazepam (Patel et al. 1995).

Oxaprozin

Oxaprozin (Daypro) is metabolized by unspecified oxidative reactions (65%) and glucuronidation (35%) and has a long half-life (Daypro 2002). It is also highly protein bound. One unique aspect of oxaprozin's metabolism is that several of the oxidative metabolites can produce false-positive results on urine benzodiazepine assays (Fraser and Howell 1998).

Piroxicam

Piroxicam (Feldene) is oxidatively metabolized through 5-hydroxylation by 2C9 (Leemann et al. 1993). However, it is also appears to go through many other oxidative reactions (Feldene 1999), reactions that may occur via other P450 enzymes and non-P450 enzymes that have not been clearly identified. Although some NSAIDs may inhibit sulfation, piroxicam did not appear to do so (Vietri et al. 2000a).

Sulindac

Sulindac (Clinoril) is structurally similar to indomethacin and has similar analgesic and antipyretic properties. It is actually a pro-drug and requires sulfation for activation (Clinoril 1998). This reaction is carried out by flavin-containing monooxygenase 3 (Hamman et al. 2000) and creates sulindac sulfoxide. Both the parent compound and the active metabolite are conjugated by unspecified UGTs. Pharmacokinetic drug interactions involving the aforementioned reactions have not been described.

Tolmetin

Tolmetin (Tolmene) is oxidatively metabolized, and both the parent compound and the metabolite are conjugated to an acyl glucuronide. Sixty percent of the oxidative metabolite, 20% of the glucuronides, and 20% of unchanged tolmetin are found in the urine 24 hours after ingestion. The exact enzymes involved in these reactions have not been elucidated. Drug interactions have not been well established.

■ REFERENCES

Aithal GP, Day CP, Leathart JB, et al: Relationship of polymorphism in CYP2C9 to genetic susceptibility to diclofenac-induced hepatitis. Pharmacogenetics 10:511–518, 2000

Ansaid (package insert). Kalamazoo, MI, Pharmacia and Upjohn Co., 2002

Berendes U, Blaschke G: Simultaneous determination of the phase II metabolites of the non steroidal anti-inflammatory drug etodolac in human urine. Enantiomer 1:415–422, 1996

Bextra (package insert). New York, Pfizer Inc., 2002

Bort R, Mace K, Boobis A, et al: Hepatic metabolism of diclofenac: role of human CYP in the minor oxidative pathways. Biochem Pharmacol 58: 787–796, 1999

Celebrex (package insert). New York, Pfizer Inc., 2002

Chesne C, Guyomard C, Guillouzo A, et al: Metabolism of meloxicam in human liver involves cytochromes P4502C9 and 3A4. Xenobiotica 28: 1–13, 1998

Clinoril (package insert). West Point, PA, Merck and Company, 1998

Court MH, Duan SX, von Moltke LL, et al: Interindividual variability in acetaminophen glucuronidation by human liver microsomes: identification of relevant acetaminophen UDP-glucuronosyltransferase isoforms. J Pharmacol Exp Ther 299:998–1006, 2001

Davies NM, McLachlan AJ: Properties and features of nabumetone (in French). Drugs 59:25–33, 2000

Daypro (package insert). Chicago, IL, GD Searle LLC, January 2002

de Wildt SN, Kearns GL, Leeder JS, et al: Glucuronidation in humans. Pharmacogenetic and developmental aspects. Clin Pharmacokinet 36:439–452, 1999

Dolobid (package insert). West Point, PA, Merck and Company, 1998

Dooley TP: Molecular biology of the human phenol sulfotransferase gene family. J Exp Zool 282:223–230, 1998

Feldene (package insert). New York, Pfizer Inc., 1999

Fraser AD, Howell P: Oxaprozin cross-reactivity in three commercial immunoassays for benzodiazepines in urine. J Anal Toxicol 22:50–54, 1998

Garnett WR: Clinical implications of drug interactions with coxibs. Pharmacotherapy 21:1223–1232, 2001

Goodman and Gilman's The Pharmacological Basis of Therapeutics, 10th Edition. Edited by Hardman JG, Limbird LE, Gilman AG. New York, McGraw-Hill, 2001

Grancharov K, Naydenova Z, Lozeva S, et al: Natural and synthetic inhibitors of UDP-glucuronosyltransferases. Pharmacol Ther 89:171–186, 2001

Green MD, King CD, Mojarrabi B, et al: Glucuronidation of amines and other xenobiotics catalyzed by expressed human UDP-glucuronosyltransferase 1A3. Drug Metab Dispos 26:507–512, 1998

Hamman MA, Haehner-Daniels BD, Wrighton SA, et al: Stereoselective sulfoxidation of sulindac sulfide by flavin-containing monooxygenases. Comparison of human liver and kidney microsomes and mammalian enzymes. Biochem Pharmacol 60:7–17, 2000

318

Humber LG, Ferdinandi E, Demerson CA, et al: Etodolac, a novel antiin-
flammatory agent. The syntheses and biological evaluation of its metabolites. J Med Chem 31:1712–1719, 1988

Ibrahim A, Karim A, Feldman J, et al: The influence of parecoxib, a parenteral
cyclooxygenase-2 specific inhibitor, on the pharmacokinetics and clinical effects of midazolam. Anesth Analg 95:667–673, 2002a

Ibrahim A, Park S, Feldman J, et al: Effects of parecoxib, a parenteral COX-
2-specific inhibitor, on the pharmacokinetics and pharmacodynamics of
propofol. Anesthesiology 96:88–95, 2002b

Indocin (package insert). West Point, PA, Merck Sharp and Dohme Inc., 1999

King C, Tang W, Ngui J, et al: Characterization of rat and human UDP-
glucuronosyltransferases responsible for the in vitro glucuronidation of
diclofenac. Toxicol Sci 61:49–53, 2001

Kirchheiner J, Meineke I, Freytag G, et al: Enantiospecific effects of cytochrome P450 2C9 amino acid variants on ibuprofen pharmacokinetics
and on the inhibition of cyclooxygenases 1 and 2. Clin Pharmacol Ther
72:62–75, 2002

Klose TS, Ibeanu GC, Ghanayem BI, et al: Identification of residues 286 and
289 as critical for conferring substrate specificity of human CYP2C9 for
diclofenac and ibuprofen. Arch Biochem Biophys 357:240–248, 1998

Leemann TD, Transon C, Bonnabry P, et al: A major role for cytochrome
P450TB (CYP2C subfamily) in the actions of non-steroidal antiinflam-
matory drugs. Drugs Exp Clin Res 19:189–195, 1993

Manyike PT, Kharasch ED, Kalhorn TF, et al: Contribution of CYP2E1 and
CYP3A to acetaminophen reactive metabolite formation. Clin Pharmacol Ther 67:275–282, 2000

McGurk KA, Remmel RP, Hosagrahara VP, et al: Reactivity of mefenamic
acid 1-o-acyl glucuronide with proteins in vitro and ex vivo. Drug Metab
Dispos 24:842–849, 1996

Miners JO: Drug interactions involving aspirin (acetylsalicylic acid) and
salicylic acid. Clin Pharmacokinet 17:327–344, 1989

Mobic (package insert). Ridgefield, CT, Boehinger Ingelheim Pharma KG,
2000

Mroszczak EJ, Jung D, Yee J, et al: Ketorolac tromethamine pharmacokinetics and metabolism after intravenous, intramuscular, and oral administration in humans and animals. Pharmacotherapy 10:33S–39S, 1990

Nakajima M, Inoue T, Shimada N, et al: Cytochrome P450 2C9 catalyzes
indomethacin O-demethylation in human liver microsomes. Drug Metab
Dispos 26:261–266, 1998

Naprosyn (package insert). Nutley, NJ, Roche Laboratories Inc., 2001

Orudis (package insert). Philadelphia, PA, Wyeth-Ayerst Co., 1997

Patel M, Tang BK, Kalow W: *(S)*oxazepam glucuronidation is inhibited by ketoprofen and other substrates of UGT2B7. Pharmacogenetics 5:43–49, 1995

Paulson SK, Hribar JD, Liu NW, et al: Metabolism and excretion of [(14)C]celecoxib in healthy male volunteers. Drug Metab Dispos 28: 308–314, 2000

Ponstel (package insert). Morris Plains, NJ, Parke-Davis, 2000

Relafen (package insert). Research Triangle Park, NC, GlaxoSmithKline, 2001

Ritter JK: Roles of glucuronidation and UDP-glucuronosyltransferases in xenobiotic bioactivation reactions. Chem Biol Interact 129:171–193, 2000

Sabolovic N, Magdalou J, Netter P, et al: Nonsteroidal anti-inflammatory drugs and phenols glucuronidation in Caco-2 cells: identification of the UDP-glucuronosyltransferases UGT1A6, 1A3 and 2B7. Life Sci 67: 185–196, 2000

Sallustio BC, Sabordo L, Evans AM, et al: Hepatic disposition of electrophilic acyl glucuronide conjugates. Curr Drug Metab 1:163–180, 2000

Sim SM, Back DJ, Breckenridge AM: The effect of various drugs on the glucuronidation of zidovudine (azidothymidine; AZT) by human liver microsomes. Br J Clin Pharmacol 32:17–21, 1991

Strickmann DR, Blaschke G: Isolation of an unknown metabolite of the non-steroidal anti-inflammatory drug etodolac and its identification as 5-hydroxy etodolac. J Pharm Biomed Anal 25:977–984, 2001

Tang C, Shou M, Rushmore TH, et al: In-vitro metabolism of celecoxib, a cyclooxygenase-2 inhibitor, by allelic variant forms of human liver microsomal cytochrome P450 2C9: correlation with CYP2C9 genotype and in-vivo pharmacokinetics. Pharmacogenetics 11:223–235, 2001

Tang W, Stearns RA, Wang RW, et al: Roles of human hepatic cytochrome P450s 2C9 and 3A4 in the metabolic activation of diclofenac. Chem Res Toxicol 12:192–199, 1999

Toradol (package insert). Humacao, Puerto Rico, Roche Laboratories Inc., 1997

Tracy TS, Marra C, Wrighton SA, et al: Involvement of multiple cytochrome P450 isoforms in naproxen O-demethylation. Eur J Clin Pharmacol 52:293–298, 1997

Tracy TS, Marra C, Wrighton SA, et al: Studies of flurbiprofen 4′-hydroxylation: additional evidence suggesting the sole involvement of cytochrome P450 2C9. Biochem Pharmacol 52(8):1305–1309, 1996

Veal GJ, Back DJ: Metabolism of zidovudine. Gen Pharmacol 26:1469–1475, 1995

Vietri M, De Santi C, Pietrabissa A, et al: Inhibition of human liver phenol sulfotransferase by nonsteroidal anti-inflammatory drugs. Eur J Clin Pharmacol 56:81–87, 2000a

Vietri M, Pietrabissa A, Mosca F, et al: Mycophenolic acid glucuronidation and its inhibition by non-steroidal anti-inflammatory drugs in human liver and kidney. Eur J Clin Pharmacol 56:659–664, 2000b

Vietri M, Pietrabissa A, Mosca F, et al: Human adult and foetal liver sulphotransferases: inhibition by mefenamic acid and salicylic acid. Xenobiotica 31(3):153–161, 2001

Vioxx (package insert). West Point, PA, Merck and Company, 2002

Voltaren (package insert). East Hanover, NJ, Novartis Pharmaceutical Corp., 2000

Werner U, Werner D, Pahl A, et al: Investigation of the pharmacokinetics of celecoxib by liquid chromatography-mass spectrometry. Biomed Chromatogr 16:56–60, 2002

Yasar U, Eliasson E, Forslund-Bergengren C, et al: The role of CYP2C9 genotype in the metabolism of diclofenac in vivo and in vitro. Eur J Clin Pharmacol 57:729–735, 2001

Yuan JJ, Yang DC, Zhang JY, et al: Disposition of a specific cyclooxygenase-2 inhibitor, valdecoxib, in human. Drug Metab Dispos 30:1013–1021, 2002

18

PAIN MANAGEMENT II: NARCOTIC ANALGESICS

Reminder: This chapter is dedicated primarily to metabolic and P-glycoprotein interactions. Interactions due to displaced protein-binding, alterations in absorption or excretion, and pharmacodynamics are not covered.

■ SYNTHETIC OPIATES: PHENYLPIPERIDINES

The phenylpiperidines are a class of chemicals that have been developed as opiate narcotic analgesics. They are synthetic in that they are not chemically related to natural-occurring morphine and are strictly created in the laboratory. Meperidine (Demerol) was the first phenylpiperidine analgesic to come on the market in the United States. The basic structure of phenylpiperidines is shown in Figure 18–1.

The very-short-acting phenylpiperidines, such as alfentanil, also change or add complex moieties at the site with the benzyl group attached. Meperidine has the simplest structure, with a $-CH_3$ (methyl) group at R_1, no moiety at R_2, and a 3-carbon ester group at R_3.

Because phenylpiperidines differ from morphine and morphine-related compounds, they are metabolized differently. 3A4 appears to metabolize most of the phenylpiperidines, but there are some notable exceptions (see "Phenylpiperidine Synthetic Opiates" table). Two phenylpiperidines, diphenoxylate and loperamide, are also known P-glycoprotein substrates. Therefore, inhibitors and inducers of 3A4 and P-glycoprotein inhibitors are likely candidates for causing drug interactions with these compounds. The phenylpiperidines do

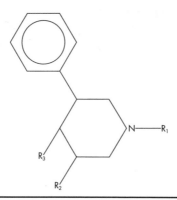

FIGURE 18–1.　**Basic structure of phenylpiperidines.**

not significantly induce any known metabolic enzymes, and none of them are known to be pro-drugs (requiring enzymatic metabolism to enhance analgesic efficacy).

Alfentanil

Alfentanil (Alfenta) is a parenteral or intrathecal synthetic opiate whose clearance has been well established as depending on 3A4 (Tateishi et al. 1996). 3A4 metabolizes alfentanil to two separate metabolites through dealkylation (Labroo et al. 1995). Alfentanil is extremely short acting in normal circumstances, having a half-life of 1–2 hours. Because it relies on 3A4 for clearance, studies have been done to determine whether 3A4 inducers and inhibitors can significantly alter alfentanil's pharmacokinetics and effectiveness. Kharasch et al. (1997) found that adding rifampin (a 3A4 inducer) or troleandomycin (a 3A4 inhibitor) significantly alters alfentanil's elimination half-life. Adding rifampin decreased the half-life from 58 to 35 minutes, but more significantly, the inhibitor troleandomycin increased the half-life to an average of 630 minutes. In addition, Palkama et al. (1998a) found that adding fluconazole (a moderate inhibitor of 3A4) decreased clearance of alfentanil by 55%.

■ PHENYLPIPERIDINE SYNTHETIC OPIATES

Drug	Enzyme(s) drug is metabolized by	Enzymes inhibited?	P-glycoprotein substrate?
Alfentanil (Alfenta)	3A4	No	No
Diphenoxylate (Lomotil)	?	No	Probable
Fentanyl (Duragesic)	3A4	?Yes/3A4	No
Loperamide (Imodium)	?	No	Yes
Meperidine (Demerol)	?3A4, ?other P450 enzymes, ?UGT1A4, ?other UGTs	?	No
Remifentanil (Ultiva)	Esterases	No	No
Sufentanil (Sufenta)	3A4, 2D6	No	No

Note. ?=unknown; UGT=uridine 5'-diphosphate glucuronosyltransferase.

Given these findings, caution is advised when alfentanil is administered with *any* 3A4 inhibitor, of which there are many (see Chapter 6 ["3A4"]). A number of confirmed cases of this interaction exist, including cases involving the commonly used drugs diltiazem (Ahonen et al. 1996) and erythromycin (Bartkowski et al. 1989). Finally, 3A4 inducers may decrease alfentanil's expected effectiveness.

Fentanyl

Fentanyl (Duragesic) is a synthetic opiate whose metabolism is similar to alfentanil's in that the predominant route of clearance is through dealkylation by 3A4 (Labroo et al. 1997; Tateishi et al. 1996). Unlike alfentanil, however, fentanyl is available by injection or in a "patch" for long-term delivery (up to 72 hours). The metabolites from 3A4 are not active. In 12 healthy volunteers, pretreatment with ritonavir, a potent 3A4 inhibitor, reduced the clearance of a single intravenous dose of fentanyl (5 mg/kg) by 67% and increased the area under the curve from 4.8 to 8.8 hours (Olkkola et al. 1999). Other findings involving 3A4 inhibitors have been inconsistent, however. For example, fentanyl pharmacokinetics did not change when the drug was administered with itraconazole, another potent 3A4 inhibitor (Palkama et al. 1998b). Nevertheless, caution is advised when fentanyl is used with any 3A4 inhibitor or inducer.

Fentanyl may be a modest competitive inhibitor of 3A4. In an in vitro study, Oda et al. (1999) demonstrated that use with midazolam slowed midazolam clearance. Further study is needed to confirm this finding in vivo.

Meperidine

Meperidine (Demerol), available both orally and parenterally, is the oldest of the synthetic opioids discussed in this section. Therefore, knowledge of its metabolism is both extensive and limited: the metabolites created by meperidine, its pharmacokinetics in terms of half-life, and its routes of elimination are all well known, but the actual enzymes responsible for these reactions are not. It is thus difficult to draw any definitive conclusions regarding meperidine's metabolism and the potential for other drugs to inhibit or induce that metabolism.

The route of meperidine metabolism is shown in Figure 18–2.

Although the actual enzymes involved in the metabolism of meperidine have not been described in the literature, one can deduce that 3A4 may be involved, because 3A4 inhibitors and inducers have been shown to alter normeperidine levels (see the discussion later in this section).

Meperidine's hydrolysis reaction may also occur via P450 enzymes, although non-P450 enzymes catalyze this type of reaction for other drugs. The uridine 5′-diphosphate glucuronosyltransferases (UGTs) that form conjugates have also not been established, although there is some evidence that UGT1A4 may be involved (Hawes 1998).

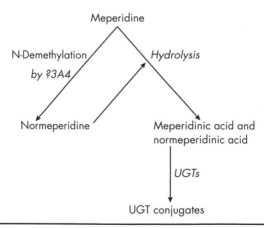

FIGURE 18–2. **Metabolism of meperidine.**

UGT=uridine 5′-diphosphate glucuronosyltransferase.

Source. Adapted from *Goodman and Gilman's The Pharmacological Basis of Therapeutics* 1980 and Demerol 2000.

Meperidine is not indicated for long-term use, because nor-meperidine has a long half-life, stimulates the central nervous system (CNS), and can lead to seizures. Theoretically, if hydrolysis (or perhaps N-demethylation) were inhibited, both meperidine and nor-meperidine levels would increase, causing CNS toxicity or excessive opioid activity. An inducer of the N-demethylation enzyme would perhaps have an even more important effect—that of directly increasing the amount of toxic normeperidine. Both chronically administered ritonavir (Piscitelli et al. 2000)—which eventually induces 3A4 and perhaps other P450 enzymes—and phenobarbital (Stambaugh et al. 1978) have been shown to decrease meperidine levels. Normeperidine's area under the curve was increased by 47% in the ritonavir study by Piscitelli et al. (2000). Stambaugh et al. (1978) showed that more N-demethylation occurs and more normeperidine is made when meperidine is used with phenobarbital. Caution is advised when meperidine is used with 3A4 inducers or "pan-inducers." The package insert also warns that these inducers could also decrease meperidine levels and cause opiate withdrawal (Demerol 2000).

Finally, there are no case reports of the use of inhibitors of 3A4 or other P450 enzymes with meperidine. One reason for this lack of data may be that use of selective serotonin reuptake inhibitors, which are notorious for P450 inhibition, with meperidine is contraindicated because of the risk of serotonin syndrome. Meperidine blocks serotonin reuptake and therefore should not be used with selective serotonin reuptake inhibitors, monoamine oxidase inhibitors, or St. John's wort.

Remifentanil

Remifentanil (Ultiva) is available as a very-short-acting anesthetic opiate with a half-life of 5–10 minutes. It is rapidly metabolized throughout the body by nonspecific esterases (Haigh 2000). There are no reports of pharmacokinetic drug-drug interactions involving this drug.

Sufentanil

Sufentanil (Sufenta), like most of the "fentanils," is a short-acting anesthetic synthetic opiate that is used only parenterally or intrathecally. Its elimination half-life is 2–3 hours. 3A4 has been shown to N-dealkylate sufentanil (Tateishi et al. 1996), but a small amount of sufentanil may be O-demethylated by 2D6. As with other fentanils that rely on 3A4 for clearance, caution is advised when sufentanil is administered with 3A4 inhibitors or inducers. To date, there are very few reports of interactions, and a potent 3A4 inhibitor had no effect on the terminal half-life of sufentanil in one small series (Bartkowski et al. 1993).

Diphenoxylate and Loperamide

Diphenoxylate and loperamide (Imodium) are phenylpiperidine derivatives, but they are not normally CNS-acting analgesics. Both compounds are used to relieve diarrhea and are taken orally. Diphenoxylate is commonly combined with atropine in a formulation called Lomotil.

Diphenoxylate and loperamide have opiate activity outside the CNS. Loperamide is a P-glycoprotein substrate (Sadeque et al. 2000), which is the major reason the drug lacks CNS opiate activity. P-glycoprotein is a major component of the blood-brain barrier, and therefore P-glycoprotein prevents substrates from entering the CNS. It is unclear whether diphenoxylate is a P-glycoprotein substrate, but we suspect that it may be. Other phenylpiperidine analogs are *not* P-glycoprotein substrates, which may be why they are effective in the CNS (Wandel et al. 2002).

In eight healthy control subjects, use of loperamide with a known P-glycoprotein inhibitor, quinidine, resulted in respiratory depression, despite the fact that serum loperamide levels were unchanged (Sadeque et al. 2000). This effect did not occur with administration of loperamide alone. The implications are clear: use of loperamide (and perhaps diphenoxylate) with a P-glycoprotein inhibitor can lead to CNS opiate effects by inhibiting or disabling the blood-brain barrier. Some P-glycoprotein inhibitors (such as cyclosporine, quinidine, ritonavir, and verapamil [Bendayan et al. 2002]) are widely available by prescription. Thus, there is the potential for an untoward drug interaction or for abuse, with use of a P-glycoprotein inhibitor and either of these two over-the-counter antidiarrheals.

■ MORPHINE AND RELATED SEMISYNTHETIC OR SYNTHETIC OPIATES

Opium, derived from seeds of the poppy plant, is a combination of several distinct alkaloids. Many of these alkaloids—including morphine, heroin, codeine, and papaverine—have pharmacological activity. Morphine and nearly all its related chemicals have some opiate receptor activity. The basic structure of morphine and all related opiates is found in Figure 18–3.

The 3-, 6-, and 17- positions are the three key sites where various substitutions by methyl, ester, and hydroxyl groups occur to form different drugs. Morphine has hydroxyl groups at carbon positions 3 and 6 and a methyl group at the 17-*N* position. Codeine is created by adding a methyl group to the 3- position hydroxyl group. (Other synthetic narcotics are made by substituting at the 3-, 6-, and 17- positions and with a single bond between carbons 7 and 8.) The 3-, 6-, and 17- positions are very important in metabolism because they are the sites oxidized by P450 enzymes. These oxidative reactions ease glucuronidation in the liver, by UGTs, at the 3- and 6- positions. The 3- and 6- positions are often referred to as the *O* and *N* sites, respectively, in regard to oxidative P450 metabolism.

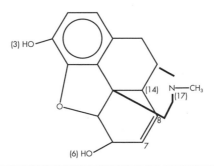

FIGURE 18–3. **Basic structure of morphine and all related opiates.**

329

■ MORPHINE-LIKE OPIATES, METHADONE-LIKE OPIATES, AND TRAMADOL

Drug	P450 enzymes drug is metabolized by	Other enzymes drug is metabolized by	Enzyme(s) inhibited	Pro-drug?[1]
Buprenorphine (Buprenex)	3A4, ?2D6	UGT2B7 metabolizes 3A4 metabolite	None	No
Codeine	3A4 (10%), 2D6 (5%)	UGT2B7 (80%)	UGT2B7	No[2]
Hydrocodone (Vicodin [with acetaminophen])	2D6, 3A4	Reduction by unknown enzymes	None	Yes[3]
Hydromorphone (Dilaudid)	None	UGT1A3, UGT2B7, others	None	No
Methadone	3A4, ?2D6	None known	3A4, ?UGT2B7	No
Morphine	Small amounts by 2D6 and 3A4	UGT2B7, UGT1A3	UGT2B7	Yes[4]
Nalbuphine (Nubain)	?Unspecified P450 enzymes	Reduction by unknown enzymes; conjugated by UGT2B7	None	No
Naloxone (Narcan)	None	UGT2B7	None	No
Naltrexone (ReVia)	?Unspecified P450 enzymes	Reduction by unknown enzymes; conjugated by UGT2B7	None	No
Oxycodone (OxyContin)	2D6, ?3A4	2D6 metabolite, oxymorphone, glucuronidated with UGT2B7	None	No[5]

■ MORPHINE-LIKE OPIATES, METHADONE-LIKE OPIATES, AND TRAMADOL (continued)

Drug	P450 enzymes drug is metabolized by	Other enzymes drug is metabolized by	Enzyme(s) inhibited	Pro-drug?[1]
Oxymorphone (Numorphan)	None	UGT2B7, others	None	No
Propoxyphene (Darvon)	3A4	None known	3A4	Yes[6]
Tramadol (Ultram)	2D6, 3A4, 2B6	Unspecified UGTs	None	Yes[7]

Note. UGT=uridine 5'-diphosphate glucuronosyltransferase.

[1]Drug is metabolized to an active analgesic metabolite.

[2]It is doubtful that codeine is a pro-drug from 2D6 activity. If codeine is a pro-drug, it may be from UGT2B7 conversion to codeine-6-glucuronide.

[3]Hydrocodone is metabolized by 2D6 to hydromorphone, which may be a significant component of hydrocodone's analgesia efficacy.

[4]Morphine is metabolized by UGT2B7 to morphine-6-glucuronide, which is more potent than morphine.

[5]Oxycodone is metabolized by 2D6 to hydrocodone; however, oxycodone is a very good analgesic independently.

[6]Propoxyphene is metabolized by 3A4 to norpropoxyphene—a potent analgesic along with the parent compound, but with central nervous system toxicity.

[7]Tramadol is metabolized by 2D6 to an active analgesic metabolite. The metabolite, M1, has been confirmed in controlled trials to be correlated with analgesic efficacy.

Some morphine-related analgesics inhibit metabolic enzymes, but none are known to be potent inhibitors (see "Morphine-like Opiates, Methadone-like Opiates, and Tramadol" table). In addition, none of the morphine-related analgesics induce any metabolic enzymes. Several of these agents are pro-drugs or are theorized to be pro-drugs. Details regarding the morphine-related analgesics are presented here.

Morphine

Morphine is the principal alkaloid obtained from unripened seed capsules of the opium poppy. It can also be made in the laboratory. Morphine is metabolized chiefly through glucuronidation. UGT2B7 (de Wildt et al. 1999) and UGT1A3 (Green et al. 1998) appear to be the major UGTs involved. The glucuronides are 3-glucuronide (50%), 6-glucuronide, and 3/6-glucuronide. Morphine-6-glucuronide (M6G) is more potent as an analgesic than is morphine itself (Lotsch and Geisslinger 2001)—possibly 50 times more potent (Christrup 1997). M6G is chiefly metabolized by UGT2B7 (Coffman et al. 1997) and has been proposed as a possible analgesic. The 3-glucuronide has few analgesic properties but may cause CNS neuroexcitatory effects (Smith 2000). Although codeine is structurally almost identical to morphine (see "Codeine," later in the chapter) and is metabolized to some extent by P450 enzymes, it is unclear whether morphine is also oxidatively metabolized by the P450 system, and any amount of P450 metabolism is probably small. Inhibition of UGT2B7 could decrease morphine's analgesia as a result of a decrease in M6G production, but there are no reports of this interaction to date.

Morphine has been shown to competitively inhibit UGTs—probably UGT2B7 (Grancharov et al. 2001)—and morphine has been shown to increase zidovudine (AZT) levels via this mechanism.

Hydromorphone and Oxymorphone

Hydromorphone (Dilaudid) and oxymorphone (Numorphan) are chemically almost identical to morphine; hydromorphone differs only in that it has an =O (keto) group at the 6- position (morphine has an –OH, hydroxyl), and oxymorphone is similar to hydromorphone except an –OH group is added to carbon position 14 in oxymorphone. In addition, unlike morphine, both hydromorphone and oxymorphone have a single bond between carbons 7 and 8.

Hydromorphone is metabolized at the 3- and 6-positions to form glucuronides via UGTs, including UGT1A3 and UGT2B7 (Green et al. 1998; Radominska-Pandya et al. 1999). Oxidative metabolism with P450 enzymes appears to be minimal. There is reduction of the 6-glucuronide to form dihydromorphone, which is not active as an analgesic in humans. Hydromorphone has not been shown to inhibit any enzymes. Similar to morphine's, hydromorphone's 3-glucuronide may be CNS toxic (Smith 2000) and has been shown to cause seizures in rats (Wright et al. 1998).

Like hydromorphone, oxymorphone is metabolized by several UGTs, with the 6-glucuronide being created primarily by UGT2B7 (Numorphan 2002; Radominska-Pandya et al. 1999). Oxymorphone is only available parenterally and is a potent analgesic.

Codeine

Codeine is very similar in structure to morphine, with the only difference being a methyl group attached to the 3-hydroxyl site of morphine. They have a methyl group at the *N*-17 site of the molecule and a hydroxyl group at the 6- position. These three sites are the main sites of metabolism of all morphinelike derivatives.

Eighty percent of codeine is glucuronidated as codeine-6-glucuronide (Vree et al. 2000), 5% is oxidatively metabolized by 2D6 via O-3-demethylation, and 10% is N-6-demethylated by 3A4. The 2D6 O-demethylation creates morphine, and the 3A4 N-demethylation creates norcodeine (Caraco et al. 1996). Norcodeine has few analgesic properties. Codeine itself is a poor analgesic, and therefore its metabolites are believed to be the key to the drug's efficacy as an analgesic.

In the early to mid-1990s, investigators hypothesized that much of codeine's analgesia is due to its conversion to morphine by 2D6.

In their review, Sindrup and Brosen (1995) further hypothesized that the analgesic effect of codeine would be lessened in 2D6 poor metabolizers (PMs) or by inhibitors of 2D6 (such as fluoxetine or paroxetine) through reduction of the amount of morphine created. However, over the last few years, several reports have seemed to indicate that this interaction may not be so significant:

- Poulsen et al. (1998) have presented the most definitive study. They looked at 81 patients with postoperative pain and found 8 genotypic PMs at 2D6. Codeine was used as the analgesic in all patients, and morphine and M6G levels were measured and compared with self-reports of analgesia. Although patients who reported poor analgesia did have lower morphine and M6G levels, the decrease in levels and analgesia did not correspond to the 2D6 phenotype.

- Wilder-Smith et al. (1998) studied a compound called dihydrocodeine. It is structurally very similar to codeine, except that it has a single bond between carbons 7 and 8, instead of a double bond as in codeine. Wilder-Smith et al. reported that dihydrocodeine is metabolized to dihydromorphine by 2D6. Similarly, dihydrocodeine is principally glucuronidated at the 6- position by UGT2B7 (Kirkwood et al. 1998). Wilder-Smith and colleagues (1998) looked at pain and heat thresholds in volunteers given dihydrocodeine alone or dihydrocodeine and the potent 2D6 inhibitor quinidine. Dihydromorphine production was decreased with quinidine coadministration, but concomitant use of the two drugs did not alter reports of dihydrocodeine-produced analgesia.

- It was also supposed that PMs at 2D6 might be at less risk for codeine dependence because no morphine is created to induce a "high." Fernandes et al. (2002) administered fluoxetine, quinidine, or placebo to 30 patients to determine whether codeine use would decrease. Codeine use decreased the same amount (roughly 50%) in all groups, including the placebo group.

- Finally, Vree et al. (2000) hypothesized that codeine-6-glucuronide (C6G), the main metabolite of codeine formed by UGT2B7, is the main compound that gives codeine its analgesia. C6G is very similar in structure to M6G, which is a very potent analgesic—much more potent than morphine itself. It has not yet been proven, however, that C6G is a potent analgesic.

Given this information, we believe that the analgesic response to codeine is not typically altered in 2D6 PMs or by 2D6 inhibitors. This mechanism has been reported to occur in individual cases, but as the findings of the study by Poulsen et al. (1998) imply, there may be other reasons for a poor analgesic response to codeine. Finally, it should be noted that if 5% of codeine is metabolized by 2D6 to morphine, that percentage is the equivalent of 3 mg of morphine from 60 mg of oral codeine—a morphine dose that is generally considered very inadequate for analgesia.

Codeine may inhibit UGT2B7, perhaps through its metabolite C6G (Grancharov et al. 2001).

Codeine has an isomer. In the *S* form, it is codeine. In the *R* form, it is the over-the-counter antitussive dextromethorphan. Dextromethorphan lacks CNS opiate activity but does have antitussive activity. Its metabolism appears to be similar to that of codeine in that dextromethorphan is O-demethylated by 2D6 and N-demethylated by 3A4. The 2D6 reaction gives rise to dextrophan, and the secretion of this product can be used to determine 2D6 activity (see Chapter 5 ["2D6"]) because no other enzyme creates dextrophan from dextromethorphan.

Hydrocodone and Oxycodone

Hydrocodone (Vicodin [with acetaminophen]) and oxycodone (Oxy-Contin) are chemically similar to codeine. They both have a single bond between carbons 7 and 8 (codeine has a double bond there). Hydrocodone has an =O (keto) instead of a hydroxyl moiety at the 6-carbon site. Oxycodone is similar to hydrocodone, with the simple addition of a hydroxyl group at the 14-carbon site.

Hydrocodone is O-3-demethylated by 2D6 to hydromorphone (Otton et al. 1993). N-6-Demethylation occurs as well, probably via 3A4. Hydrocodone is also reduced at the 6- position to a keto group by an unknown enzyme or enzymes that create active metabolites.

Hydromorphone has more affinity at the μ receptor than does hydrocodone. Therefore, it is theorized that poorer analgesic responses to hydrocodone will occur in PMs at 2D6 or with coadministration of 2D6 inhibitors (a theory similar to one regarding codeine). Results of studies conducted to test this theory are conflicting. One small study showed that being an extensive metabolizer or PM at 2D6 does not predict hydrocodone abuse liability (Kaplan et al. 1997). In contrast, Tyndale et al. (1997) showed that PMs are underrepresented as opiate abusers. Unfortunately, the study did not distinguish between the three codeinelike drugs. The only published study of inhibition of 2D6 in analgesia was by Lelas et al. (1999). In that study, use of 2D6 inhibitors did change the analgesic response to hydrocodone, but the study was performed in rhesus monkeys, and the findings are not easily applied to humans. Nevertheless, it is plausible that hydrocodone's transformation in humans by 2D6 is more important for analgesic efficacy than codeine's similar transformation, because hydrocodone's clearance is more dependent on oxidative reactions than is codeine's and because little glucuronidation of hydrocodone occurs (Cone et al. 1978). Thus, we believe that there is some evidence that hydrocodone's effectiveness could be affected by 2D6 inhibitors or in PMs at 2D6.

Oxycodone is a potent analgesic itself, so inhibition of its metabolism should not decrease its effectiveness, but inhibition could increase its effectiveness or cause excessive CNS opioid effects. Oxycodone is O-3-demethylated by 2D6 to oxymorphone and probably N-6-demethylated by 3A4 to noroxycodone. In a study involving concomitant use of quinidine, a potent 2D6 inhibitor, oxycodone's metabolism to oxymorphone was completely stopped (Heiskanen et al. 1998). However, the effects of oxycodone (by subjective measures and in terms of psychomotor functions) did not differ in subjects who received quinidine and those who did not. We would argue that 2D6 inhibitors or PMs taking oxycodone could, however, have *increased* opiate effects over time, because oxy-codone is often prescribed for long periods, unlike in this study.

Ultimately, oxycodone's oxidative metabolites are glucuroni-dated. The 2D6 metabolite of oxycodone, oxymorphone, is known to be glucuronidated with UGT2B7 (see "Hydromorphone and Oxy-morphone," earlier in the chapter).

Buprenorphine

Buprenorphine (Buprenex) is a powerful semisynthetic morphine-like drug with mixed agonist/antagonist properties. It is extensively metabolized by 3A4 via N-6-dealkylation (Kobayashi et al. 1998). These metabolites are further conjugated by UGTs—most likely UGT2B7 and UGT1A3 (Green et al. 1998). Because of buprenor-phine's reliance on 3A4, caution is advised when the drug is used with 3A4 inhibitors and 3A4 inducers (Buprenex 2001).

Nalbuphine

Nalbuphine (Nubain) is a semisynthetic morphine-like mixed opi-ate agonist/antagonist. Because of extensive first-pass elimination, it is used only parenterally. The enzyme or enzymes responsible for clearance have not been well characterized, but clearance appears to involve both oxidative enzymes and glucuronidation (Yoo et al. 1995). Pharmacokinetic drug-drug interactions involving nalbuphine have been little studied.

Naloxone

Naloxone (Narcan) is a semisynthetic opioid compound with a structure similar to that of morphine but with opiate antagonist properties. It is chiefly metabolized by UGT2B7 (Coffman et al. 2001; de Wildt et al. 1999). Because naloxone does not rely on P450 enzymes for metabolism, untoward pharmacokinetic drug-drug in-teractions have *not* been reported. The main concern is that a phar-macodynamic event might occur with inadvertent use in a patient who is dependent on opiates.

Naltrexone

Naltrexone (ReVia) is a semisynthetic opiate antagonist. It is very similar in structure to naloxone, but naltrexone has a much longer half-life and is effective orally, whereas naloxone is not effective orally because of extensive first-pass metabolism. Naltrexone is oxidatively metabolized to several metabolites by unknown enzymes. These products are then glucuronidated, presumably by UGT2B7 (Radominska-Pandya et al. 1999). Very little study has been done of pharmacokinetic drug-drug interactions involving naltrexone.

■ METHADONE AND PROPOXYPHENE

Methadone

Methadone's structure does not resemble that of morphine or morphinelike compounds. Steric factors appear to force the molecule into a pseudopiperidine ring, thought to be essential to its opioid activity.

Methadone is a powerful opiate agonist. It is N-demethylated by 3A4 (Iribarne et al. 1996) and perhaps secondarily by 2D6 (DeVane and Nemeroff 2002). When this agent is administered with an inducer of 3A4, opiate withdrawal may occur. Altice et al. (1999) reported on a series of seven HIV-positive patients in a methadone maintenance program who were administered the antiviral nevirapine (Viramune), an inducer of 3A4. The patients developed opiate withdrawal symptoms. There are also reports of methadone withdrawal with coadministration of rifampin, another potent 3A4 inducer (Holmes 1990; Kreek et al. 1976). Altice and colleagues (1999) suggested that methadone and rifampin may be coadministered if higher doses of methadone are prescribed. Caution is needed if patients discontinue taking the inducing medication (nevirapine, rifampin, carbamazepine, phenobarbital, phenytoin), because it may take several weeks for the effects of induction to diminish, and opiate toxicity may gradually develop if patients are not simultaneously weaned from opiate therapy.

Methadone is also subject to inhibition by potent 3A4 inhibitors, but these findings have been inconsistent. Fluvoxamine, not a particularly strong 3A4 inhibitor, increased methadone levels (DeMaria and Serota 1999; Eap et al. 1997). In a double-blind study, chronic methadone users counterintuitively increased their use of methadone with concomitant administration of ketoconazole (Kosten et al. 2002). Iribarne et al. (1997) reported in vitro evidence that methadone is an inhibitor at 3A4 as well. Finally, methadone may inhibit UGT2B7 (Trapnell et al. 1998).

Propoxyphene

Propoxyphene (Darvon) is a synthetic opiate agonist with a structure similar to that of methadone. Its metabolism is not well defined, and most that is known about it is in question. It appears to be oxidatively metabolized by N-dealkylation to norpropoxyphene (Spina et al. 1996), and this reaction is believed to be catalyzed by 3A4 and may inhibit 3A4 (Spina et al. 1996). Norpropoxyphene is an active metabolite with a long half-life (30 hours), whereas the parent compound's half-life is only 6–12 hours. Norpropoxyphene, like normeperidine, has CNS stimulatory effects. Although no definitive studies or cases have been reported at the time of this writing, caution is advised when propoxyphene is used with 3A4 inhibitors or inducers.

■ TRAMADOL

Tramadol (Ultram) is an analgesic with a low affinity for opioid receptors. It is chemically related to codeine but has unique features that make it a very weak opiate agonist. Its mechanism of action with regard to analgesia is unclear.

Tramadol may be an inactive pro-drug that requires phase I metabolism to become efficacious.

Tramadol is O-demethylated by 2D6 from parent drug to active metabolite, called M1. The (+)-M1 isomer is associated with better pain control (Sindrup et al. 1999). 3A4 and 2B6 are involved in the metabolism of tramadol to other metabolites, and the drug is also conjugated by UGTs (Subrahmanyam et al. 2001; Ultram 2000).

PMs at 2D6 may have little or no analgesic response to tramadol. Poulsen et al. (1996) showed that a distinct difference in analgesic response could be detected in PMs at 2D6 compared with extensive metabolizers. We believe that evidence for the reliance of tramadol on 2D6 for efficacy is fairly strong. Tramadol may truly be a pro-drug, requiring 2D6 activity for adequate efficacy. However, tram-adol and its 2D6 metabolite, M1, are very poor μ agonists. The ac-tual mechanism behind tramadol's analgesia is unclear. Serotonin and norepinephrine receptor effects with M1 and other metabolites probably contribute greatly to tramadol's analgesic effects. Despite this caveat, we urge clinicians to use caution when administering tramadol with potent 2D6 inhibitors. Patients who have a poor anal-gesic response to tramadol may be phenotypic PMs at 2D6.

■ REFERENCES

Ahonen J, Olkkola KT, Salmenpera M, et al: Effect of diltiazem on midazo-lam and alfentanil disposition in patients undergoing coronary artery by-pass grafting. Anesthesiology 85:1246–1252, 1996

Altice FL, Friedland GH, Cooney EL: Nevirapine induced opiate with-drawal among injection drug users with HIV infection receiving metha-done. AIDS 13:957–962, 1999

Bartkowski RR, Goldberg ME, Larijani GE, et al: Inhibition of alfentanil metabolism by erythromycin. Clin Pharmacol Ther 46:99–102, 1989

Bartkowski RR, Goldberg ME, Huffnagle S, et al: Sufentanil disposition. Is it affected by erythromycin administration? Anesthesiology 78:260–265, 1993

Bendayan R, Lee G, Bendayan M: Functional expression and localization of P-glycoprotein at the blood brain barrier. Microsc Res Tech 57:365–380, 2002

Buprenex (package insert). Hull, England, Reckitt Benckiser Healthcare (UK) Ltd, 2001

Caraco Y, Tateishi T, Guengerich FP, et al: Microsomal codeine N-demeth-ylation: cosegregation with cytochrome P4503A4 activity. Drug Metab Dispos 24:761–764, 1996

Christrup LL: Morphine metabolites. Acta Anaesthesiol Scand 41:116–122, 1997

Coffman BL, Rios GR, King CD, et al: Human UGT2B7 catalyzes morphine glucuronidation. Drug Metab Dispos 25:1–4, 1997

Coffman BL, Kearney WR, Green MD, et al: Analysis of opioid binding to UDP-glucuronosyltransferase 2B7 fusion proteins using nuclear resonance spectroscopy. Mol Pharmacol 59(6):1464–1469, 2001

Cone EJ, Darwin WD, Gorodetzky CW, et al: Comparative metabolism of hydrocodone in man, rat, guinea pig, rabbit, and dog. Drug Metab Dispos 6:488–493, 1978

DeMaria PA Jr, Serota RD: A therapeutic use of the methadone fluvoxamine drug interaction. J Addict Dis 18:5–12, 1999

Demerol (package insert). New York, NY, Sanofi-Synthelabo, 2000

DeVane CL, Nemeroff CB: 2002 guide to psychotropic drug interactions. Primary Psychiatry 9:28–57, 2002

de Wildt SN, Kearns GL, Leeder JS, et al: Glucuronidation in humans. Pharmacogenetic and developmental aspects. Clin Pharmacokinet 36:439–452, 1999

Eap CB, Bertschy G, Powell K, et al: Fluvoxamine and fluoxetine do not interact in the same way with the metabolism of the enantiomers of methadone. J Clin Psychopharmacol 17:113–117, 1997

Fernandes LC, Kilicarslan T, Kaplan HL, et al: Treatment of codeine dependence with inhibitors of cytochrome P450 2D6. J Clin Psychopharmacol 22:326–329, 2002

Goodman and Gilman's The Pharmacological Basis of Therapeutics, 6th Edition. New York, Macmillan, 1980

Grancharov K, Naydenova Z, Lozeva S, et al: Natural and synthetic inhibitors of UDP-glucuronosyltranferase. Pharmacol Ther 89:171–186, 2001

Green MD, King CD, Mojarrabi B, et al: Glucuronidation of amines and other xenobiotics catalyzed by expressed human UDP-glucuronosyltransferase 1A3. Drug Metab Dispos 26:507–512, 1998

Haigh CG: Drug development in anaesthesia: the remifentanil. Minerva Anestesiol 66:414–416, 2000

Hawes EM: N+-Glucuronidation, a common pathway in human metabolism of drugs with a tertiary amine group. Drug Metab Dispos 26:830–837, 1998

Heiskanen T, Olkkola KT, Kalso E: Effects of blocking CYP2D6 on the pharmacokinetics and pharmacodynamics of oxycodone. Clin Pharmacol Ther 64:603–611, 1998

Holmes VF: Rifampin-induced methadone withdrawal in AIDS (letter). J Clin Psychopharmacol 10:443–444, 1990

Iribarne C, Berthou F, Baird S, et al: Involvement of cytochrome P450 3A4 enzyme in the N-demethylation of methadone in human liver microsomes. Chem Res Toxicol 9:365–373, 1996

Iribarne C, Dreano Y, Bardou LG, et al: Interaction of methadone with substrates of human hepatic cytochrome P450 3A4. Toxicology 117:13–23, 1997

Kaplan HL, Busto UE, Baylon GJ, et al: Inhibition of cytochrome P450 2D6 metabolism of hydrocodone to hydromorphone does not importantly affect abuse liability. J Pharmacol Exp Ther 281:103–108, 1997

Kharasch ED, Russell M, Mautz D, et al: The role of cytochrome P450 3A4 in alfentanil clearance. Implications for interindividual variability in disposition and perioperative drug interactions. Anesthesiology 87:36–50, 1997

Kirkwood LC, Nation RL, Somogyi AA: Glucuronidation of dihydrocodeine by human liver microsomes and the effect of inhibitors. Clin Exp Pharmacol Physiol 25:266–270, 1998

Kobayashi K, Yamamoto T, Chiba K, et al: Human buprenorphine N-dealkylation is catalyzed by cytochrome P450 3A4. Drug Metab Dispos 26:818–821, 1998

Kosten TR, Oliveto A, Sevarino KA, et al: Ketoconazole increases cocaine and opioid use in methadone maintained patients. Drug Alcohol Depend 66:173–180, 2002

Kreek MJ, Garfield JW, Gutjahr CL, et al: Rifampin-induced methadone withdrawal. N Engl J Med 294:1104–1106, 1976

Labroo RB, Thummel KE, Kunze KL, et al: Catalytic role of cytochrome P4503A4 in multiple pathways of alfentanil metabolism. Drug Metab Dispos 23:490–496, 1995

Labroo RB, Paine MF, Thummel KE, et al: Fentanyl metabolism by human hepatic and intestinal cytochrome P450 3A4: implications for interindividual variability in disposition, efficacy, and drug interactions. Drug Metab Dispos 25:1072–1080, 1997

Lelas S, Wegert S, Otton SV, et al: Inhibitors of cytochrome P450 differentially modify discriminative-stimulus and antinociceptive effects of hydrocodone and hydromorphone in rhesus monkeys. Drug Alcohol Depend 54:239–249, 1999

Lotsch J, Geisslinger G: Morphine-6-glucuronide: an analgesic of the future? Clin Pharmacokinet 40:485–499, 2001

342

Numorphan (package insert). Chadds Ford, PA, Endo Pharmaceuticals Inc., 2002

Oda Y, Mizutani K, Hase I, et al: Fentanyl inhibits metabolism of midazolam: competitive inhibition of CYP3A4 in vitro. Br J Anaesth 82:900–903, 1999

Olkkola KT, Palkama VJ, Neuvonen PJ: Ritonavir's role in reducing fentanyl clearance and prolonging its half-life. Anesthesiology 91:681–685, 1999

Otton SV, Schadel M, Cheung SW, et al: CYP2D6 phenotype determines the metabolic conversion of hydrocodone to hydromorphone. Clin Pharmacol Ther 54:463–472, 1993

Palkama VJ, Isohanni MH, Neuvonen PJ, et al: The effect of intravenous and oral fluconazole on the pharmacokinetics and pharmacodynamics of intravenous alfentanil. Anesth Analg 87:190–194, 1998a

Palkama VJ, Neuvonen PJ, Olkkola KT: The CYP 3A4 inhibitor itraconazole has no effect on the pharmacokinetics of i.v. fentanyl. Br J Anaesth 81:598–600, 1998b

Piscitelli SC, Kress DR, Bertz RJ, et al: The effect of ritonavir on the pharmacokinetics of meperidine and normeperidine. Pharmacotherapy 20: 549–553, 2000

Poulsen L, Arendt-Nielsen L, Brosen K, et al: The hypoalgesic effect of tramadol in relation to CYP2D6. Clin Pharmacol Ther 60:636–644, 1996

Poulsen L, Riishede L, Brosen K, et al: Codeine in post-operative pain. Study of the influence of sparteine phenotype and serum concentrations of morphine and morphine-6-glucuronide. Eur J Clin Pharmacol 54: 451–454, 1998

Radominska-Pandya A, Czernik PJ, Little JM, et al: Structural and functional studies of UDP-glucuronosyltransferases. Drug Metab Rev 31:817–899, 1999

Sadeque AJ, Wandel C, He H, et al: Increased drug delivery to the brain by P-glycoprotein inhibition. Clin Pharmacol Ther 68:231–237, 2000

Sindrup SH, Brosen K: The pharmacogenetics of codeine hypoalgesia. Pharmacogenetics 5:335–346, 1995

Sindrup SH, Madsen C, Brosen K, et al: The effect of tramadol in painful polyneuropathy in relation to serum drug and metabolite levels. Clin Pharmacol Ther 66:636–641, 1999

Smith MT: Neuroexcitatory effects of morphine and hydromorphone: evidence implicating the 3-glucuronide metabolites. Clin Exp Pharmacol Physiol 27:524–528, 2000

Spina E, Pisani F, Perucca E: Clinically significant pharmacokinetic drug interactions with carbamazepine: an update. Clin Pharmacokinet 31:198–214, 1996

Stambaugh JE, Wainer IW, Schwartz I: The effect of phenobarbital on the metabolism of meperidine in normal volunteers. J Clin Pharmacol 18: 482–490, 1978

Subrahmanyam V, Renwick AB, Walters DG, et al: Identification of cytochrome P-450 isoforms responsible for cis-tramadol metabolism in human liver microsomes. Drug Metab Dispos 29:1146–1155, 2001

Tateishi T, Krivoruk Y, Ueng YF, et al: Identification of human liver cytochrome P-450 3A4 as the enzyme responsible for fentanyl and sufentanil N-dealkylation. Anesth Analg 82:167–172, 1996

Trapnell CB, Klecker RW, Jamis-Dow C, et al: Glucuronidation of 3'-azido-3'-deoxythymidine (zidovudine) by human liver microsomes: relevance to clinical pharmacokinetic interactions with atovaquone, fluconazole, methadone, and valproic acid. Antimicrob Agents Chemother 42:1592–1596, 1998

Tyndale RF, Droll KP, Sellers EM: Genetically deficient CYP2D6 metabolism provides protection against oral opiate dependence. Pharmacogenetics 7:375–379, 1997

Ultram (package insert). Raritan, NJ, Ortho-McNeil Pharmaceutical Inc., 2000

Umehara K, Shimokawa Y, Miyamoto G: Inhibition of human drug metabolizing cytochrome P450 by buprenorphine. Biol Pharm Bull 25:682–685, 2002

Vree TB, van Dongen RT, Koopman-Kimenai PM: Codeine analgesia is due to codeine-6-glucuronide, not morphine. Int J Clin Pract 54:395–398, 2000

Wandel C, Kim R, Wood M, et al: Interaction of morphine, fentanyl, sufentanil, alfentanil, and loperamide with the efflux drug transporter P-glycoprotein. Anesthesiology 96:913–920, 2002

Wilder-Smith CH, Hufschmid E, Thorman W: The visceral and somatic antinociceptive effects of dihydrocodeine and its metabolite, dihydromorphine. A cross-over study with extensive and quinidine-induced poor metabolizers. Br J Pharmacol 45:575–581, 1998

Wright AW, Nocente ML, Smith MT: Hydromorphone-3-glucuronide: biosynthesis and preliminary pharmacological evaluation. Life Sci 63: 401–411, 1998

Yoo YC, Chung HS, Kim IS, et al: Determination of nalbuphine in drug abuser's urine. J Anal Toxicol 19:120–123, 1995

19

PSYCHIATRY

Tricyclic antidepressants (TCAs), typical antipsychotics, lithium, and benzodiazepines were the mainstay of psychiatric interventions until the last 20 years, when many new drugs became available. Surprisingly little is known about the metabolism of the older drugs. Fifteen years ago, P450 bench techniques were in their infancy, and U.S. Food and Drug Administration requirements were less stringent. Currently, there is little incentive for drug companies to conduct research on older drugs after their patents have expired. In this chapter, we review the psychotropic drugs in groups: antidepressants (selective serotonin reuptake inhibitors [SSRIs], other commonly used antidepressants, and tricyclics), anxiolytics and hypnotics (benzodiazepines and others), antipsychotics, and drugs to treat attention-deficit/hyperactivity disorder (ADHD). Drugs used for the treatment of seizure disorders are often used as mood stabilizers, and they are discussed in Chapter 15 ("Neurology").

> **Reminder:** This chapter is dedicated primarily to metabolic and P-glycoprotein interactions. Interactions due to displaced protein-binding, alterations in absorption or excretion, and pharmacodynamics are not covered.

■ ANTIDEPRESSANTS

Selective Serotonin Reuptake Inhibitors

Each of the six selective serotonin reuptake inhibitors (SSRIs) has unique P450 metabolisms and inhibitions. Their active metabolites also contribute to drug interactions (e.g., norfluoxetine is a mild to moderate inhibitor of 3A4, whereas its parent compound has less inhibitory ability). Because norfluoxetine has a long half-life (7–17 days [Brunswick et al. 2001]), P450 inhibitions continue after treatment with fluoxetine (Prozac) has been discontinued. Because many of the SSRI-drug interactions are discussed at length in other chapters, only basic information about SSRI P450 metabolism and inhibition is included here.

Citalopram and S-*Citalopram*

Citalopram (Celexa) is a chiral drug. Its more pharmacologically active enantiomer, *S*-citalopram (Lexapro), was introduced into the United States market as an antidepressant in its own right. Both citalopram and *S*-citalopram undergo a series of demethylation steps at 2C19, 2D6, and 3A4. Both drugs mildly inhibit 2D6 (Greenblatt et al. 1999; von Moltke et al. 2001). Because of the diversity of metabolic pathways and the relative lack of P450 inhibition, there are few drug interactions involving either citalopram or *S*-citalopram (Brosen and Naranjo 2001). However, drug concentrations of both can decrease when carbamazepine or another "pan-inducer" is coadministered (Steinacher et al. 2002).

Fluoxetine

Fluoxetine (Prozac) is also a chiral drug. In clinical trials, however, use of the *R*-enantiomer as an antidepressant resulted in cardiac toxicity. Fluoxetine and its long-lived metabolite norfluoxetine are substrates of 2C9, 2C19, 3A4, and 2D6 (Greenblatt et al. 1999; Ring et al. 2001). Together, they are potent inhibitors of 2D6 and mild to moderate inhibitors of 2B6, 2C9, 2C19, and 3A4 (Greenblatt et al. 1999; Hesse et al. 2000). Because of fluoxetine's multiple metabolic pathways, levels are not usually altered by P450 inhibitors. However, metabolism of the drug can be vulnerable to the older anticonvulsants that are P450 pan-inducers. Fluoxetine's potent inhibition of 2D6 means that patients taking fluoxetine and 2D6 substrates are particularly at risk for increased concentrations of the substrates (e.g., desip-

■ SELECTIVE SEROTONIN REUPTAKE INHIBITORS

Drug	Major metabolism site(s)	Enzyme(s)/process inhibited
Citalopram (Celexa)	2C19, 2D6, 3A4	2D6[c]
S-Citalopram (Lexapro)	2C19, 2D6, 3A4	2D6[c]
Fluoxetine (Prozac)	2C9, 2C19, 2D6, 3A4	1A2,[c] 2B6,[b] 2C9,[b] **2C19, 2D6**,[a] 3A4[b]
Fluvoxamine (Luvox)	1A2, 2D6	**1A2**,[a] 2B6,[b] 2C9,[b] **2C19**,[a] 2D6,[b] 3A4[b]
Paroxetine (Paxil)	2D6	1A2,[c] **2B6**,[a] 2C9,[c] 2C19,[c] **2D6**,[a] 3A4[b]
Sertraline (Zoloft)	2B6, 2C9, 2C19, 2D6, 3A4	1A2,[c] 2B6,[b] 2D6,[a,b*] 3A4,[b] glucuronidation

Note. Data presented relate to parent drug and metabolites combined.

*Sertraline is a potent 2D6 inhibitor at high concentrations (typically at dosages > 200 mg/day).

[a]Potent (**bold** type).

[b]Moderate.

[c]Mild.

ramine's [Norpramin's] concentration is increased fourfold [Preskorn et al. 1994] (see Chapter 5 ["2D6"]). Because fluoxetine inhibits other P450 enzymes in addition to 2D6, clinicians treating patients receiving fluoxetine should be cautious about adding drugs that are metabolized via 2D6 and other affected P450 enzymes. When fluoxetine and risperidone (Risperdal) are coadministered, the concentration of risperidone increases 75% because both fluoxetine and norfluoxetine inhibit 2D6 and 3A4 (Spina et al. 2002).

Fluvoxamine

Fluvoxamine (Luvox) is an achiral drug that has no significant metabolites. It is a substrate of 2D6 and 1A2 (Spigset et al. 2001). Fluvoxamine is best described as a "pan-inhibitor" because it is a potent inhibitor of 1A2 and 2C19 even at low doses (Christensen et al. 2002), a mild to moderate inhibitor of 2B6, 2C9, and 3A4, and a mild inhibitor of 2D6 (Hesse et al. 2000). The possible drug interactions associated with fluvoxamine's P450 inhibitions are legion. Particularly important are interactions with drugs that have narrow therapeutic indices, such as theophylline (see Chapter 7 ["1A2"]), warfarin (see Chapter 8 ["2C9"]), phenytoin (see Chapters 8 ["2C9"] and 9 ["2C19"]), and the tertiary TCAs. When adding *any* drug to fluvoxamine therapy, clinicians are advised to be cautious—"starting low and going slow," measuring blood levels, and watching carefully for signs of toxicity. Concentrations of fluvoxamine, a substrate of 1A2, may be decreased when 1A2 is induced by cigarette smoke (Yoshimura et al. 2002) (see Chapter 7 ["1A2"] for a discussion of tobacco smoke as a 1A2 inducer).

Paroxetine

Paroxetine (Paxil) is marketed as the *S*-enantiomer. It has no significant metabolites, and it is principally a 2D6 substrate, with a minor contribution by 3A4 (Hemeryck and Belpaire 2002). Paroxetine is a potent inhibitor of 2B6 and 2D6 and a mild inhibitor of 1A2, 2C9, 2C19, and 3A4. Patients taking substrates of 2B6 (see Chapter 11 ["Other Relevant P450 Enzymes"]) and 2D6 (see Chapter 5 ["2D6"]) may be at particular risk for significant drug interactions when these drugs are combined with paroxetine (e.g., desipramine concentrations increased 360% with coadministration of paroxetine [Alderman et al. 1997]). Paroxetine is vulnerable to drug interactions only with 2D6 inhibitors more potent than itself, such as quinidine, because paroxetine occupies the P450 site and "pushes off" other drugs with less affinity for 2D6 (Bloomer et al. 1992).

Sertraline

Sertraline (Zoloft) is marketed as the *S*-enantiomer. Its active metabolite, desmethylsertraline, has an inhibitory profile that is similar to (albeit milder than) that of its parent compound (Greenblatt et al. 1999). Both are modest inhibitors of 2C9, 2C19, and 3A4, which accounts for scattered case reports of increased concentrations of phenytoin, warfarin, and cyclosporine when these drugs are combined with sertraline (Lill et al. 2000; Sayal et al. 2000). A recent drug warning sent on October 2002 by Pfizer highlights sertraline's ability to inhibit these P450 enzymes (Zoloft 2002). Sertraline was shown to slightly increase the maximum concentration of diazepam and, more importantly, to increase the maximum concentration of pimozide (Orap). In this letter, it is stated that "concomitant administration of Zoloft and pimozide should be contraindicated." There exists extensive documentation of sertraline's inhibition of 2D6 substrates when sertraline is given at higher doses (e.g., desipramine's concentration is increased 44% [Alderman et al. 1997]; see Chapter 5 ["2D6"]). In vitro evidence supports moderate 2B6 inhibition by sertraline, but in vivo evidence is lacking (Hesse et al. 2002). Sertraline is known to be an inhibitor of glucuronidation, and it has precipitated toxic lamotrigine concentrations (Kaufman and Gerner 1998). Sertraline and desmethylsertraline are substrates of several P450 enzymes, including 2B6, 2C9, 2C19, 2D6, and 3A4 (Greenblatt et al. 1999; Hemeryck and Belpaire 2002; Wang et al. 2001), and their metabolisms are therefore vulnerable only to drugs that are pan-inducers, such as carbamazepine and phenytoin (Pihlsgard and Eliasson 2002).

Non–Selective Serotonin Reuptake Inhibitors

Bupropion

Bupropion (Wellbutrin) is metabolized mainly by 2B6 (Faucette et al. 2001) (see Chapter 11 ["Other Relevant P450 Enzymes"]); it is also handled by 1A2, 2A6, 2C9, 2E1, 3A4, and glucuronidation (Wellbutrin 2002). Neither smoking nor cimetidine alters bupropion's pharmacokinetics (Desai et al. 2001; Kustra et al. 1999). Ritonavir, efavirenz, nelfinavir, paroxetine, sertraline, and other 2B6 inhibitors may interact with bupropion (Hesse et al. 2000, 2002), but clinical documentation is lacking. Because carbamazepine induces several P450 enzymes, bupropion concentrations are reduced with coadministration of carbamazepine (Popli et al. 1995).

Bupropion is a modest inhibitor of 2D6. It can increase concentrations of venlafaxine (Effexor) (Kennedy et al. 2002), nortriptyline (Pamelor) (Weintraub 2001), and desipramine (Wellbutrin 2002). When added to treatment with paroxetine or fluoxetine (substrates of 2D6), sustained-release bupropion did not increase the concentration of either SSRI, probably because SSRIs have lower Ki's and will occupy the P450 site and "push off" bupropion from 2D6 (Kennedy et al. 2002). When adding 2D6 substrates with narrow therapeutic indices to bupropion therapy, clinicians should start with low doses (see Chapter 5 ["2D6"]). Although bupropion does not interact with lamotrigine, it may interact with other glucuronidation substrates (Odishaw and Chen 2000).

Mirtazapine

Mirtazapine (Remeron) is metabolized to several metabolites by 1A2, 2D6, 3A4, and glucuronidation (Stormer et al. 2000) and is not a potent P450 inhibitor. Because fluvoxamine is an inhibitor of all three of mirtazapine's P450 pathways, mirtazapine's concentration is increased up to fourfold when the two drugs are combined (Anttila et al. 2001). As a modest P450 inhibitor, cimetidine increases the concentration of mirtazapine by only 22% (Sitsen et al.

351

■ OTHER ANTIDEPRESSANTS

Drug	Major metabolism site(s)	Enzyme(s) inhibited
Bupropion (Wellbutrin)	2B6	**2D6**[a]
Mirtazapine (Remeron)	1A2, 2D6, 3A4	None known
Nefazodone (Serzone)	3A4, 2D6	**3A4**[a]
Trazodone (Desyrel)	3A4, 2D6	None known
Venlafaxine (Effexor)	2D6	2D6[c]

Note. Data presented relate to parent drug and metabolites combined.

[a]Potent (**bold** type).
[b]Moderate.
[c]Mild.

2000). As a P450 pan-inducer, carbamazepine decreases mirtazapine's concentration significantly (Sitsen et al. 2001).

Nefazodone and Trazodone

Nefazodone (Serzone) is metabolized to three active metabolites via 3A4 (Serzone 2002). One of these, m-chlorophenylpiperazine (m-CPP), is anxiogenic and is further metabolized by 2D6 (von Moltke et al. 1999a). The concentration of m-CPP may be increased in poor metabolizers at 2D6 and by potent inhibitors of 2D6, such as fluoxetine and paroxetine. Metabolisms of nefazodone and its metabolites are vulnerable to 3A4 inhibitors and inducers (see Chapter 6 ["3A4"]). Nefazodone itself is a potent inhibitor of 3A4. It can increase concentrations of other 3A4 substrates, such as carbamazepine, simvastatin, cyclosporine, tacrolimus, alprazolam (Xanax), and triazolam (Halcion) (see Chapter 6 ["3A4"]). Nefazodone is contraindicated with pimozide (Serzone 2002). Trazodone (Desyrel) is not a potent 3A4 inhibitor. It is also metabolized by 3A4 to m-CPP (Rotzinger et al. 1998), and trazodone's metabolism, like the metabolism of nefazodone, is vulnerable to 3A4 inducers and inhibitors.

Venlafaxine

Venlafaxine (Effexor) is a mild inhibitor of 2D6 and is metabolized to an active metabolite, O-desmethylvenlafaxine, by 2D6 (Ball et al. 1997). An inactive metabolite is handled by 3A4 and 2C19 (Greenblatt et al. 1999; Otton et al. 1996). Although drug interactions involving venlafaxine have not been well studied, inhibitors of 2D6—such as quinidine, paroxetine, diphenhydramine, and bupropion—have been shown to increase venlafaxine concentrations (Fogelman et al. 1999; Kennedy et al. 2002; Lessard et al. 2001). As a mild 2D6 inhibitor itself, venlafaxine has been shown to increase concentrations of imipramine (Tofranil) (Ball et al. 1997), desipramine, haloperidol (Haldol), and risperidone (Effexor 2002). It may increase concentrations of other 2D6 substrates in extensive metabolizers.

Tricyclic Antidepressants

Tricyclic antidepressants (TCAs) can be divided into two groups. The tertiary TCAs—which include amitriptyline (Elavil), clomipramine (Anafranil), doxepin (Adapin, Sinequan), imipramine (Tofranil), and trimipramine (Surmontil)—contain a tertiary amine side chain. The secondary TCAs—desipramine (Norpramin), nortriptyline (Pamelor), and protriptyline (Vivactil)—contain a secondary amine side chain. The metabolism of TCAs is very complex. Tertiary TCAs are first demethylated into secondary TCAs: amitriptyline to nortriptyline, imipramine to desipramine, doxepin to desmethyldoxepin, trimipramine to desmethyltrimipramine, and clomipramine to desmethylclomipramine. These compounds are then hydroxylated and finally are conjugated with glucuronic acid. Secondary TCAs are hydroxylated and glucuronidated. Extensive enterohepatic "recycling" of the glucuronidated TCA compounds may occur. As a general rule, 2D6 is responsible for hydroxylations, and other P450 enzymes are responsible for demethylations. In some cases, 2D6 may also act as a minor pathway for demethylation, and 3A4 may act as a "sink" or "reservoir" for hydroxylations (this is true of nortriptyline, for example [Venkatakrishnan et al. 1999]). TCA hydroxymetabolites exist as enantiomers, and they are psychoactive.

Before SSRIs entered the United States market, it had been well established that phenothiazines could increase TCA concentrations (e.g., thioridazine [Mellaril] increases nortriptyline levels [Jerling et al. 1994a]), but it was TCA-SSRI interactions that ushered in the modern age of physician interest in P450 enzymes (see Chapter 5 ["2D6"]). Because the hydroxylation step of TCA metabolism is rate limited, significant increases in TCA concentrations can occur when potent 2D6 inhibitors are coadministered (Leucht et al. 2000). The C_{max} of desipramine is increased 360% when paroxetine is added and 44% when sertraline is added (Alderman et al. 1997). When fluoxetine is administered with amitriptyline, the concentration of amitriptyline increases up to twofold, but nortriptyline levels are increased up to ninefold (el-Yazigi et al. 1995). Whether a drug

■ TRICYCLIC ANTIDEPRESSANTS

Drug	Major metabolism site(s)	Enzyme(s) inhibited
Amitriptyline (Elavil)	2C19, 2D6, 3A4, UGT1A4	2C19,[b] 2D6[c]
Clomipramine (Anafranil)	2C19, 2D6, 3A4	2D6[c]
Desipramine (Norpramin)	2D6	2D6[c]
Doxepin (Adapin, Sinequan)	1A2, 2D6, 3A4, UGT1A4, UGT1A3	None known
Imipramine (Tofranil)	1A2, 2C19, 2D6, 3A4, UGT1A4, UGT1A3	2C19,[c] 2D6[c]
Nortriptyline (Pamelor)	2D6	2D6,[b]
Protriptyline (Vivactil)	?2D6	?
Trimipramine (Surmontil)	2C19, 2D6, 3A4	?

Note. Data presented relate to parent drug and metabolites combined. ?=unknown.

interaction will occur at the demethylation step of a TCA depends on whether the coadministered drug is a *potent* inhibitor or inducer of the major P450 enzyme responsible for TCA demethylation and whether the added drug inhibits or induces *all* demethylation sites. Smoking cigarettes decreases concentrations of imipramine and clomipramine because smoking significantly induces 1A2, an important demethylation pathway (Desai et al. 2001). Fluvoxamine increases clomipramine concentrations up to eightfold because it inhibits all of clomipramine's demethylation pathways (Wagner and Vause 1995).

Clinicians should be aware that TCAs are P450 inhibitors. Amitriptyline and imipramine are inhibitors of 2C19, and they and nortriptyline and desipramine are mild to moderate inhibitors of 2D6 (Shin et al. 2002). Imipramine and nortriptyline can increase concentrations of chlorpromazine (Thorazine) and other phenothiazines (Loga et al. 1981; Rasheed et al. 1994). Olanzapine (Zyprexa) concentrations are increased by 20% with the addition of imipramine (Callaghan et al. 1997).

■ ANXIOLYTICS AND HYPNOTICS

Benzodiazepines

There are many benzodiazepines marketed, and the metabolisms of less than half have been elucidated (see the table entitled "Benzodiazepines"). Some are marketed as anxiolytics and others as hypnotics. Many benzodiazepines are metabolized principally or in part by 3A4, among them alprazolam (Xanax) (Venkatakrishnan et al. 1998), midazolam (Versed) (Wandel et al. 1994), and triazolam (Halcion) (von Moltke et al. 1996). Diazepam (Valium) is metabolized by 2C19 and 3A4 (major pathways) and by 2B6 and perhaps 2C9 (minor pathways) (Ono et al. 1996). Flunitrazepam (Rohypnol, or "Roofies") is a substrate of 2C19 and 3A4 (Kilicarslan et al. 2001). All these benzodiazepines are glucuronidated. Clonazepam (Klonopin) undergoes part of its metabolism via 3A4 and is then acetylated (Seree et al. 1993).

■ BENZODIAZEPINES

Drug	Metabolism
Alprazolam (Xanax)	**3A4**, glucuronidation
Clonazepam (Klonopin)	**3A4**, acetylation
Diazepam (Valium)	2C19, **3A4**, 2B6, 2C9, glucuronidation
Flunitrazepam (Rohypnol ["Roofies"])	2C19, **3A4**
Lorazepam (Ativan)	**UGT2B7**, ?other UGTs
Midazolam (Versed)	**3A4, glucuronidation**
Oxazepam (Serax)	*S*-Oxazepam: UGT2B15
	R-Oxazepam: UGT1A9, UGT2B7
Temazepam (Restoril)	**UGT2B7**, ?other UGTs, 2C19, 3A4
Triazolam (Halcion)	**3A4**, glucuronidation

Note. **Bold** type indicates major pathway. UGT=uridine 5'-diphosphate glucuronosyltransferase.

Three benzodiazepines are handled primarily by glucuronidation. Lorazepam (Ativan), oxazepam (Serax), and temazepam (Restoril) are conjugated by uridine 5′-diphosphate glucuronosyltransferase UGT2B7 (Liston et al. 2001) (see Chapter 3 ["Metabolism in Depth"]. A portion of the metabolism of temazepam occurs via 3A4, and the drug may be partially metabolized to oxazepam before glucuronidation (Azzam et al. 1998).

Metabolisms of only those benzodiazepines that are 3A4 substrates are vulnerable to potent 3A4 inhibitors (nefazodone, erythromycin, and others) and potent 3A4 inducers (carbamazepine and others) (see Tanaka 1999 and Chapter 6 ["3A4"] for reviews of benzodiazepine interactions). For example, fluconazole increases the concentration of midazolam up to fourfold (Ahonen et al. 1999). Diltiazem increases the concentration of triazolam twofold (Varhe et al. 1996), and rifampin decreases triazolam's clearance to only 12% (Villikka et al. 1997a). Even though temazepam undergoes some 3A4 metabolism, its glucuronidation pathway protects it from drug interactions via potent 3A4 inhibitors such as itraconazole (Ahonen et al. 1996). Diazepam may be protected from drug interactions via potent 3A4 inhibitors such as itraconazole by 2C19 (Ahonen et al. 1996). When omeprazole, a potent 2C19 inhibitor, is administered with diazepam, clearance of diazepam is decreased only 26% in 2C19 extensive metabolizers (Andersson et al. 1990) (see Chapter 9 ["2C19"]). Obviously, if a coadministered drug inhibits both 2C19 and 3A4 (e.g., oral contraceptives), diazepam metabolism may be more significantly affected (see Chapter 12 ["Gynecology"]).

Drug interactions involving lorazepam, oxazepam, and temazepam through glucuronidation interactions are not yet well delineated, although it is known that oral contraceptives can induce benzodiazepine glucuronidation (see Chapter 12 ["Gynecology"]) and that probenecid and valproate can inhibit lorazepam glucuronidation (Samara et al. 1997; von Moltke et al. 1993). It is likely that drugs conjugated via UGT2B7 may competitively inhibit each other.

Nonbenzodiazepines

None of the nonbenzodiazepine anxiolytics and hypnotics are P450 inhibitors, and all are partially or completely dependent on 3A4 for metabolism.

Buspirone

Buspirone (BuSpar) is metabolized by 3A4 to an active metabolite, 1-pyrimidinylpiperazine (BuSpar 2002). Inhibitors of 3A4 can increase the C_{max} of buspirone: nefazodone up to 20-fold (BuSpar 2002), itraconazole up to 13-fold (Kivisto et al. 1997, 1999), erythromycin 5-fold (Kivisto et al. 1997), grapefruit juice and diltiazem 4-fold (Lamberg et al. 1998b; Lilja et al. 1998), verapamil 3-fold (Lamberg et al. 1998b), and fluvoxamine 2-fold (Lamberg et al. 1998a). Other potent 3A4 inhibitors may also have the same effect (see Chapter 6 ["3A4"]). 3A4 inducers such as rifampin can reduce the plasma concentration of buspirone by 85% (Kivisto et al. 1999), as can dexamethasone, the older pan-inducing anticonvulsants (BuSpar 2002), and other potent 3A4 inducers.

Zaleplon

Zaleplon (Sonata) is metabolized principally by aldehyde oxidase and, to a lesser extent, by 3A4 (Lake et al. 2002; Renwick et al. 1998). Potent inducers of 3A4 such as rifampin can reduce zaleplon's maximum concentration by 80% and should be avoided (Sonata 2002). Other potent 3A4 inducers are likely to have similar actions (see Chapter 6 ["3A4"]). Potent 3A4 inhibitors such as erythromycin increase zaleplon concentration by 34% (Sonata 2002), and other potent 3A4 inhibitors may, also (see Chapter 6 ["3A4"]). Cimetidine, which inhibits both 3A4 and aldehyde oxidase, has been shown to increase zaleplon's maximum concentration by 85% (Renwick et al. 2002; Sonata 2002), and if the drugs are coadministered, zaleplon's dosing should be substantially reduced. Other substrates of xanthine oxidase (e.g., ziprasidone) should be avoided.

■ NONBENZODIAZEPINES

Drug	Metabolism
Buspirone (BuSpar)	3A4
Zaleplon (Sonata)	**Aldehyde oxidase, 3A4**
Zolpidem (Ambien)	**3A4**, 1A2, 2C9
Zopiclone (Imovane)	2C8, **3A4; excreted through kidneys, lungs, and liver**

Note. **Bold** type indicates major pathway.

Zolpidem

Zolpidem (Ambien) is metabolized principally via 3A4; 1A2 and 2C9 also participate in its metabolism (von Moltke et al. 1999b). The most potent inhibitors of 3A4 reduce zolpidem clearance 70% (ritonavir [Ambien 2002]), 60% (ketoconazole [Greenblatt et al. 1998]), and 34% (itraconazole [Ambien 2002]). Sertraline, a less potent 3A4 inhibitor, increases the C_{max} of zolpidem 43% (Ambien 2002), and fluoxetine and cimetidine have minimal effects (Allard et al. 1998; Hulhoven et al. 1988). These interactions contrast with the much more significant interaction involving buspirone (see the section entitled "Buspirone"), which is totally dependent on 3A4 for its metabolism. Potent inducers of 3A4 reduce the efficacy of zolpidem (e.g., rifampin reduces the peak plasma concentration of zolpidem by 58% [Villikka et al. 1997c]).

Zopiclone

Zopiclone (Imovane) is a chiral drug with an active metabolite. It has a complicated metabolism and may be excreted through the kidneys, lungs, and liver, where it is a substrate of 2C8 and 3A4 (Becquemont et al. 1999; Fernandez et al. 1995). Potent 3A4 inhibitors such as nefazodone and erythromycin can significantly increase zopiclone's plasma concentration and side effects (Aranko et al. 1994). Itraconazole increases zopiclone's peak plasma concentration by 77% (Jalava et al. 1996). There is no information on possible drug interactions with other 2C8 substrates or inhibitors (see Chapter 11 ["Other Relevant P450 Enzymes"]). Potent inducers of 3A4 reduce zopiclone's clinical effectiveness (e.g., rifampin reduces zopiclone levels to one-third of C_{max} [Villikka et al. 1997b]).

■ ANTIPSYCHOTICS

Atypical Antipsychotics

Aripiprazole

Aripiprazole (Abilify) is a quinolone derivative, the first in a new class of atypical antipsychotics, released in 2002. It is metabolized

■ ATYPICAL ANTIPSYCHOTICS

Drug	Major metabolism site(s)	Enzyme(s) inhibited
Aripiprazole (Abilify)	2D6, 3A4	None known
Clozapine (Clozaril)	1A2, 3A4, 2D6, 2C19, UGT1A4, UGT1A3	2D6[c]
Olanzapine (Zyprexa)	1A2, 2D6, UGT1A4, ?other UGTs, ?FMO$_3$	None known
Quetiapine (Seroquel)	3A4, sulfation	None known
Risperidone (Risperdal)	2D6, 3A4	2D6[b]
Ziprasidone (Geodon)	Aldehyde oxidase, 3A4, 1A2	None known

Note. Data presented relate to parent drug and metabolites combined. FMO$_3$=flavin monooxygenase; UGT=uridine 5'-diphosphate glucuronosyltransferase.

[a]Potent (**bold** type).
[b]Moderate.
[c]Mild.

by 2D6 and 3A4 to an active metabolite, dehydroaripiprazole (Abilify 2002). According to its manufacturer, aripiprazole is vulnerable to 2D6 inhibitors (e.g., paroxetine, fluoxetine, quinidine) (see Chapter 5 ["2D6"]), 3A4 inhibitors (e.g., ketoconazole), and 3A4 inducers (e.g., carbamazepine) (see Chapter 6 ["3A4"]).

Clozapine

Clozapine (Clozaril) is principally metabolized to its active metabolite, norclozapine, via 1A2 and (to a lesser extent) 3A4, 2D6, 2C9, and 2C19. Clozapine is also metabolized to clozapine-*N*-oxide, an inactive metabolite, through 3A4 and possibly flavin-containing monooxygenase 3 (Linnet and Olesen 1997). Both active compounds are further glucuronidated by UGT1A4, UGT1A3, and possibly other UGTs (Breyer-Pfaff and Wachsmuth 2001; Green et al. 1998). On the basis of the abundance of liver P450 enzymes, it has been estimated that about 35% of clozapine is metabolized by 2C19, 35% by 3A4, and 10% by 1A2 (Shader and Greenblatt 1998). In contrast to these in vitro studies, in vivo studies have supported the importance of 1A2 as the principal pathway of clozapine metabolism (see Chapter 7 ["1A2"]).

The most repeatedly reviewed drug interaction involves clozapine and fluvoxamine (Heeringa et al. 1999; Lu et al. 2001; Shader and Greenblatt 1998; Szegedi et al. 1999). This interaction is predictable because fluvoxamine is a potent inhibitor of 1A2 and 2C19 and a milder inhibitor of 2D6, 3A4, 2C9, and 2B6. Therefore, all of clozapine's P450 pathways are blocked. Although the extent of this interaction varies greatly because of interindividual variability in the amounts of P450 enzymes, the increase in clozapine levels may be as high as two- to threefold (Wetzel et al. 1998). Other potent inhibitors of 2C19 can also decrease clozapine clearance (e.g., modafinil [Dequardo 2002]). As inhibitors of 2C19 and 1A2, oral contraceptives containing ethinyl estradiol may also affect clozapine metabolism, and one case of this interaction has been reported (Gabbay et al. 2002). Inhibitors of 1A2 (see Chapter 7 ["1A2"]), such as caffeine and ciprofloxacin (see Carrillo and Benitez 2000;

Markowitz et al. 1997; Raaska and Neuvonen 2000), can be expected to decrease clozapine clearance. Potent inhibitors of 2D6 (paroxetine [Spina et al. 2000] and fluoxetine [Spina et al. 1998]) have also been reported to variably decrease clozapine and norclozapine clearance.

Clinical studies of potent 3A4 inhibitors such as ketoconazole and grapefruit juice (Lane et al. 2001), itraconazole (Raaska and Neuvonen 1998), and nefazodone (Taylor et al. 1999) have failed to show decreased clozapine clearance (a few cases of decreased clearance have been reported). At first glance, this is puzzling. A likely explanation involves the important distinction between low-capacity, high-affinity P450 enzymes (e.g., 2D6) and low-affinity, high-capacity P450 enzymes (e.g., 3A4, the reservoir of the P450 system). Because clozapine is a substrate of so many "possible" P450 enzymes—2D6, 2C9, and 2C19—the drug fills these high-affinity P450 enzymes first. 1A2, though it is only 10% of the total liver P450 capacity, "expands" when cigarette smokers induce it (see Chapter 7 ["1A2"]). Therefore, except in the case of a clozapine overdose, clozapine does not "fill" 3A4, and thus no drug interaction occurs.

There are a number of interactions involving clozapine that are not well documented. A single case has been reported of a plasma clozapine concentration increase associated with lamotrigine therapy (Kossen et al. 2001). Both drugs use UGT1A4, and competitive inhibition of the conjugate may occur. Case and clinical studies have found both increased and decreased clozapine clearance with the addition of valproate (Conca et al. 2000; Facciola et al. 1999); the mechanism remains obscure. Several cases have been reported of respiratory distress or delirium in association with coadministration of clozapine and lorazepam, clonazepam, or diazepam, but similar cases have been reported with administration of clozapine alone (Cobb et al. 1991).

Potent pan-inducers of P450 enzymes, such as phenobarbital, carbamazepine, rifampin, and phenytoin, reduce the concentration of clozapine (Facciola et al. 1998; Jerling et al. 1994b; Miller 1991). Cigarette smoking is known to increase clearance of clozapine (Mookhoek and Loonen 2002). When these potent P450 inducers are withdrawn, clozapine toxicity can result (Zullino et al. 2002). Finally, clozapine is a modest 2D6 inhibitor, and concentrations of 2D6 substrates such as nortriptyline can be increased in patients taking clozapine (Smith and Riskin 1994).

Olanzapine

Olanzapine (Zyprexa, Zydis) is not a significant P450 inhibitor or inducer (Ring et al. 1996a), but it has a complex metabolism. The most important pathway quantitatively is glucuronidation, and UGT1A4 has been identified as an important conjugate. Probenecid, a broadly potent UGT inhibitor, has been shown to decrease clearance of olanzapine (Markowitz et al. 2002). Carbamazepine has been shown to increase the clearance of the glucuronidation of olanzapine (Linnet and Olesen 2002). It is likely that many other UGT-based drug-drug interactions involving olanzapine will be found.

The second most important pathway for metabolism of olanzapine is through 1A2 (Kassahun et al. 1997). Potent inhibitors of 1A2, such as ciprofloxacin, caffeine, and fluvoxamine (see Chapter 7 ["1A2"]), increase olanzapine concentrations (de Jong et al. 2001; Markowitz and DeVane 1999). Potent 1A2 inducers such as cigarette smoking reduce olanzapine concentrations (Lucas et al. 1998; Skogh et al. 2002). Cessation of smoking in individuals receiving olanzapine will lead to gradual increases in olanzapine concentrations, with resultant side effects or toxicity (Zullino et al. 2002).

Although 2D6 is a minor pathway of olanzapine metabolism, potent inhibitors such as fluoxetine (see Chapter 5 ["2D6"]) increase olanzapine concentrations by about 30% (Gossen et al. 2002). Flavin monooxygenase may play a minor role in olanzapine metabolism (Ring et al. 1996b).

Quetiapine

Quetiapine (Seroquel) is metabolized principally by 3A4 (Potkin et al. 2002a). Its metabolism is vulnerable to all potent 3A4 inhibitors:

ketoconazole (which increases C_{max} more than 300% [Seroquel 2001]), erythromycin, clarithromcyin, diltiazem, nefazodone, and others (see Chapter 6 ["3A4"]). Two drugs with less inhibitory effects on 3A4 have minimal effects on quetiapine: cimetidine had modest effects on quetiapine clearance (Strakowski et al. 2002), and fluoxetine decreased quetiapine clearance by only 11% (Potkin et al. 2002a). Similarly, all potent 3A4 inducers, such as phenytoin (Wong et al. 2001) and carbamazepine, increase clearance of quetiapine (DeVane and Nemeroff 2001a).

Surprisingly, thioridazine has also been shown to increase clearance of quetiapine (Potkin et al. 2002b). The mechanism of this interaction is unknown. Thioridazine may induce a heretofore-unknown quetiapine P450 pathway or induce 3A4 (Potkin et al. 2002b). Further studies are needed.

Risperidone

Not a P450 inducer and only a modest 2D6 inhibitor (Shin et al. 1999), risperidone (Risperdal) is metabolized predominantly by 2D6 and 3A4 to its major metabolite, 9-hydroxyrisperidone (DeVane and Nemeroff 2001a; Eap et al. 2001). Risperidone clearance is likely decreased by potent 2D6 inhibitors such as paroxetine and fluoxetine (see Chapter 5 ["2D6"]) and potent 3A4 inhibitors such as erythromycin and nefazodone (see Chapter 6 ["3A4"]). As information about P450-based drug interactions has become more available, and clinicians have been able to predict such interactions, use of these combinations has become less likely. As a result, reports of interactions between risperidone and these potent inhibitors (e.g., nefazodone) are absent from the literature.

An argument has been made that because the major metabolite of risperidone, 9-hydroxyrisperidone, has pharmacological characteristics that are almost identical to those of its parent, risperidone interactions may be irrelevant (DeVane and Nemeroff 2001b). However, it has been shown that when paroxetine is coadministered, the combined plasma concentration of risperidone and 9-hydroxyrisperidone increases 45% (Spina et al. 2001). The clinical result of increased risperidone concentrations may be the onset of extrapyramidal side effects. Inducers of 3A4 such as carbamazepine and phenytoin (see Chapter 6 ["3A4"]) increase risperidone clearance and can result in decreased or absent efficacy. When treatment with these inducers is discontinued and risperidone therapy is continued, the concentration of risperidone increases over time, and side effects may ensue (Takahashi et al. 2001).

Carbamazepine concentrations can be increased by risperidone, which suggests that risperidone or its metabolites inhibit the cytochromal paths of carbamazepine or that there is another, unknown mechanism (Mula and Monaco 2002). Concentrations of both risperidone and valproate, when coadministered, have been found to remain the same or to be increased or decreased (DeVane and Nemeroff 2001a). A recent study has questioned the existence of any drug interactions between risperidone and valproate (Sund et al. 2003). As with clozapine and valproate, the mechanism is obscure. However, the clinical take-home lesson is clear: When another drug is added to risperidone therapy, plasma concentrations should be measured if possible.

Ziprasidone

The major pathway for metabolism of ziprasidone (Geodon) is through a molybdoflavoprotein, aldehyde oxidase. Other substrates of aldehyde oxidase include zaleplon, citalopram, famciclovir, acyclovir, quinine, methotrexate, cyclophosphamide, and nicotine (Al-Salmy 2001; Heydorn 2000; Krenitsky et al. 1984; Rochat et al. 1998; Wierzchowski et al. 1996). Only one-third of ziprasidone's metabolic clearance occurs through the P450 enzymes, and 3A4 is the major and 1A2 a minor pathway (Geodon 2002). Ziprasidone has no inhibitory P450 activity. As a result, pharmacokinetic drug interactions through P450 pathways are restricted to coadministered potent 3A4 inhibitors and inducers (Caley and Cooper 2002). Ketoconazole, the most potent 3A4 inhibitor, increases the C_{max} of ziprasidone by only about 40% (Miceli et al. 2000b), and carbamazepine increases its clearance about 35% (Miceli et al. 2000a).

Although P450-based drug interactions that involve ziprasidone might be clinically important because of ziprasidone's potential to increase the QTc interval, there is no evidence that even the most potent 3A4 inhibitor, ketoconazole, can increase the QTc (Geodon 2002).

However, the danger of coadministration of ziprasidone and other drugs known to increase the QTc interval also is well recognized, and use of drugs such as mesoridazine (Serentil), thioridazine, pimozide (Orap), droperidol, halofantrine, and all class IA and III antiarrhythmics must be avoided to prevent this pharmacodynamic-based interaction (Geodon 2002). It is not known whether drugs with the capacity to inhibit aldehyde oxidase will further increase the QTc when they are administered with ziprasidone. Although no clinical data support a drug interaction, it has been shown that chlorpromazine, cimetidine, hydralazine, and methadone can inhibit aldehyde oxidase, and administration of these drugs with ziprasidone is best avoided until there is further clinical clarification (Johnson et al. 1985; Jordan et al. 1999; Renwick et al. 2002; Robertson and Gamage 1994).

Typical Antipsychotics

Because the typical antipsychotics are older, few relevant studies of their phase I and phase II status have been done since sophisticated technology became available. The table entitled "Typical antipsychotics" summarizes what is known.

■ PSYCHOSTIMULANTS AND ATOMOXETINE

Psychostimulants can be grouped into three categories: methylphenidates (Concerta, Focalin, Metadate ER, Metadate CR, Ritalin, Ritalin-SR, Ritalin-LA); amphetamines (dextroamphetamine sulfate, Dexedrine-SR, Adderall, Adderall-XR); and pemoline (Cylert). No drug interactions of pemoline have been reported (Markowitz and Patrick 2001). Atomoxetine (Strattera) is not a psychostimulant; it is a selective norepinephrine reuptake inhibitor, new to the U.S.

■ TYPICAL ANTIPSYCHOTICS

Drug	Metabolism site(s)[1]	Enzyme(s) inhibited[2]	Enzyme(s) induced
Chlorpromazine (Thorazine)	**2D6**, 1A2, 3A4, UGT1A4, UGT1A3	**2D6**	None known
Fluphenazine (Prolixin)	**2D6**, 1A2	**2D6**, 1A2	None known
Haloperidol (Haldol)	**2D6**, **3A4**, 1A2	**2D6**	None known
Loxapine (Loxitane)	?2D6, ?3A4, ?1A2, UGT1A4, UGT1A3	None known	None known
Mesoridazine (Serentil)	2D6, 1A2	?	?
Perphenazine (Trilafon)	**2D6**, **3A4**, 1A2, 2C19	**2D6**, 1A2	None known
Pimozide (Orap)	**3A4**, 1A2	**2D6**, 3A4	None known
Thioridazine (Mellaril)	**2D6**, 1A2, 2C19, FMO₃	**2D6**	?3A4

Note. Data presented relate to parent drug and metabolites combined. FMO₃=flavin monooxygenase.

[1]**Bold** type indicates major pathway.

[2]**Bold** type indicates potent inhibition.

market. It is the first nonstimulant drug to be approved by the FDA for treatment of ADHD.

Methylphenidate and Amphetamines

Methylphenidate (Ritalin) has a complex metabolism that has not been completely elucidated, but it is generally believed that most of its inactive metabolite, ritalinic acid, is produced by plasma esterases and other phase I and phase II systems. Although 2D6 has been postulated to be a partial source of methylphenidate's metabolism, a recent study failed to show that a potent 2D6 inhibitor, quinidine, had any effect on methylphenidate or ritalinic acid (DeVane et al. 2000). In the past 30 years, there have been reports of drug interactions between methylphenidate and imipramine, haloperidol, phenytoin, and others, which suggests that methylphenidate may be a P450 inhibitor (Markowitz et al. 1999). Amphetamines also have a complex metabolism, and the major metabolite is benzoic acid. 2D6 has been shown to be involved in amphetamine's metabolism (Bach et al. 1999). There is no clinical evidence that amphetamines are P450 inhibitors (Markowitz et al. 1999).

Atomoxetine

Although it is not a P450 inhibitor, atomoxetine (Strattera) is metabolized principally by 2D6 (Strattera 2002). Potent 2D6 inhibitors such as fluoxetine, paroxetine, and quinidine can increase the maximum plasma concentration of atomoxetine as much as fourfold, and the manufacturer recommends that its dosing be adjusted upward only after 4 weeks instead of within the first week (Strattera 2002). Other potent 2D6 inhibitors (see Chapter 5 ["2D6"]) should also be used with caution, and the dosing of atomoxetine should be reduced.

■ REFERENCES

Abilify (package insert). Princeton, NJ, Bristol-Myers Squibb Company, 2002

Ahonen J, Olkkola KT, Neuvonen PJ: Lack of effect of antimycotic itraconazole on the pharmacokinetics or pharmacodynamics of temazepam. Ther Drug Monit 18:124–127, 1996

Ahonen J, Olkkola KT, Takala A, et al: Interaction between fluconazole and midazolam in intensive care patients. Acta Anaesthesiol Scand 43:509–514, 1999

Alderman J, Preskorn SH, Greenblatt DJ, et al: Desipramine pharmacokinetics when coadministered with paroxetine or sertraline in extensive metabolizers. J Clin Psychopharmacol 17:284–291, 1997

Allard S, Sainati S, Roth-Schechter B, et al: Minimal interaction between fluoxetine and multiple-dose zolpidem in healthy women. Drug Metab Dispos 26:617–622, 1998

Al-Salmy HS: Individual variation in hepatic aldehyde oxidase activity. IUBMB Life 51:249–253, 2001

Ambien (package insert). New York, NY, Sanofi-Synthelabo Inc, 2002

Andersson T, Cederberg C, Edvardsson G, et al: Effect of omeprazole treatment on diazepam plasma levels in slow versus normal rapid metabolizers of omeprazole. Clin Pharmacol Ther 47:79–85, 1990

Anttila AK, Rasanen L, Leinonen EV: Fluvoxamine augmentation increases mirtazapine concentrations three- to fourfold. Ann Pharmacother 35:1221–1223, 2001

Aranko K, Luurila H, Backman JT, et al: The effect of erythromycin on the pharmacokinetics and pharmacodynamics of zopiclone. Br J Clin Pharmacol 38:363–367, 1994

Azzam RM, Notarianni LJ, Ali HM: Rapid and simple chromatographic method for the determination of diazepam and its major metabolites in human plasma and urine. J Chromatogr B Biomed Sci Appl 708:304–309, 1998

Bach MV, Coutts RT, Baker GB: Involvement of CYP2D6 in the in vitro metabolism of amphetamine, two N-alkylamphetamines and their 4-methoxylated derivatives. Xenobiotica 29:719–732, 1999

Ball SE Ahern D, Scatina J, et al: Venlafaxine: in vitro inhibition of CYP2D6 dependent imipramine and desipramine metabolism: comparative studies with selected SSRIs, and effects on human hepatic CYP3A4, CYP2C9 and CYP1A2. Br J Clin Pharmacol 43:619–626, 1997

Becquemont L, Mouajjah S, Escaffre O, et al: Cytochrome P-450 3A4 and 2C8 are involved in zopiclone metabolism. Drug Metab Dispos 27:1068–1073, 1999

Bloomer JC, Woods FR, Haddock RE, et al: The role of cytochrome P4502D6 in the metabolism of paroxetine by human liver microsomes. Br J Clin Pharmacol 33:521–523, 1992

Breyer-Pfaff U, Wachsmuth H: Tertiary *N*-glucuronides of clozapine and its metabolite desmethylclozapine in patient urine. Drug Metab Dispos 29: 1343–1348, 2001

Brosen K, Naranjo CA: Review of pharmacokinetic and pharmacodynamic interaction studies with citalopram. Eur Neuropsychopharmacol 11: 275–283, 2001

Brunswick DJ, Amsterdam JD, Fawcett J, et al: Fluoxetine and norfluoxetine plasma levels after discontinuing fluoxetine therapy. J Clin Psychopharmacol 21:616–618, 2001

BuSpar (package insert). Princeton, NJ, Bristol-Myers Squibb Company, 2002

Caley CF, Cooper CK: Ziprasidone: the fifth atypical antipsychotic. Ann Pharmacother 36:839–851, 2002

Callaghan JT, Cerimele BJ, Kassahun KJ, et al: Olanzapine: interaction study with imipramine. J Clin Pharmacol 37:971–978, 1997

Carrillo JA, Benitez J: Clinically significant pharmacokinetic interactions between dietary caffeine and medications. Clin Pharmacokinet 39:127–153, 2000

Christensen M, Tybring G, Mihara K, et al: Low daily 10-mg and 20-mg doses of fluvoxamine inhibit the metabolism of both caffeine (cytochrome P4501A2) and omeprazole (cytochrome P4502C19). Clin Pharmacol Ther 71:141–152, 2002

Cobb CD, Anderson CB, Seidel DR: Possible interaction between clozapine and lorazepam (letter). Am J Psychiatry 148:1606–1607, 1991

Conca A, Beraus W, Konig P, et al: A case of pharmacokinetic interference in comedication of clozapine and valproic acid. Pharmacopsychiatry 33: 234–235, 2000

Court MH, Duan SX, Guillemette C, et al: Stereoselective conjugation of oxazepam by human UDP-glucuronosyltransferases (UGTs): S-oxazepam is glucuronidated by UGT2B15, while R-oxazepam is glucuronidated by UGT2B7 and UGT1A9. Drug Metab Dispos 30:1257–1265, 2002

de Jong J, Hoogenboom B, van Troostwijk LD, et al: Interaction of olanzapine with fluvoxamine. Psychopharmacology (Berl) 155:219–220, 2001

Dequardo JR: Modafinil-associated clozapine toxicity (letter). Am J Psychiatry 159:1243–1244, 2002

Desai HD, Seabolt J, Jann MW: Smoking in patients receiving psychotropic medications: a pharmacokinetic perspective. CNS Drugs 15:469–494, 2001

DeVane CL, Nemeroff CB: Clinical pharmacokinetics of quetiapine: an atypical antipsychotic. Clin Pharmacokinet 40:509–522, 2001a

DeVane CL, Nemeroff CB: An evaluation of risperidone drug interactions. J Clin Psychopharmacol 21:408–416, 2001b

DeVane CL, Markowitz JS, Carson SW, et al: Single-dose pharmacokinetics of methylphenidate in CYP2D6 extensive and poor metabolizers. J Clin Psychopharmacol 20:347–349, 2000

Eap CB, Bondolfi G, Zullino D, et al: Pharmacokinetic drug interaction potential of risperidone with cytochrome p450 isozymes as assessed by the dextromethorphan, the caffeine, and the mephenytoin test. Ther Drug Monit 23:228–231, 2001

Effexor (package insert). Philadelphia, PA, Wyeth Laboratories, 2002

el-Yazigi A, Chaleby K, Gad A, et al: Steady-state kinetics of fluoxetine and amitriptyline in patients treated with a combination of these drugs as compared with those treated with amitriptyline alone. J Clin Pharmacol 35:17–21, 1995

Facciola G, Avenoso A, Spina E, et al: Inducing effect of phenobarbital on clozapine metabolism in patients with chronic schizophrenia. Ther Drug Monit 20:628–630, 1998

Facciola G, Avenoso A, Scordo MG, et al: Small effects of valproic acid on the plasma concentrations of clozapine and its major metabolites in patients with schizophrenic or affective disorders. Ther Drug Monit 21: 341–345, 1999

Faucette SR, Hawke RL, Shord SS, et al: Evaluation of the contribution of cytochrome P450 3A4 to human liver microsomal bupropion hydroxylation. Drug Metab Dispos 29:1123–1129, 2001

Fernandez C, Martin C, Gimenez F, et al: Clinical pharmacokinetics of zopiclone. Clin Pharmacokinet 29:431–441, 1995

Fogelman SM, Schmider J, Venkatakrishnan K, et al: O- and N-demethylation of venlafaxine in vitro by human liver microsomes and by microsomes from cDNA-transfected cells: effect of metabolic inhibitors and SSRI antidepressants. Neuropsychopharmacology 20:480–490, 1999

Gabbay V, O'Dowd MA, Mamamtavrishvili M, et al: Clozapine and oral contraceptives: a possible drug interaction. J Clin Psychopharmacol 22: 621–622, 2002

Geodon (package insert). New York, NY, Pfizer Inc, 2002

Gossen D, de Suray JM, Vandenhende F, et al: Influence of fluoxetine on olanzapine pharmacokinetics. AAPS PharmSci 4:E11, 2002

Green MD, King CD, Mojarrabi B, et al: Glucuronidation of amines and other xenobiotics catalyzed by expressed human UDP-glucuronosyl-transferase 1A3. Drug Metab Dispos 26:507–512, 1998

Greenblatt DJ, von Moltke LL, Harmatz JS, et al: Kinetic and dynamic interaction study of zolpidem with ketoconazole, itraconazole, and fluconazole. Clin Pharmacol Ther 64:661–671, 1998

Greenblatt DJ, von Moltke LL, Harmatz JS, et al: Human cytochromes and some newer antidepressants: kinetics, metabolism, and drug interactions. J Clin Psychopharmacol 19:23S–35S, 1999

Heeringa M, Beurskens R, Schouten W, et al: Elevated plasma levels of clozapine after concomitant use of fluvoxamine. Pharm World Sci 21: 243–244, 1999

Hemeryck A, Belpaire FM: Selective serotonin reuptake inhibitors and cytochrome P-450 mediated drug-drug interactions: an update. Curr Drug Metab 3:13–37, 2002

Hesse LM, Venkatakrishnan K, Court MH, et al: CYP2B6 mediates the in vitro hydroxylation of bupropion: potential drug interactions with other antidepressants. Drug Metab Dispos 28:1176–1183, 2000

Hesse LM, von Moltke LL, Shader RI, et al: Ritonavir, efavirenz, and nelfinavir inhibit CYP2B6 activity in vitro: potential drug interactions with bupropion. Drug Metab Dispos 29:100–102, 2002

Heydorn WE: Zaleplon—a review of a novel sedative hypnotic used in the treatment of insomnia. Expert Opin Investig Drugs 9:841–858, 2000

Hulhoven R, Desager JP, Harvengt C, et al: Lack of interaction between zolpidem and H_2 antagonists, cimetidine and ranitidine. Int J Clin Pharmacol Res 8:471–476, 1988

Jalava KM, Olkkola KT, Neuvonen PJ: Effect of itraconazole on the pharmacokinetics and pharmacodynamics of zopiclone. Eur J Clin Pharmacol 51:331–334, 1996

Jerling M, Bertilsson L, Sjoqvist F: The use of therapeutic drug monitoring data to document kinetic drug interactions: an example with amitriptyline and nortriptyline. Ther Drug Monit 16:1–12, 1994a

Jerling M, Lindstrom L, Bondesson U, et al: Fluvoxamine inhibition and carbamazepine induction of the metabolism of clozapine: evidence from a therapeutic drug monitoring service. Ther Drug Monit 16:368–374, 1994b

Johnson C, Stubley-Beedham C, Stell JG: Hydralazine: a potent inhibitor of aldehyde oxidase activity in vitro and in vivo. Biochem Pharmacol 34: 4251–4256, 1985

Jordan CG, Rashidi MR, Laljee H, et al: Aldehyde oxidase-catalysed oxidation of methotrexate in the liver of guinea-pig, rabbit and man. J Pharm Pharmacol 51:411–418, 1999

Kassahun K, Mattiuz E, Nyhart E Jr, et al: Disposition and biotransformation of the antipsychotic agent olanzapine in humans. Drug Metab Dispos 25:81–93, 1997

Kaufman KR, Gerner R: Lamotrigine toxicity secondary to sertraline. Seizure 7:163–165, 1998

Kennedy SH, McCann SM, Masellis M, et al: Combining bupropion SR with venlafaxine, paroxetine, or fluoxetine: a preliminary report on pharmacokinetic, therapeutic, and sexual dysfunction effects. J Clin Psychiatry 63:181–186, 2002

Kilicarslan T, Haining RL, Rettie AE, et al: Flunitrazepam metabolism by cytochrome P450s 2C19 and 3A4. Drug Metab Dispos 29:460–465, 2001

Kivisto KT, Lamberg TS, Kantola T, et al: Plasma buspirone concentrations are greatly increased by erythromycin and itraconazole. Clin Pharmacol Ther 62:348–354, 1997

Kivisto KT, Lamberg TS, Neuvonen PJ: Interactions of buspirone with itraconazole and rifampicin: effects on the pharmacokinetics of the active 1-(2-pyrimidinyl)-piperazine metabolite of buspirone. Pharmacol Toxicol 84:94–97, 1999

Kossen M, Selten JP, Kahn RS: Elevated clozapine plasma level with lamotrigine (letter). Am J Psychiatry 158:1930, 2001

Krenitsky TA, Hall WW, de Miranda P, et al: 6-Deoxyacyclovir: a xanthine oxidase-activated prodrug of acyclovir. Proc Natl Acad Sci U S A 81:3209–3213, 1984

Kustra R, Corrigan B, Dunn J, et al: Lack of effect of cimetidine on the pharmacokinetics of sustained-release bupropion. J Clin Pharmacol 39: 1184–1188, 1999

Lake BG, Ball SE, Kao J, et al: Metabolism of zaleplon by human liver: evidence for involvement of aldehyde oxidase. Xenobiotica 32:835–847, 2002

Lamberg TS, Kivisto KT, Laitila J, et al: The effect of fluvoxamine on the pharmacokinetics and pharmacodynamics of buspirone. Eur J Clin Pharmacol 54:761–766, 1998a

Lamberg TS, Kivisto KT, Neuvonen PJ: Effects of verapamil and diltiazem on the pharmacokinetics and pharmacodynamics of buspirone. Clin Pharmacol Ther 63:640–645, 1998b

Lane HY, Chiu CC, Kazmi Y, et al: Lack of CYP3A4 inhibition by grapefruit juice and ketoconazole upon clozapine administration in vivo. Drug Metabol Drug Interact 18:263–278, 2001

Lessard E, Yessine MA, Hamelin BA, et al: Diphenhydramine alters the disposition of venlafaxine through inhibition of CYP2D6 activity in humans. J Clin Psychopharmacol 21:175–184, 2001

Leucht S, Hackl HJ, Steimer W, et al: Effect of adjunctive paroxetine on serum levels and side-effects of tricyclic antidepressants in depressive inpatients. Psychopharmacology (Berl) 147:378–383, 2000

Lilja JJ, Kivisto KT, Backman JT, et al: Grapefruit juice substantially increases plasma concentrations of buspirone. Clin Pharmacol Ther 64: 655–660, 1998

Lill J, Bauer LA, Horn JR, et al: Cyclosporine-drug interactions and the influence of patient age. Am J Health Syst Pharm 57:1579–1584, 2000

Linnet K, Olesen OV: Metabolism of clozapine by cDNA-expressed human cytochrome P450 enzymes. Drug Metab Dispos 25:1379–1382, 1997

Linnet K, Olesen OV: Free and glucuronidated olanzapine serum concentrations in psychiatric patients: influence of carbamazepine comedication. Ther Drug Monit 24:512–517, 2002

Liston HL, Markowitz JS, DeVane CL: Drug glucuronidation in clinical psychopharmacology. J Clin Psychopharmacol 21:500–515, 2001

Loga S, Curry S, Lader M: Interaction of chlorpromazine and nortriptyline in patients with schizophrenia. Clin Pharmacokinet 6:454–462, 1981

Lu ML, Lane HY, Chang WH: Differences between in vitro and in vivo determinations of fluvoxamine-clozapine interaction (letter). J Clin Psychopharmacol 21:625–626, 2001

Lucas RA, Gilfillan DJ, Bergstrom RF: A pharmacokinetic interaction between carbamazepine and olanzapine: observations on possible mechanism. Eur J Clin Pharmacol 54:639–643, 1998

Markowitz JS, DeVane CL: Suspected ciprofloxacin inhibition of olanzapine resulting in increased plasma concentration (letter). J Clin Psychopharmacol 19:289–291, 1999

Markowitz JS, Patrick KS: Pharmacokinetic and pharmacodynamic drug interactions in the treatment of attention-deficit hyperactivity disorder. Clin Pharmacokinet 40:753–772, 2001

Markowitz JS, Gill HS, DeVane CL, et al: Fluoroquinolone inhibition of clozapine metabolism (letter). Am J Psychiatry 154:881, 1997

Markowitz JS, Morrison SD, DeVane CL: Drug interactions with psycho-stimulants. Int Clin Psychopharmacol 14:1–18, 1999

Markowitz JS, DeVane CL, Liston HL, et al: The effects of probenecid on the disposition of risperidone and olanzapine in healthy volunteers. Clin Pharmacol Ther 71:30–38, 2002

Miceli JJ, Anziano RJ, Robarge L, et al: The effect of carbamazepine on the steady-state pharmacokinetics of ziprasidone in healthy volunteers. Br J Clin Pharmacol 49 (suppl 1):65S–70S, 2000a

Miceli JJ, Smith M, Robarge L, et al: The effects of ketoconazole on ziprasidone pharmacokinetics—a placebo-controlled crossover study in healthy volunteers. Br J Clin Pharmacol 49 (suppl 1):71S–76S, 2000b

Miller DD: Effect of phenytoin on plasma clozapine concentrations in two patients. J Clin Psychiatry 52:23–25, 1991

Mookhoek EJ, Loonen AJ: Does the change of omeprazole to pantoprazole affect clozapine plasma concentrations? Br J Clin Pharmacol 53:545, 2002

Mula M, Monaco F: Carbamazepine-risperidone interactions in patients with epilepsy. Clin Neuropharmacol 25:97–100, 2002

Odishaw J, Chen C: Effects of steady-state bupropion on the pharmaco-kinetics of lamotrigine in healthy subjects. Pharmacotherapy 20:1448–1453, 2000

Ono S, Hatanaka T, Miyazawa S, et al: Human liver microsomal diazepam metabolism using cDNA-expressed cytochrome P450s: role of CYP2B6, 2C19 and the 3A subfamily. Xenobiotica 26:1155–1166, 1996

Otton SV, Ball SE, Cheung SW, et al: Venlafaxine oxidation in vitro is catalysed by CYP2D6. Br J Clin Pharmacol 41:149–156, 1996

Pihlsgard M, Eliasson E: Significant reduction of sertraline plasma levels by carbamazepine and phenytoin. Eur J Clin Pharmacol 57:915–916, 2002

Popli AP, Tanquary J, Lamparella V, et al: Bupropion and anticonvulsant drugs. Ann Clin Psychiatry 7:99–101, 1995

Potkin SG, Thyrum PT, Alva G, et al: Effect of fluoxetine and imipramine on the pharmacokinetics and tolerability of the antipsychotic quetiapine. J Clin Psychopharmacol 22:174–182, 2002a

Potkin SG, Thyrum PT, Alva G, et al: The safety and pharmacokinetics of quetiapine when coadministered with haloperidol, risperidone, or thio-ridazine. J Clin Psychopharmacol 22:121–130, 2002b

Preskorn SH, Alderman J, Chung M, et al: Pharmacokinetics of desipramine coadministered with sertraline or fluoxetine. J Clin Psychopharmacol 14:90–98, 1994

Raaska K, Neuvonen PJ: Serum concentrations of clozapine and *N*-desmethylclozapine are unaffected by the potent CYP3A4 inhibitor itraconazole. Eur J Clin Pharmacol 54:167–170, 1998

Raaska K, Neuvonen PJ: Ciprofloxacin increases serum clozapine and *N*-desmethylclozapine: a study in patients with schizophrenia. Eur J Clin Pharmacol 56:585–589, 2000

Rasheed A, Javed MA, Nazir S, et al: Interaction of chlorpromazine with tricyclic anti-depressants in schizophrenic patients. J Pak Med Assoc 44: 233–234, 1994

Renwick AB, Mistry H, Ball S, et al: Metabolism of zaleplon by human hepatic microsomal cytochrome P450 isoforms. Xenobiotica 28:337–348, 1998

Renwick AB, Ball SE, Tredger JM, et al: Inhibition of zaleplon metabolism by cimetidine in the human liver: in vitro studies with subcellular fractions and precision-cut liver slices. Xenobiotica 32:849–862, 2002

Ring BJ, Binkley SN, Vandenbranden M, et al: In vitro interaction of the antipsychotic agent olanzapine with human cytochromes P450 CYP2C9, CYP2C19, CYP2D6 and CYP3A. Br J Clin Pharmacol 41:181–186, 1996a

Ring BJ, Catlow J, Lindsay TJ, et al: Identification of the human cytochromes P450 responsible for the in vitro formation of the major oxidative metabolites of the antipsychotic agent olanzapine. J Pharmacol Exp Ther 276:658–666, 1996b

Ring BJ, Eckstein JA, Gillespie JS, et al: Identification of the human cytochromes P450 responsible for in vitro formation of *R*- and *S*-norfluoxetine. J Pharmacol Exp Ther 297:1044–1050, 2001

Robertson IG, Gamage RS: Methadone: a potent inhibitor of rat liver aldehyde oxidase. Biochem Pharmacol 47:584–587, 1994

Rochat B, Kosel M, Boss G, et al: Stereoselective biotransformation of the selective serotonin reuptake inhibitor citalopram and its demethylated metabolites by monoamine oxidases in human liver. Biochem Pharmacol 56:15–23, 1998

Rotzinger S, Fang J, Baker GB: Trazodone is metabolized to *m*-chlorophenylpiperazine by CYP3A4 from human sources. Drug Metab Dispos 26: 572–575, 1998

Samara EE, Granneman RG, Witt GF, et al: Effect of valproate on the pharmacokinetics and pharmacodynamics of lorazepam. J Clin Pharmacol 37:442–450, 1997

378

Sayal KS, Duncan-McConnell DA, McConnell HW, et al: Psychotropic interactions with warfarin. Acta Psychiatr Scand 102:250–255, 2000

Seree EJ, Pisano PJ, Placidi M, et al: Identification of the human and animal hepatic cytochromes P450 involved in clonazepam metabolism. Fundam Clin Pharmacol 7:69–75, 1993

Seroquel (package insert). Wilmington, DE, AstraZeneca Pharmaceuticals LP, 2001

Serzone (package insert). Princeton, NJ, Bristol-Myers Squibb Company, 2002

Shader RI, Greenblatt DJ: Clozapine and fluvoxamine, a curious complexity (editorial). J Clin Psychopharmacol 18:101–102, 1998

Shin JG, Soukhova N, Flockhart DA: Effect of antipsychotic drugs on human liver cytochrome P-450 (CYP) isoforms in vitro: preferential inhibition of CYP2D6. Drug Metab Dispos 27:1078–1084, 1999

Shin JG, Park JY, Kim MJ, et al: Inhibitory effects of tricyclic antidepressants (TCAs) on human cytochrome p450 enzymes in vitro: mechanism of drug interaction between TCAs and phenytoin. Drug Metab Dispos 30:1102–1107, 2002

Sitsen JM, Maris FA, Timmer CJ: Concomitant use of mirtazapine and cimetidine: a drug-drug interaction study in healthy male subjects. Eur J Clin Pharmacol 56:389–394, 2000

Sitsen J[M], Maris F, Timmer C: Drug-drug interaction studies with mirtazapine and carbamazepine in healthy male subjects. Eur J Drug Metab Pharmacokinet 26:109–121, 2001

Skogh E, Reis M, Dahl ML, et al: Therapeutic drug monitoring data on olanzapine and its N-demethyl metabolite in the naturalistic clinical setting. Ther Drug Monit 24:518–526, 2002

Smith T, Riskin J: Effect of clozapine on plasma nortriptyline concentration. Pharmacopsychiatry 27:41–42, 1994

Sonata (package insert). Philadelphia, PA, Wyeth Laboratories, 2002

Spigset O, Axelsson S, Norstrom A, et al: The major fluvoxamine metabolite in urine is formed by CYP2D6. Eur J Clin Pharmacol 57:653–658, 2001

Spina E, Avenoso A, Facciola G, et al: Effect of fluoxetine on the plasma concentrations of clozapine and its major metabolites in patients with schizophrenia. Int Clin Psychopharmacol 13:141–145, 1998

Spina E, Avenoso A, Salemi M, et al: Plasma concentrations of clozapine and its major metabolites during combined treatment with paroxetine or sertraline. Pharmacopsychiatry 33:213–217, 2000

Spina E, Avenoso A, Facciola G, et al: Plasma concentrations of risperidone and 9-hydroxyrisperidone during combined treatment with paroxetine. Ther Drug Monit 23:223–237, 2001

Spina E, Avenoso A, Scordo MG, et al: Inhibition of risperidone metabolism by fluoxetine in patients with schizophrenia: a clinically relevant pharmacokinetic drug interaction. J Clin Psychopharmacol 22:419–423, 2002

Steinacher L, Vandel P, Zullino DF, et al: Carbamazepine augmentation in depressive patients non-responding to citalopram: a pharmacokinetic and clinical pilot study. Eur Neuropsychopharmacol 12:255–260, 2002

Stormer E, von Moltke LL, Shader RI, et al: Metabolism of the antidepressant mirtazapine in vitro: contribution of cytochromes P-450 1A2, 2D6, and 3A4. Drug Metab Dispos 28:1168–1175, 2000

Strakowski SM, Keck PE Jr, Wong YW, et al: The effect of multiple doses of cimetidine on the steady-state pharmacokinetics of quetiapine in men with selected psychotic disorders. J Clin Psychopharmacol 22:201–205, 2002

Strattera (package insert). Indianapolis, IN, Eli Lilly and Company, 2002

Sund JK, Aamo T, Spigset O: Valproic acid and risperidone: a drug interaction? J Am Acad Child Adolesc Psychiatry 42:1–2, 2003

Szegedi A, Anghelescu I, Wiesner J, et al: Addition of low-dose fluvoxamine to low-dose clozapine monotherapy in schizophrenia: drug monitoring and tolerability data from a prospective clinical trial. Pharmacopsychiatry 32:148–153, 1999

Takahashi H, Yoshida K, Higuchi H, et al: Development of parkinsonian symptoms after discontinuation of carbamazepine in patients concurrently treated with risperidone: two case reports. Clin Neuropharmacol 24:358–360, 2001

Tanaka E: Clinically significant pharmacokinetic drug interactions with benzodiazepines. J Clin Pharm Ther 24:347–355, 1999

Taylor D, Bodani M, Hubbeling A, et al: The effect of nefazodone on clozapine plasma concentrations. Int Clin Psychopharmacol 14:185–187, 1999

Varhe A, Olkkola KT, Neuvonen PJ: Diltiazem enhances the effects of triazolam by inhibiting its metabolism. Clin Pharmacol Ther 59:369–375, 1996

Venkatakrishnan K, Greenblatt DJ, von Moltke LL, et al: Alprazolam is another substrate for human cytochrome P450-3A isoforms (letter). J Clin Psychopharmacol 18:256, 1998

Venkatakrishnan K, von Moltke LL, Greenblatt DJ: Nortriptyline E-10-hydroxylation in vitro is mediated by human CYP2D6 (high affinity) and CYP3A4 (low affinity): implications for interactions with enzyme-inducing drugs. J Clin Pharmacol 39:567–577, 1999

Villikka K, Kivisto KT, Backman JT, et al: Triazolam is ineffective in patients taking rifampin. Clin Pharmacol Ther 61:8–14, 1997a

Villikka K, Kivisto KT, Lamberg TS, et al: Concentrations and effects of zopiclone are greatly reduced by rifampicin. Br J Clin Pharmacol 43: 471–474, 1997b

Villikka K, Kivisto KT, Luurila H, et al: Rifampin reduces plasma concentrations and effects of zolpidem. Clin Pharmacol Ther 62:629–634, 1997c

von Moltke LL, Manis M, Harmatz JS, et al: Inhibition of acetaminophen and lorazepam glucuronidation in vitro by probenecid. Biopharm Drug Dispos 14:119–130, 1993

von Moltke LL, Greenblatt DJ, Harmatz JS, et al: Triazolam biotransformation by human liver microsomes in vitro: effects of metabolic inhibitors and clinical confirmation of a predicted interaction with ketoconazole. J Pharmacol Exp Ther 276:370–379, 1996

von Moltke LL, Greenblatt DJ, Granda BW, et al: Nefazodone, meta-chlorophenylpiperazine, and their metabolites in vitro: cytochromes mediating transformation, and P450-3A4 inhibitory actions. Psychopharmacology (Berl) 145:113–122, 1999a

von Moltke LL, Greenblatt DJ, Granda BW, et al: Zolpidem metabolism in vitro: responsible cytochromes, chemical inhibitors, and in vivo correlations. Br J Clin Pharmacol 48:89–97, 1999b

von Moltke LL, Greenblatt DJ, Giancarlo GM, et al: Escitalopram (S-citalopram) and its metabolites in vitro: cytochromes mediating biotransformation, inhibitory effects, and comparison to R-citalopram. Drug Metab Dispos 29:1102–1109, 2001

Wagner W, Vause EW: Fluvoxamine. A review of global drug-drug interaction data. Clin Pharmacokinet 29 (suppl 1):26–31, 1995

Wandel C, Bocker R, Bohrer H, et al: Midazolam is metabolized by at least three different cytochrome P450 enzymes. Br J Anaesth 73:658–661, 1994

Wang JH, Liu ZQ, Wang W, et al: Pharmacokinetics of sertraline in relation to genetic polymorphism of CYP2C19. Clin Pharmacol Ther 70:42–47, 2001

Weintraub D: Nortriptyline toxicity secondary to interaction with bupropion sustained-release. Depress Anxiety 13:50–52, 2001

Wellbutrin (package insert). Research Triangle Park, NC, GlaxoSmithKline, 2002

Wetzel H, Anghelescu I, Szegedi A, et al: Pharmacokinetic interactions of clozapine with selective serotonin reuptake inhibitors: differential effects of fluvoxamine and paroxetine in a prospective study. J Clin Psychopharmacol 18:2–9, 1998

Wierzchowski J, Wroczynski P, Interewicz E: Selective assay of the cytosolic forms of the aldehyde dehydrogenase in rat, with possible significance for the investigations of cyclophosphamide cytotoxicity. Acta Pol Pharm 53:203–208, 1996

Wong YW, Yeh C, Thyrum PT: The effects of concomitant phenytoin administration on the steady-state pharmacokinetics of quetiapine. J Clin Psychopharmacol 21:89–93, 2001

Yoshimura R, Ueda N, Nakamura J, et al: Interaction between fluvoxamine and cotinine or caffeine. Neuropsychobiology 45:32–35, 2002

Zullino DF, Delessert D, Eap CB, et al: Tobacco and cannabis smoking cessation can lead to intoxication with clozapine or olanzapine. Int Clin Psychopharmacol 17:141–143, 2002

20

TRANSPLANT SURGERY AND RHEUMATOLOGY

Immunosuppressants

Elisabeth A. Pimentel, B.S.

Immunosuppressants are used to prevent organ transplant rejection and to treat patients with autoimmune disorders. They can be classified by their mechanism or mechanisms of actions. Many immunosuppressants are administered in other disease processes; for example, cyclophosphamide is used in cancer chemotherapy, and steroids are prescribed for numerous inflammatory medical conditions.

> **Reminder:** This chapter is dedicated primarily to metabolic and P-glycoprotein interactions. Interactions due to displaced protein-binding, alterations in absorption or excretion, and pharmacodynamics are not covered.

■ GLUCOCORTICOIDS

The synthetic glucocorticoids methylprednisolone, prednisolone, and prednisone are all used for a variety of purposes, including immunosuppression in organ transplant recipients and in patients with autoimmune disorders. Prednisone is actually a pro-drug and is metabolized by the liver to prednisolone, the active glucocorticoid.

■ IMMUNOSUPPRESSANTS

Drug	Enzyme(s) drug is metabolized by	Enzyme(s) inhibited	Enzyme(s) induced	P-glycoprotein substrate?
Azathioprine (Imuran)[1]	Unknown enzymes metabolize to mercaptopurine	?	?	?
Cyclophosphamide (Cytoxan)[1]	2A6, 2B6, 2C19, 3A4	?	2B6, 3A4	No
Cyclosporine (Sandimmune)	3A4	3A4,[2] P-glycoprotein[3]	None	Yes
Mercaptopurine (Purinethol)	TPMT	?	?	?
Methotrexate	Non-P450 oxidative enzymes	?	?	?
Methylprednisolone	3A4	3A4[2]	3A4	No
Mitoxantrone (Novantrone)	Unknown oxidative enzymes and UGTs	?	?	?
Muromonab-CD3 (Orthoclone OKT3)	Not phase I or phase II enzymes	?	None	No
Mycophenolate mofetil (CellCept)[1]	Hydrolysis, UGTs	?	?	?
Prednisolone	3A4	None	3A4	?

■ IMMUNOSUPPRESSANTS *(continued)*

Drug	Enzyme(s) drug is metabolized by	Enzyme(s) inhibited	Enzyme(s) induced	P-glycoprotein substrate?
Prednisone[1]	3A4	None	3A4	Possibly
Sirolimus (Rapamune)	3A4	3A4[4]	None	Yes
Tacrolimus (Prograf)	3A4	3A4,[2] UGT1A1, P-glycoprotein	None	Yes

Note. ?=unknown; TPMT=thiopurine methyltransferase; UGT=uridine 5′-diphosphate glucuronosyltransferase.
[1]Drug is a pro-drug and requires enzymatic activity to produce active pharmacological compound.
[2]Moderate inhibition.
[3]Cyclosporine is a P-glycoprotein inhibitor. The ability of other immunosuppressants to inhibit P-glycoprotein is less clear.
[4]Mild inhibition.

Because these three drugs are very old, there is little information on their precise metabolic pathways. The naturally occurring glucocorticoids—cortisone and hydrocortisone—are metabolized in part by 3A4 (Lin et al. 1999) via 6β-hydroxylation, so it is believed that synthetic glucocorticoids are metabolized in a similar fashion.

Use of 3A4 inhibitors may alter the pharmacokinetics of glucocorticoids. Imani et al. (1999) demonstrated that when prednisone is used with the potent 3A4 inhibitor diltiazem, the latter actually enhances prednisone's effect—in part by inhibiting prednisone's active metabolite, prednisolone, from being metabolized by 3A4. This reaction could lead to toxic levels of prednisone or prednisolone. Phenobarbital and phenytoin, inducers of 3A4, have been noted in multiple case reports to decrease transplant survival and to necessitate higher doses of prednisolone to maintain efficacy (Gambertoglia et al. 1982; Wassner et al. 1977). The glucocorticoids are reportedly inducers of 3A4 themselves, but few cases of related interactions have been presented in the literature.

■ CYCLOSPORINE

Cyclosporine (Sandimmune) is a cyclic polypeptide of 11 amino acids that is produced by a fungus (Sandimmune 2001). It suppresses immune responses by inhibiting the first phase of T-cell activation by binding with a natural immunosuppressant protein, cyclophilin. This complex then inhibits calcineurin, a calcium/calmodulin–activated phosphatase. It is considered a mainstay medication for preventing rejection of organ transplants.

Cyclosporine is given both intravenously and orally. A significant first-pass effect occurs with oral administration, primarily because the drug is metabolized and cleared extensively by 3A4 (Fahr 1993). There is also some evidence that it is a moderate inhibitor of 3A4, but the literature contains few reports of cyclosporine increasing the levels of 3A4-dependent drugs. This agent is also a substrate and inhibitor of P-glycoprotein (Lo and Burckart 1999). Other enzymes may be involved in cyclosporine clearance, because multiple metabolites are found in the urine after oral administration, but these other enzymes are not well identified (Sandimmune 2001).

Because cyclosporine is dependent on 3A4 for clearance and is a P-glycoprotein substrate, there are numerous reports of drug-drug interactions. Cyclosporine has a narrow therapeutic index. Inadequate serum levels may lead to organ failure, and toxic levels may lead to delirium, nephrotoxicity, and organ failure. The following agents have been shown to significantly inhibit cyclosporine metabolism (often in vivo) through inhibition of 3A4: clarithromycin (Biaxin), diltiazem (Cardizem), erythromycin, fluconazole (Diflucan), fluvoxamine (Luvox), grapefruit juice, indinavir (Crixivan), itraconazole (Sporanox), ketoconazole (Nizoral), nefazodone (Serzone), quinupristin/dalfopristin (Synercid), ritonavir (Norvir), and troleandomycin (Tao). Indeed, the list of drugs that can increase cyclosporine levels reads nearly like a list of all known 3A4 inhibitors—including modest ones, such as fluoxetine and fluvoxamine. In one case, a 20-mg dose of fluoxetine (Prozac) doubled cyclosporine levels (Horton and Bonser 1995). In another case, a 100-mg dose of fluvoxamine increased serum cyclosporine levels from 200 to 380 ng/mL (Vella and Sayegh 1998).

Cyclosporine is an expensive drug, and some have advocated exploiting the inhibition of cyclosporine metabolism to reduce the drug's cost. Grapefruit juice was given to healthy volunteers taking cyclosporine, and the effect was hypothesized to be cost saving (Min et al. 1996; Yee et al. 1995). There are risks to this strategy; for example, the concentration of the chemical that inhibits 3A4 and P-glycoprotein is inconsistent. Diltiazem and verapamil were found to have cyclosporine-sparing effects through their inhibition of 3A4 (Leibbrandt and Day 1992; Sketris et al. 1994). In a review of these strategies, Jones (1997) noted the potential risk of toxicity due to increased pill burden and side effects, factors that may outweigh the economic benefit. Vella and Sayegh (1998) and Wright et al. (1999) presented cases in which nefazodone and fluvoxamine increased serum cyclosporine and creatinine levels. Although lower doses of the expensive cyclosporine were possible, patients were subjected to more frequent monitoring and blood sampling, procedures that may be particularly poorly tolerated by depressed or anxious patients. Patients may also experience organ rejection if treatment with the inhibiting agent is stopped suddenly, which will rapidly decrease serum cyclosporine concentrations (Moore et al. 1996).

Because cyclosporine is a substrate of P-glycoprotein, inhibitors of P-glycoprotein can increase cyclosporine levels as well. It can be difficult to pinpoint this mechanism, however, because there is so much overlap with 3A4 and P-glycoprotein substrates, inhibitors, and inducers. In one report, the authors suggested that a P-glycoprotein-related interaction between azithromycin and cyclosporine might have occurred (Page et al. 2001), because azithromycin is only a mild inhibitor of 3A4. However, azithromycin's inhibition of P-glycoprotein is not well established. Cyclosporine's inhibition of P-glycoprotein may be responsible for increases in levels of other drugs, such as cancer chemotherapy agents (Theis et al. 1998), but again, the overlap with 3A4 makes it difficult to draw definite conclusions.

Drugs that induce 3A4 (or P-glycoprotein) can decrease cyclosporine levels and bring about transplant rejection. Well-known inducers of 3A4 have all been reported, in multiple cases, to significantly decrease levels of cyclosporine; such drugs include carbamazepine, phenobarbital, phenytoin, and rifampin. In one case, cyclosporine levels decreased 50% after 1 month of coadministration of the modest 3A4 inducer modafinil (Provigil) at 200 mg/day (Provigil 1999).

St. John's wort has been publicized as a safe and natural alternative for treating modest depression; therefore, its use in medically complicated recipients of organ transplants is not surprising. This herbal supplement is considered an inducer of 3A4 and perhaps P-glycoprotein (Durr et al. 2000). Since the first report of heart transplant rejection from the use of the supplement with cyclosporine (Ruschitzka et al. 2000), 11 more case reports on this interaction have been published (Ernst 2002). Thus, St. John's wort should not be used with cyclosporine unless cyclosporine levels are vigorously monitored.

■ DNA CROSS-LINKING AGENTS

Cyclophosphamide

Cyclophosphamide is discussed in Chapter 16 ["Oncology"].

Mitoxantrone

Mitoxantrone (Novantrone) is a parenteral antineoplastic agent similar to anthracyclines, such as doxorubicin. Although approved for use in treating a variety of neoplasms, in 2000 the U.S. Food and Drug Administration (FDA) approved its use in multiple sclerosis. Mitoxantrone is cleared by oxidative metabolism, glucuronidation, and excretion (some of the drug is excreted unchanged) (Novantrone 2001). Very little is known about any pharmacokinetic drug-drug interactions, although pharmacodynamic interactions are a known potential problem—particularly with other drugs that may affect bleeding times.

■ FOLATE INHIBITORS

Methotrexate

Methotrexate is discussed in Chapter 16 ("Oncology").

■ INHIBITORS AND ANALOGS OF DNA BASE PAIRS

Azathioprine

Azathioprine (Imuran), first released by the FDA in 1968, is used in a host of autoimmune disorders and is administered to prevent renal transplant rejection. Few drug interactions involving azathioprine are known (Haagsma 1998), but azathioprine is a pro-drug and is metabolized to its active purine analog by unknown liver enzymes to mercaptopurine (see "Mercaptopurine"). In this sense, azathioprine's drug-drug interaction profile is similar to that of mercapto-purine.

Mercaptopurine

Mercaptopurine (6-MP; Purinethol) was approved by the FDA in 1953 and is used in a wide variety of disorders, including Crohn's disease, ulcerative colitis, and several forms of leukemia. Some of it is excreted unchanged. It is also metabolized by thiopurine methyltransferase (TPMT), an oxidative enzyme in the liver that metabolizes other endogenous thiopurines. For years it has been known that TPMT is polymorphic and that 1 in 300 individuals essentially lack the enzyme (Lennard et al. 1989). Normal doses of azathioprine or 6-MP in patients with low TPMT activity can cause severe toxicity, resulting in acute myelosuppression. It is current practice for genetic screening to be performed before azathioprine or 6-MP is prescribed, to determine whether the patient has diminished TPMT activity (Schwartz 2002).

Mycophenolate Mofetil

Mycophenolate mofetil (CellCept) is a parenteral or oral immunosuppressive agent that works by inhibiting an enzyme necessary for purine synthesis. It is actually a pro-drug and is quickly metabolized to mycophenolic acid. It is approved for use in a variety of organ transplantation procedures, for the purpose of preventing graft rejection. The pro-drug is rapidly hydrolyzed, and 5 minutes after intravenous injection, levels of mycophenolate mofetil are undetectable. Mycophenolic acid, the metabolite, is metabolized through glucuronidation, and most excreted mycophenolic acid is in the form of its glucuronide conjugate. Although pharmacodynamic drug-drug interactions involving mycophenolate mofetil are known, there are no reports of pharmacokinetic drug interactions with mycophenolate mofetil that relate to its rapid hydrolysis or its conjugation with glucuronic acid (CellCept 2000).

■ MACROLIDES

Sirolimus

Sirolimus (Rapamune) is a macrolide immunosuppressant that inhibits the second phase of T-cell activation (Rapamune 2002). This mechanism is different than that of cyclosporine or tacrolimus (Prograf). Unlike cyclosporine and tacrolimus, sirolimus appears not to produce end-organ toxicity. Therefore, higher levels of sirolimus are rarely associated with cognitive impairment or nephrotoxicity.

Sirolimus is metabolized by 3A4 and is also a P-glycoprotein substrate (Rapamune 2002). Inhibitors of 3A4 (including cyclosporine, diltiazem, and ketoconazole) have been shown to increase sirolimus levels. Of greater concern is the possibility of a decrease in sirolimus levels when the drug is administered with a 3A4 or P-glycoprotein inducer. Fourteen days of rifampin therapy was shown to increase sirolimus clearance 5.5-fold (Rapamune 2002). The manufacturer has indicated that other typical 3A4 inducers, such as carbamazepine, phenobarbital, and phenytoin, can decrease sirolimus levels (Rapamune 2002). Therefore, when sirolimus is used with any 3A4 inducer, sirolimus concentrations should be monitored, to avoid graft rejection due to decreased levels.

Tacrolimus

Tacrolimus (Prograf), formerly known as FK-506, is a macrolide immunosuppressant that inhibits the first phase of T-cell activation, a mechanism similar to that of cyclosporine (Prograf 1998). It appears to be a substrate of 3A4 (Prograf 1998) and P-glycoprotein (Arima et al. 2001), as well as an inhibitor of P-glycoprotein (Naito et al. 1992). Tacrolimus has narrow safety and therapeutic windows. Excessive levels can lead to cognitive impairment and nephrotoxicity, and low levels can lead to organ transplant rejection.

Multiple cases have been reported of increased serum tacrolimus levels with coadministration of the 3A4 inhibitors clarithromycin, diltiazem, erythromycin, fluconazole, indinavir, itraconazole, ketoconazole, nefazodone, and ritonavir. It is also suspected that grapefruit juice (Kane and Lipsky 2000) and quinupristin (Synercid 2000) may significantly increase tacrolimus levels by inhibiting 3A4 or P-glycoprotein or both.

Clotrimazole, a modest inhibitor of 3A4, was shown to increase tacrolimus levels in a series of 17 renal transplant recipients (Vasquez et al. 2001). The drug was used prophylactically to prevent oral thrush. Nystatin, which was given to control subjects, did not have an effect on tacrolimus levels. Felodipine, a calcium-channel blocker with modest 3A4 inhibition, increased tacrolimus levels in one case (Butani et al. 2002).

Homma et al. (2002) reported that a patient who was a poor metabolizer at 2C19 had increased levels of tacrolimus when prescribed lansoprazole, a proton pump inhibitor. Most proton pump inhibitors are metabolized by 3A4 and 2C19. It was theorized that in this patient, who was deficient in 2C19, the responsibility for lansoprazole clearance shifted to 3A4, which resulted in competitive inhibition of tacrolimus clearance.

Tacrolimus appears to be a moderate inhibitor of 3A4, and tacrolimus use has led to increases in serum levels of cyclosporine in vitro (Omar et al. 1991). Generally, these drugs are combined cautiously because even if tacrolimus does not increase cyclosporine levels, coadministration may increase the risk of nephrotoxicity. Tacrolimus also increased simvastatin levels in one case, leading to rhabdomyolysis and renal failure (Kotanko et al. 2002). It is presumed that tacrolimus inhibited simvastatin clearance via 3A4.

Like cyclosporine, tacrolimus is a substrate of P-glycoprotein, and therefore inhibitors and inducers of P-glycoprotein may change serum tacrolimus levels. Evidence of these interactions is scant, in part because of the overlap between 3A4 and P-glycoprotein substrates, inhibitors, and inducers.

Uridine 5'-diphosphate glucuronosyltransferase (UGT) enzymes may be involved in the metabolism of tacrolimus, and tacrolimus may inhibit UGTs. Taber et al. (2000) reported a fivefold increase in tacrolimus levels when the drug was used with chloramphenicol, and the investigators hypothesized that the increase was due to inhibition of UGTs. In one patient, use of tacrolimus with the anticancer agent CPT-11, a pro-drug that is catalyzed to SN-38 by UGT1A1, resulted in decreased SN-38 levels, perhaps because tacrolimus inhibited UGT1A1 (Gornet et al. 2001).

Induction of 3A4 has been demonstrated to decrease tacrolimus levels. Rifampin was shown to induce tacrolimus metabolism in a 61-year-old renal transplant recipient (Chenhsu et al. 2000). The patient required 10 times the dose of tacrolimus when taking rifampin. St. John's wort, a known inducer of 3A4 and P-glycoprotein, also has been shown to decrease tacrolimus levels (Bolley et al. 2002). As with cyclosporine, patients receiving tacrolimus should not use St. John's wort without careful monitoring of serum tacrolimus levels.

■ MONOCLONAL ANTIBODIES

Three monoclonal antibodies are used as immunosuppressant agents in recipients of allografts: basiliximab (Simulect), daclizumab (Zenapax), and muromonab-CD3 (Orthoclone OKT3). Basiliximab and daclizumab are produced by DNA technology (Simulect 2001; Zenapax 1999). They are immunoglobulin G monoclonal antibodies with half-lives similar to those of endogenous immunoglobulin G (several weeks). Muromonab-CD3 is a monoclonal antibody of murine origin. It recognizes and binds to CD3 antigens of human T lymphocytes, inhibiting their function (Orthoclone OKT3 2001). Its clearance is dependent on the amount of available CD3 molecules. Although there are reports of pharmacodynamic interactions involving these drugs and, particularly, other immunosuppressants, pharmacokinetic drug-drug interactions have not been reported.

■ SUMMARY

Potent inhibitors and inducers of 3A4 metabolism may greatly affect immunosuppressants, leading to nephrotoxicity or organ failure. The addition of a potent inhibitor may make it possible to decrease the dose of an administered immunosuppressant—and thus reduce the cost of immunosuppressant therapy—but the risks of exploitation of the drug interaction may outweigh the benefits. Nefazodone and fluvoxamine have been implicated in interactions with these drugs. Most authors recommend serial monitoring of serum immunosuppressant and creatinine levels.

■ REFERENCES

Arima H, Yunomae K, Hirayama F, et al: Contribution of P-glycoprotein to the enhancing effects of dimethyl-beta-cyclodextrin on oral bioavailability of tacrolimus. J Pharmacol Exp Ther 297:547–555, 2001

Bolley R, Zulke C, Kammerl M, et al: Tacrolimus-induced nephrotoxicity unmasked by induction of the CYP3A4 system with St John's wort (letter). Transplantation 73:1009, 2002

Butani L, Berg G, Makker SP: Effect of felodipine on tacrolimus pharmacokinetics in a renal transplant recipient. Transplantation 73:159–160, 2002

CellCept (package insert). Nutley, NJ, Roche Laboratories, 2000

Chenhsu RY, Loong CC, Chou MH, et al: Renal allograft dysfunction associated with rifampin-tacrolimus interaction. Ann Pharmacother 34:27–31, 2000

Durr D, Stieger B, Kullak-Ublick GA, et al: St John's wort induces intestinal P-glycoprotein/MDR1 and intestinal and hepatic CYP3A4. Clin Pharmacol Ther 68:598–604, 2000

Ernst E: St. John's wort supplements endanger the success of organ transplantation. Arch Surg 137:316–319, 2002

Fahr A: Cyclosporin clinical pharmacokinetics. Clin Pharmacokinet 24:472–495, 1993

Gambertoglia JG, Frey FJ, Holferd NH, et al: Prednisone and prednisolone bioavailability in renal transplant patients. Kidney Int 21(4):621–626, 1982

Gornet JM, Lokiec F, Duclos-Vallee JC, et al: Severe CPT-11 induced diarrhea in the presence of FK-506 following liver transplantation for hepatocellular injury. Anticancer Res 21:4203–4206, 2001

Haagsma CJ: Clinically important drug interactions with disease-modifying antirheumatic drugs. Drugs Aging 13:281–289, 1998

Homma M, Itagaki F, Yuzawa K, et al: Effects of lansoprazole and rabeprazole on tacrolimus blood concentrations: case of a renal transplant recipient with *CYP2C19* gene mutation. Transplantation 73:303–304, 2002

Horton RC, Bonser RS: Interaction between cyclosporin and fluoxetine. BMJ 311:422, 1995

Imani S, Jusko WJ, Steiner R: Diltiazem retards the metabolism of oral prednisone with effects on T-cell markers. Pediatr Transplant 3:126–130, 1999

Jones TE: The use of other drugs to allow a lower dosage of cyclosporin to be used. Therapeutic and pharmacoeconomic considerations. Clin Pharmacokinet 32:357–367, 1997

Kane GC, Lipsky JJ: Drug-grapefruit juice interactions. Mayo Clin Proc 75: 933–942, 2000

Kotanko P, Kirisits W, Skrabel F: Rhabdomyolysis and acute renal graft impairment in a patient treated with simvastatin, tacrolimus and fusidic acid. Nephron 90:234–235, 2002

Leibbrandt DM, Day RO: Cyclosporin and calcium channel blockers: an exploitable drug interaction? Med J Aust 157:296–297, 1992

Lennard L, Van Loon JA, Weinshilboum RM: Pharmacogenetics of acute azathioprine toxicity: relationship to thiopurine methyltransferase genetic polymorphism. Clin Pharmacol Ther 46:149–154, 1989

Lin Y, Anderson GD, Kantor E, et al: Differences in the urinary excretion of 6-beta-hydroxycortisol/cortisol between Asian and Caucasian women. J Clin Pharmacol 39:578–582, 1999

Lo A, Burckart GJ: P-glycoprotein and drug therapy in organ transplantation. J Clin Pharmacol 39:995–1005, 1999

Min DI, Ku YM, Perry PJ, et al: Effect of grapefruit juice on cyclosporine pharmacokinetics in renal transplant patients. Transplantation 62:123–125, 1996

Moore LW, Alloway RR, Vera SR, et al: Clinical observations of metabolic changes occurring in renal transplant recipients receiving ketoconazole. Transplantation 61:537–541, 1996

Naito M, Oh-hara T, Yamazaki A, et al: Reversal of multidrug resistance by an immunosuppressive agent FK-506. Cancer Chemother Pharmacol 29:195–200, 1992

Novantrone (package insert). Seattle, WA, Immunex Corp., 2001

Omar G, Shah IA, Thomson AW, et al: FK 506 inhibition of cyclosporine metabolism by human liver microsomes. Transplant Proc 23:934–935, 1991

Orthoclone OKT3 (package insert). Raritan, NJ, Ortho Biotech Products, 2001

Page RL 2nd, Ruscin JM, Fish D, et al: Possible interaction between intravenous azithromycin and oral cyclosporine. Pharmacotherapy 21:1436–1443, 2001

Prograf (package insert). Deerfield, IL, Fujisawa Healthcare Inc., 1998

Provigil (package insert). West Chester, PA, Cephalon, Inc., 1999

Rapamune (package insert). Philadelphia, PA, Wyeth-Ayerst Pharmaceuticals Inc., 2002

Ruschitzka F, Meier PJ, Turina M, et al: Acute heart transplant rejection due to Saint John's wort. Lancet 355:548–549, 2000

Sandimmune (package insert). East Hanover, NJ, Novartis, 2001

Schwartz JB: Pharmacogenetics: has it reached the clinic? Journal of Gender Specific Medicine 5:13–18, 2002

Simulect (package insert). East Hanover, NJ, Novartis Pharmaceuticals Corp., 2001

Sketris IS, Methot ME, Nicol D, et al: Effect of calcium-channel blockers on cyclosporine clearance and use in renal transplant patients. Ann Pharmacother 28:1227–1231, 1994

Synercid (package insert). Bridgewater, NJ, Aventis Pharmaceuticals Products, Inc., 2000

Taber DJ, Dupuis RE, Hollar KD, et al: Drug-drug interaction between chloramphenicol and tacrolimus in a liver transplant recipient. Transplant Proc 32:660–662, 2000

Theis JG, Chan HS, Greenberg ML, et al: Increased systemic toxicity of sarcoma chemotherapy due to combination with the P-glycoprotein inhibitor cyclosporin. Int J Clin Pharmacol Ther 36:61–64, 1998

Vasquez E, Pollak R, Benedetti E: Clotrimazole increases tacrolimus blood levels: a drug interaction in kidney transplant patients. Clin Transplant 15:95–99, 2001

Vella JP, Sayegh MH: Interactions between cyclosporine and newer antidepressant medications. Am J Kidney Dis 31:320–323, 1998

Wassner SJ, Malekzadeh MH, Dennis AJ, et al: Allograft survival in patients receiving anticonvulsant medications. Clin Nephrol 8(1):293–297, 1977

Wright DH, Lake KD, Bruhn PS, et al: Nefazodone and cyclosporine drug-drug interaction. J Heart Lung Transplant 18:913–915, 1999

Yee GC, Stanley DL, Pessa LJ, et al: Effect of grapefruit juice on blood cyclosporin concentration. Lancet 345:955–956, 1995

Zenapax (package insert). Nutley, NJ, Roche Laboratories, 1999

Part IV

Practical Matters

21

GUIDELINES

- ■ **GUIDELINES FOR CATEGORIZING DRUG INTERACTIONS**

- ■ **GUIDELINES FOR PRESCRIBING IN A POLYPHARMACY ENVIRONMENT**

Given the modern polypharmacy environment, clinicians may feel hindered in making prescribing decisions. Because there are so many interactions and potential interactions to watch for, clinicians often feel "frozen" when facing polypharmacy. The use of multiple physicians and pharmacies by patients increases the risk of insufficient clinical coordination of complicated medication regimens. The five basic principles that follow can help guide clinicians and prevent the occurrence of most metabolism-mediated drug interactions. We hope the rest of this book frees clinicians up even further, allowing for safer prescribing of "difficult" drugs.

- ■ **GUIDELINES FOR ASSESSING AND MANAGING DRUG INTERACTIONS**

Polypharmacy cannot be avoided. It is important to remain watchful and to understand the steps for identification and management of drug interactions should they arise. A useful algorithm for attending to drug interactions is found here.

■ SIX PATTERNS OF PHARMACOKINETIC DRUG INTERACTIONS

Pattern 1: Inhibitor added to a substrate

This pattern generally results in increased substrate levels. If the substrate has a low therapeutic index, toxicity may result unless care is exercised (such as close monitoring of blood levels and/or decreasing of parent drug doses in anticipation of the interaction).

Example: Paroxetine (2D6 inhibitor) added to nortriptyline (2D6 substrate with a narrow therapeutic window), leading to tricyclic toxicity

Corollary: If a drug or substrate needs to be activated at a particular enzyme (i.e., is a pro-drug) and the necessary enzyme is inhibited, there will be a loss of efficacy, not toxicity, because the active metabolite will not be produced (e.g., tramadol [pro-drug requiring activation at 2D6] administered with paroxetine [2D6 inhibitor]). If the parent compound has a narrow therapeutic index and accumulates, toxicity may result (e.g., terfenadine [cardiotoxic 3A4 substrate pro-drug] administered with ketoconazole [3A4 inhibitor], leading to terfenadine's being unable to form noncardiotoxic yet active fexofenadine).

Pattern 2: Substrate added to an inhibitor

This pattern may cause difficulties if the substrate has a low therapeutic index and is titrated according to preset guidelines that do not take into account the presence of an inhibitor. If the substrate is titrated to specific blood levels or to therapeutic effect, or with appreciation that an inhibitor is present, toxicity is less likely.

Example: Nortriptyline (2D6 substrate) added to quinidine (2D6 inhibitor) rapidly (i.e., not slowly and at low doses, or without checking levels)

■ SIX PATTERNS OF PHARMACOKINETIC DRUG INTERACTIONS (continued)

Pattern 3: Inducer added to a substrate

This pattern generally results in decreased substrate levels after 7–10 days, which may lead to a loss of substrate efficacy, unless levels are monitored and/or substrate doses are increased in anticipation of the interaction.

Example: Carbamazepine (3A4 inducer) added to oral contraceptives or cyclosporine (3A4 substrates), leading to contraceptive or organ transplant failure

Corollary: If an inducer is added to a compound with a more active or toxic metabolite, toxicity rather than loss of efficacy may result (e.g., acetaminophen is metabolized at 2E1 to a hepatotoxic metabolite, which normally is detoxified by the liver, but if acute acetaminophen overdose is associated with chronic ethanol use or with use of another "pan-inducer," hepatotoxic effects are produced).

Pattern 4: Substrate added to an inducer

This pattern may lead to ineffective dosing if preset dosing guidelines are followed that do not take into account the presence of a chronic inducer. If the substrate is titrated to a therapeutic blood level or to clinical effect, or with an appreciation that an inducer is present, dosing is more likely to be effective.

Example: Cyclosporine (3A4 substrate) added to St. John's wort (3A4 inducer)

Pattern 5: Reversal of inhibition

A substrate and an inhibitor are coadministered, equilibrium is achieved, and then treatment with the inhibitor is discontinued. This leads to a resumption of normal enzyme function and immediately results in lower levels of substrate, increased metabolite formation, and possibly loss of efficacy of the substrate.

Example: Cimetidine ("pan-inhibitor"; enzymes inhibited include 2D6) and nortriptyline (2D6 substrate) are simultaneously administered to good effect. When treatment with cimetidine is abruptly discontinued, subtherapeutic nortriptyline levels and loss of efficacy result.

■ SIX PATTERNS OF PHARMACOKINETIC DRUG INTERACTIONS *(continued)*

Pattern 6: Reversal of induction

A substrate and an inducer are simultaneously administered, equilibrium is achieved, and then treatment with the inducer is abruptly discontinued. This gradually results (over 2–3 weeks) in decreased amounts of available enzyme, leading to increased substrate levels, decreased metabolite formation, slower metabolism, and possibly to substrate toxicity.

Example: A chronic smoker (1A2 inducer in smoke) with therapeutic clozapine levels (1A2 substrate) stops smoking abruptly (during a hospitalization). Several weeks later, clozapine levels increase to the point of toxicity.

Source. N.B. Sandson, M.D. Adapted with permission.

■ PRESCRIBING GUIDELINES

If at all clinically possible:

1. **Avoid prescribing medications that either significantly inhibit or significantly induce enzymes.**

2. **Prescribe medications that are eliminated by multiple pathways (phase I metabolism, phase II metabolism, and/or renal excretion).**

Principles 1 and 2 should be weighed concurrently. By following the first principle, a clinician can avoid trouble. The serum levels of medications a patient is already taking will not be altered appreciably by the newly introduced medication, and if the patient is later prescribed a new medication by another physician, the prescribing clinician can feel relatively confident that potential drug interactions are less likely.

Similarly, if a clinician follows Principle 2 by prescribing a medication that is eliminated by multiple pathways, drugs later introduced—drugs with the potential to inhibit or induce one or two enzymes—will not cause as much of a problem with the original drug. In addition, phenotypic variability may be less of an issue; if the patient lacks full activity of one enzyme, other enzymes will help clear the drug.

3. **Prescribe medications that do not have serious consequences if their metabolisms are prolonged either because of concomitant use of a substrate inhibitor or because the patient being treated is a phenotypic poor metabolizer.**

Some psychotropic drugs have narrow margins of safety. Pimozide, clozapine, tricyclic antidepressants, many typical antipsychotics, and some antiseizure medications may have serious untoward effects if their metabolisms are significantly prolonged by substrate inhibitors or because of phenotypic variability. Some of these effects are severe cardiac toxicity, seizures, extreme sedation, and extrapyramidal symptoms.

■ PRESCRIBING GUIDELINES *(continued)*

4. Monitor serum drug levels often if you are concerned about potential P450-mediated interactions.

Although it is not necessary to obtain serum drug levels at all times, drug level monitoring can often be of great assistance when multiple drugs are being administered. Some examples of the practical use of serum drug levels are given in the study cases in Part II.

5. Remind patients to tell you when other physicians prescribe medications for them.

Educating patients about the possibilities of drug interactions often reduces the risk of such interactions. *All patients receiving medications with narrow therapeutic windows or severe toxicities should be given this instruction.* A prescribing clinician can keep up with possible interactions by asking patients to contact him or her any time a new medication has been prescribed by another clinician. Patients appreciate being given the responsibility of monitoring the effects of their medications (with their providers' assistance); and side effects, toxicities, and potentially fatal outcomes have been prevented many, many times with this approach.

There are two other important issues to consider when making prescribing decisions:

1. Metabolism by P450 enzymes does not always inactivate compounds. Some drugs are pro-drugs and are activated by enzymatic action to active or more active compounds.

Tramadol and some alkylating agents are examples of such medications. Additionally, some drugs, such as bupropion, haloperidol, fluoxetine, and risperidone, are metabolized to equally effective pharmacologically active metabolites.

2. Generally, the older the drug (particularly if the drug was released in the United States before 1990), the less is known about its metabolism.

Older information on drug-drug interactions is often based on case reports, whereas newer drugs have been better profiled by the manufacturers to improve their chances of approval by the U.S. Food and Drug Administration. Much of this change occurred after unexpected interactions associated with fluoxetine and with nonsedating antihistamines were reported in the 1980s and 1990s.

■ ALGORITHM FOR ASSESSING AND MANAGING DRUG INTERACTIONS

1. Identify interaction

Consult pertinent resources: Resources include literature identified through *PubMed* or other citation databases, drug interaction textbooks or newsletters, commercial drug interaction software programs, and abstracts from conferences. Important information may be obtained from researchers or the manufacturer directly.

Anticipate or predict likely interactions: On the basis of the pharmacology and pharmacokinetics of the suspected medications, would you anticipate a potential interaction? (For example, are the drugs metabolized by the same subset of P450 enzymes? Do they have enzyme-inhibiting or -inducing properties? Is drug absorption pH dependent or susceptible to cation binding?)

2. Verify existence of interaction

In the literature

How was the interaction described? Was it noted retrospectively, in a study of a single case, an in vitro study, preclinical testing, or a controlled pharmacokinetic human study? In healthy volunteers or in a target patient population?

Can the data be applied to your patient population? Was the study population similar to your own? What were the doses and duration of the agent used? Did the subjects have coexisting disease states? Were the subjects taking concomitant medications?

In a clinical situation

What is the time course of the interaction? How long will it take for the interaction to develop? What clinical consequences do you expect to see? Has the interaction already occurred?

Do the clinical signs and symptoms support your assumptions?

Is the objective evidence, such as drug concentrations, available?

Have other potentiating factors been ruled out?

■ ALGORITHM FOR ASSESSING AND MANAGING DRUG INTERACTIONS (*continued*)

3. Assess clinical significance of interaction

Do the agents involved have a narrow therapeutic index? Are the drugs associated with dose-related efficacy or toxicity?

Is there risk of therapeutic failure or of development of resistance?

4. Evaluate available therapeutic alternatives

Space doses: Can doses be spaced in a practical and/or convenient way for the patient?

Increase dose: Is increasing the dose affordable? Are appropriate dosage forms available?

Decrease dose: Are appropriate dosage forms available?

Discontinue administration of one drug: What are the therapeutic consequences of temporarily or permanently discontinuing treatment with one agent?

Change agent: What are the comparative efficacy, adverse effects, cost, availability, compliance issues, and drug interactions associated with a new agent?

Add another agent to counteract effect of interaction: What are the comparative efficacy, adverse effects, cost, availability, compliance issues, and drug interactions associated with a new agent?

Take no action: In certain situations (e.g., when the likelihood of an interaction occurring is low or when the clinical effect of a potential interaction would be minor or insignificant), the practitioner may want to maintain the patient's current regimen and monitor the patient's condition. Should evidence of a clinically significant interaction be detected, one of the above-mentioned management options may then be considered.

Source. Adapted from Tseng AL, Foisy MM: "Management of Drug Interactions in Patients With HIV." *Annals of Pharmacotherapy* 31:1040–1058, 1997. Used with permission.

MEDICOLEGAL IMPLICATIONS OF DRUG-DRUG INTERACTIONS

David M. Benedek, M.D.

Ethical principles of beneficence and nonmalfeasance dictate that physicians keep abreast of research on drug-drug interactions so that they can provide the best care for their patients. Moreover, legally defined standards of care necessitate that physicians not only incorporate this knowledge into their clinical practice but also share this information with patients, so that patient and clinician can collaborate in decision making.

In this chapter, legal standards and landmark medicolegal cases defining the scope of these responsibilities are reviewed. The extent to which drug interactions have been implicated in malpractice cases and other forensic arenas are explored. Finally, guidelines for risk management are outlined, and case vignettes illustrate the potential for application of these recommendations.

■ MEDICATION THERAPY AND MALPRACTICE

A malpractice suit is an action in tort: a request for compensation for damage to one party caused by the tortious (noncriminal) act or omission of another. Tradition, common law, and case law have upheld the idea that a physician, by virtue of his or her fiduciary relationship with the patient, has special duties—beyond those reasonably expected between other members of society—to prevent harm. In a malpractice suit, a plaintiff must establish, by a preponderance of the evidence, dereliction (by act or omission) of this special duty—dereliction resulting in physical or emotional damage. Notably, the standard of proof (often defined as 51% of the evidence) is markedly lower than that necessary for determination of criminal culpability. Malpractice suits may result from various aspects of care, ranging from misdiagnosis to inadequate performance of surgical procedures to failure to establish or provide adequate follow-up. However, negligent use of medications (excessive or inadequate dosing, failure to monitor levels, failure to select appropriate medications) and failure to obtain appropriate informed consent are causes of action that may result from a physician's lack of awareness of drug interactions or failure to address this potential in treatment decisions.

■ LEGAL PRINCIPLES AND LANDMARK CASES

The courts determine the degree to which a physician's care represents appropriate treatment versus dereliction of duty by considering the standard of care as it applies to particular practices (acts or omissions). Exact definitions vary from jurisdiction to jurisdiction, but this benchmark is generally regarded as "the custom of the profession, as reflected in the standard of care common to other professionals of the practitioner's training and theoretical orientation" (Gutheil and Appelbaum 2000, p. 142). The courts most commonly rely on medical expert testimony to determine whether a specific practice represents a deviation from the standard of care. However, if a clinician chooses a medication for an unapproved use, prescribes medication in doses beyond those recommended, or fails to monitor levels as specifically required by the U.S. Food and Drug Administration or recommended by the manufacturer, these actions are viewed as prima facie evidence of negligence (under the legal principle of *res ipsa loquitur*—"the thing speaks for itself"). The burden of proof in such circumstances shifts from the plaintiff to the physician, who must now establish that his or her care was not negligent. In cases in which drug interactions are known to result in inhibition of a specific agent's metabolism, prescribing a medication in otherwise appropriate doses might be viewed by the court as excessive use. Failure to monitor drug levels appropriately (when therapeutic and toxic levels have been established) would similarly represent negligent care if an adverse drug reaction resulted from drug toxicity.

Cases involving death or permanent injury have resulted in multimillion-dollar awards for plaintiffs even when both agents involved in the interaction were prescribed within recommended dosing guidelines. In 1999, for example, the Oregon Court of Appeals awarded $23 million (in a case against a physician and a pharmaceutical company) when permanent brain damage resulted from seizures precipitated by theophylline toxicity 1 week after appropriately dosed ciprofloxacin was added to the patient's chronic asthma treatment (*Bocci v. Key Pharmaceuticals* 1999). Ciprofloxacin potently inhibits 1A2, an enzyme on which theophylline depends for clearance.

Legal decisions have also established more precisely the nature of the information that a physician must provide to the patient in obtaining informed consent for treatment (including medication management). If treatment is initiated without voluntary, competent, and knowing (informed) consent, this care would constitute an unconsented touching or battery as defined by common law, even if the intent was benevolent. The idea reflects the degree to which law attempts to protect bodily autonomy as a part of the fundamental right to liberty. In *Natanson v. Kline* (1960), the Kansas Supreme Court opined that "the physician should explain the nature of the ailment, the nature of the proposed treatment, the probability of success or alternatives, and perhaps, the risks of unfortunate results" (p. 1093) in response to a complaint in which the patient alleged negligent care after radiation therapy following radical mastectomy. The court was not sympathetic to Dr. Kline's argument that the prevailing standard of care did not require the provision of any information about the significant risks associated with the procedure.

Decisions in other jurisdictions have further amplified the need to inform patients of risk potential. After a plaintiff sought damages when a surgeon failed to inform him of the 1% risk of paraplegia associated with an orthopedic procedure, the U.S. Court of Appeals for the District of Columbia held that the scope of a physician's communications regarding potential risks must be "measured by the patient's need" (*Canterbury v. Spence* 1972, p. 773). This opinion, and subsequent decisions in other jurisdictions, established the idea that the patient must be informed of the material risks of treatment: those risks that are most common, and those that are most severe. In a 1996 case, after a subtotal thyroidectomy, a patient with Graves' disease received calcitriol (Rocaltrol; a synthetic vitamin D analog) and calcium carbonate (Os-Cal) for postoperative hypoparathyroidism and hypocalcemia. Shortly thereafter, he presented to the emergency room with decreased appetite, nausea, emesis, headache, ataxia, weakness, and lethargy. Then he experienced seizures, respiratory arrest, and loss of consciousness. In the subsequent malpractice suit, he alleged that he was improperly advised of his potential to develop hypocalcemia or early warning signs of hypocalcemia on this regimen and that his physician failed to monitor calcium levels properly. He was awarded more than $8 million in damages (*Brown v. Pepe et al.* 1996). Because patients must be warned about potentially severe reactions to their medications, informed consent for treatment with an agent known to interact adversely with another of the patient's medications must include provision of information about the risks of this interaction, if the adverse interaction is either common or severe. Multiple jurisdictions have upheld the principle that whereas others must exercise due care and diligence in the delivery of medications, the responsibility for warnings and informed consent rests primarily with the physician (*Kintigh v. Abbott Pharmacy* 1993; *Leesley v. West* 1988).

■ DRUG INTERACTIONS, ADVERSE OUTCOMES, AND MALPRACTICE: SCOPE OF THE PROBLEM

If physical or emotional damage result directly from a drug interaction that a physician knew or should have known about, or if an interaction-related injury was a material risk about which the patient should have been informed during the informed consent process, malpractice actions may ensue. The extent to which this type of malpractice occurs is not easy to establish. However, recent studies have shed light on the scope of these problems.

In August 2001, Kelly reviewed case reports of adverse drug reactions published in *Clin-Alert,* an established compendium of adverse drug reactions reported in medical, legal, and pharmacy journals. He found that 9% of the 1,520 reported events over a 20-year period resulted in a fatal outcome, a life-threatening event, or permanent disability. Although causality was not clearly established in all cases, and adverse drug reactions and allergies were the reported causes for the majority of adverse events, nearly one-third of the adverse drug reactions resulted from medication errors (dosing or administration) or drug interactions. Thirteen percent of the adverse drug reactions resulted in financial penalties (either via settlement or verdict) against health care providers, and the mean award amount was $3,127,890 (Kelly 2001). Data on awards stemming directly from drug-drug interactions were not reported. However, reasons for lawsuits were noted generally as overdoses, poor or no monitoring, or improper treatment (Kelly 2001). Drug interactions may figure into each of these reasons, because interactions affect dosing and monitoring. In cases in which there is known to be a high risk of a drug-drug interaction, even the choice of a medication that the Food and Drug Administration approved for use in a specific illness could constitute improper treatment (when more reasonable alternatives are available).

Actual medicolegal significance may be considerably greater than that indicated by the study. Kelly (2001) noted that *Clin-Alert* abstracted adverse drug reactions from only one legal journal, and it was not necessarily clear whether a lawsuit evolved from cases reported in the medical or pharmacological journals. In addition, clinicians have noted experience in cases involving drug interaction damage awards or settlements that have not been reported in published format (R.C. Hall, personal communication, March 2001; R.S. Simon, personal communication, May 2001).

More recently, Preskorn (2002) reported on case series and case reports of deaths presumed to be due to intentional overdoses of psychotropic medications. He noted that in some of these cases, drug-drug interactions with other prescribed medications appeared to have resulted in truly accidental deaths. In other cases, the drug-drug interaction—rather than the toxic effects of the psychotropic agent intentionally taken in excess—actually caused the (intended) death by suicide. He concluded that in such cases, although the outcome is recognized as a suicide, the extent to which a drug-drug interaction contributed to the outcome may be underappreciated.

Although courts have traditionally been hesitant to recognize legal duties of pharmacists beyond the duty to dispense medications accurately, recent cases have established the principle that pharmacists may share some responsibility for informing a patient of potential interactions, particularly if they voluntarily assume such a burden by advertising a capability to detect them (Cacciatore 1996). Nonetheless, the deference the courts have shown to the physician-patient relationship indicates that even in these circumstances, physicians will continue to bear much of the burden for knowing about, when prudent avoiding, or informing patients about potential drug interactions.

■ REDUCING LIABILITY RISK

Clearly, the physician must keep abreast of data regarding dangerous drug interactions. Continuous review of medical journals and bulletins for reports of drug-drug interactions is one way to keep pace with the knowledge that eventually shapes the standard of care. Participation in continuing medical education programs addressing these issues is certainly another. Recent technological advances such as computerized order entry and medication screening are gaining increased recognition as means to reduce medication errors and will likely represent the standard of care in hospitals in the near future. Pharmacy literature has advocated for such institutional changes for years (Cacciatore 1996). For individual providers, low-cost and free computer programs are available to aid the physician in rapidly establishing patient medication profiles for known interactions. This software includes Internet update capability that permits frequent updates. Tens of thousands of physicians are availing themselves of these programs, but the extent to which appropriate use of such software may become the standard of care is an area provoking considerable speculation.

The sharing of this increased knowledge of drug interactions with the patient when obtaining informed consent, and the documentation of such discussions in the treatment record in informed consent notes, will reduce the likelihood of liability in the event of an adverse drug interaction. Moreover, by virtue of the thorough review of medications these discussions entail, the discussions may actually modify treatment decisions and therefore decrease the potential for such interactions. Discussions with patients about the possibility that new data may emerge regarding the safety of potential medications, as well as reminders to consult clinicians and pharmacists before medication changes or use of over-the-counter medications, furthers patient confidence and trust in the care providers and decreases the risk of litigation when adverse events occur. The active development of an environment of trust and collaboration reduces the patient's propensity for litigation even when adverse events result from clinician error. Finally, because patients with psychiatric illness are often at increased risk for suicide attempts, medication decisions must take into account not only the safety in overdose of the prescribed psychotropic agent, but also the potential for a drug-drug interaction resulting in death or disability when an otherwise "safe" psychotropic medication is taken in intentional overdose.

■ CASE EXAMPLES

The following vignettes have been adapted from cases with which the author is familiar. The cases have been sufficiently altered to disguise facts and identities without altering the salient points with regard to medicolegal principles or risk management.

Case 1: Loss of the "Therapeutic Benefit" of a Drug-Drug Interaction

Mr. A, a 58-year-old man with chronic knee pain, was referred to a psychiatrist by his family physician after no improvement in depressed mood, irritability, and somatic complaints despite treatment with fluoxetine (Prozac) titrated to 80 mg/day over 8 weeks. When the psychiatrist obtained a history of worsening insomnia, increased migraine headaches, and gastrointestinal disturbance (heartburn), she recommended decreasing the fluoxetine dose to 40 mg/day to reduce activation and gastrointestinal side effects, adding amitriptyline (Elavil) 50 mg at night (to augment the selective serotonin reuptake inhibitor [SSRI], improve sleep, and potentially reduce the knee pain component of the patient's depressive syndrome), and adding cimetidine (Tagamet), 300 mg four times a day, to alleviate the patient's heartburn. The family physician followed these recommendations.

Three weeks later, Mr. A informed his family physician that he was indeed feeling significantly improved. His mood had lifted, his sleep had returned to normal, and his gastrointestinal symptoms had fully resolved. The family physician continued treatment with amitriptyline and fluoxetine but discontinued cimetidine therapy. Three weeks later, Mr. A was found at home dead. Autopsy revealed a toxic amitriptyline level, and the manner of death was considered suicide by overdose.

Mr. A's wife sued both physicians, alleging failure to monitor tricyclic antidepressant (TCA) levels and failure to warn of the potential interactions between the TCA and the SSRI *as well as the potential interaction between these medications and cimetidine*. In a deposition, an expert in clinical psychopharmacology opined that Mr. A's response to the combination of TCA and SSRI occurred at blood levels higher than expected by the dosing strategy, because of competitive inhibition of their hepatic metabolism by each other and cimetidine. He concluded that when treatment with cimetidine was discontinued, depressive symptoms returned because the antidepressant concentrations returned to subtherapeutic levels. The defendant physicians argued that the relatively low dose of amitriptyline did not necessitate therapeutic drug level monitoring and that fluoxetine levels are not routinely measured in clinical care. Both claimed that they warned the patient about the potential for reoccurrence of depressive symptoms, but both acknowledged that they did not specifically warn the patient that discontinuation of cimetidine therapy could result in a decrease in antidepressant blood levels or efficacy. The case was eventually settled out of court.

This vignette serves to illustrate several important points with regard to the medicolegal significance of drug-drug interactions. Although it is unclear whether the physicians involved recognized the potential "therapeutic benefit" of the cimetidine-TCA-SSRI interaction, available records and the physicians' testimony indicate that when making the decision to discontinue cimetidine therapy, they did not warn the patient about the potential effect of this interaction. Because the duty to obtain informed consent regarding treatment includes a requirement for the physician to provide information concerning the risk, benefits, and alternatives to treatment, it might have been successfully argued that failure to warn of the risks of discontinuing treatment breached this duty. If either physician discussed the risk of discontinuation of cimetidine with the patient and documented the counseling in the medical records, this argument would be invalidated. The fact that the widow brought suit suggests that she believed that treatment decisions were not made in a collaborative and informed manner. There is no legal obligation to involve other family members in treatment decisions concerning competent patients. However, if patient consent can be obtained, informing family members regarding warning signs for reoccurrence of depression may facilitate return to care before an untoward outcome and may reduce the extent to which grieving family members, feeling isolated from the treatment process, seek to blame physicians in the face of tragedy. Finally, although the cause of death in this case was ruled suicide by intentional overdose, whether the overdose would have proven fatal if it were not for the inhibition of TCA metabolism resulting from the prescribed fluoxetine remains an unanswered question.

Case 2: Treatment Decisions Taking Into Account the Natural Course of Comorbid Conditions

Mrs. B, a 47-year-old woman with a history of alcohol dependence and hypertension, sought additional care for intermittent symptoms of anxiety from her internist at the recommendation of her Alcoholics Anonymous sponsor. Verapamil (Calan), 180 mg twice a day, had provided fair control of her hypertension for more than a year, and she was taking no other medications. Her doctor initiated treatment for panic disorder, prescribing sertraline (Zoloft) (50 mg each morning). Cognizant of the potential for insomnia early in treatment, but cautious because of her history of alcohol dependence, he prescribed a 7-day supply of triazolam (Halcion) 0.25 mg, to be used nightly as needed for sleep if the sertraline resulted in sleep disturbance. Days later, the patient relapsed in her alcohol use and called her sponsor while intoxicated. The sponsor drove to the patient's home and found her unconscious. The sponsor then summoned emergency services, and the patient was hospitalized. The diagnosis was acute alcohol and benzodiazepine intoxication that resulted in respiratory compromise and transient coma.

On recovery, the patient sued her physician for failing to warn her about the potential interaction between the triazolobenzodiazepine triazolam and the calcium-channel blocker verapamil. She stated that had she been properly warned of this interaction, she would have continued taking verapamil but would have elected not to take triazolam. Her physician argued that her respiratory compromise and coma resulted from her voluntary alcohol ingestion rather than the medications he prescribed, but the patient's attorney countered that the physician was aware of her alcohol dependence. Indeed, medical records indicated that the internist's decision to prescribe only a minimal quantity of triazolam supported the notion that he was aware of the patient's potential for addiction, and the court ruled in favor of the patient.

Although hepatic inhibition of 3A4 by verapamil contributed to the increased central nervous system toxicity of the triazolam and subsequent respiratory collapse, so too did the patient's use of alcohol. The court, however, determined that the preponderance of evidence supported the patient's contention that she was improperly warned about the potential interactions between triazolam and verapamil and that she would not have taken the benzodiazepine if warned about this potentially serious interaction. Although the court recognized that the patient's own behavior contributed to the outcome, it apportioned a degree of responsibility to the physician in awarding damages. This vignette also illustrates the idea that when making medication decisions, physicians must remain aware of their patients' other illnesses (in Mrs. B's case, alcohol dependence), associated behavior (tendency toward relapse), and the potential effect of this behavior on drug-drug interactions. In this case, knowledge of the patient's potential for misuse of medications (given her history of alcohol dependence) and for use of medications in combination with alcohol necessitated consideration of alternative treatment choices for antidepressant-associated insomnia.

■ SUMMARY AND CONCLUSIONS

Keeping abreast of information regarding drug interactions poses significant challenges for the physician: new medications are rapidly introduced, and drug interactions are reported in a variety of forums, including legal journals, pharmacy journals, and pharmacological journals—sources to which clinicians do not frequently refer. Nonetheless, the law has established standards of physician conduct that necessitate assimilating this information into therapeutic decisions. Attention to these issues as they are reported in the medical literature, participation in relevant continuing medical education programs, use of technology that aids in identifying potential interactions, and respecting the patient's need to be aware of material risks when consenting to treatment are means by which the physician may reduce the risk of drug interaction–related liability.

418

■ REFERENCES

Armstrong SC, Cozza KL, Benedek DM: Med-psych drug-drug interactions update. Psychosomatics 43:245–247, 2002

Cacciatore GG: Advertising, computers, and pharmacy liability. A Michigan court's decision has ramifications for pharmaceutical care. J Am Pharm Assoc NS36:651–654, 1996

Gutheil TG, Appelbaum PS: Malpractice and other forms of liability, in Clinical Handbook of Psychiatry and the Law, 3rd Edition. Philadelphia, PA, Lippincott Williams & Wilkins, 2000, p 142

Kelly WN: Potential risks and prevention, part 4: reports of significant adverse drug events. Am J Health Syst Pharm 58:1406–1412, 2001

Preskorn SH: Fatal drug-drug interactions as a differential consideration in apparent suicides. Journal of Psychiatric Practice 8:233–238, 2002

Termini RB, The pharmacist duty to warn revisited: the changing role of pharmacy in health care and the resultant impact on the obligation of a pharmacist to warn, 4 OHIO N.U.L. REV. 551–566 (1998)

Winkelaar PG: Medicolegal file. Tacit approval of alternative therapy. Can Fam Physician 45:905, 1999

■ LEGAL CITATIONS

Bocci v Key Pharmaceuticals, 14 Pharmaceutical Litigation Reporter 13–14 (1999)

Brown v Pepe et al, Pharmaceutical Litigation Reporter 11781–11782 (1996)

Canterbury v Spence, 464 F2d 772 (DC Cir 1972)

Kintigh v Abbott Pharmacy, Mich Ct App, 503 NW2d 657, 661 (1993)

Leesley v West, Ill Ct App, 518 NE2d 758 (1988)

Natanson v Kline, 350 P2d 1093 (1960)

HOW TO RETRIEVE AND REVIEW THE LITERATURE

We believe it is important to help readers update this Concise Guide and maintain provider-specific lists themselves. Keeping abreast of the literature may seem daunting, but as providers in the setting of polypharmacy, physicians must do so.

■ SEARCHING THE INTERNET

The Internet is the most powerful, speedy, and all-encompassing way to keep up. How to interface with the Internet is changing daily. Many journals now provide "citation managers" that alert on-line subscribers when topics in which subscribers are interested are cited. Many of these services carry subscription fees.

Web browsers and Web sites are also evolving. Currently, our favorite search engines are *PubMed* (http://www.ncbi.nlm.nih.gov/pubmed) and that found in Physicians' Online (http://www.pol.net). *PubMed* taps directly into *MEDLINE*. Physicians' Online is a Web site with a particularly good drug-interaction tool, the Drug Therapy Monitoring System by Medi-Span, that feeds directly into *PubMed*. Physicians' Online also provides a brief review of the interaction literature and lists all interactions, not just P450-mediated interactions. There are some lapses in the provided data, however, particularly in terms of potential or predictable drug interactions. Dr. Oesterheld's Web site (http://www.mhc.com/Cytochromes) has up-to-date P450, uridine 5′-diphosphate glucuronosyltransferase

(UGT), and P-glycoprotein lists, and the optional drug interaction program is thorough, is updated regularly, and provides individualized interaction checks. This program also makes predictions about potential drug interactions, even if there are no available published reports. This drug-interaction tool provides selected references so that the reader can research why an interaction may occur.

Another interactive table is the Cytochrome P450 Drug Interaction Table (http://www.drug-interactions.com). This table is monitored by the University of Indiana Department of Medicine, is updated fairly often, and has hyperlinks to literature sources via *PubMed*. The table is restricted to P450-mediated interactions but is quite complete. *Physicians' Desk Reference* is on-line (http://www.pdr.net) and is a useful, though somewhat static, tool for reviewing drugs available in the United States. The drug interaction findings are limited to what is reported in the *Physicians' Desk Reference*. The U.S. Food and Drug Administration's Web site (http://www.fda.gov) provides the latest information on drugs, safety, and product approvals.

These sites have our seal of approval because rather than limiting the prescriber's options, they expand his or her knowledge and prescribing power. We believe that there are currently no personal digital assistant (PDA) programs with the power of these Web sites behind them. Most handheld programs do not provide the reasons or the references necessary to make an educated prescription choice. Many PDA programs simply state that an interaction exists, which may lead the user to *not* prescribe in situations in which it may be helpful to the patient to do so.

For a thorough search, we suggest going directly to one of the *MEDLINE* services mentioned earlier, which permits a review of the original research on one's own. We have found that the best MeSH terms to use to find literature on P450-mediated drug interactions are *pharmacokinetics, drug interaction, cytochrome,* and the names of the drugs being investigated. In a search for information on phase II–related interactions, using the drug name followed by the term *glucuronidation* or *metabolism* works well. Entering *P-glycoprotein* and the drug name yields references to literature on interactions involving P-glycoproteins. We search for articles published from 1985 on and in English, broadening the search by extending the year span and accepting publications in other languages only when several initial tries are fruitless or when we are researching an older drug. We restrict our searches to reports on human studies, because findings of animal studies are often not translatable to humans or are too preliminary to be useful clinically.

A "great" search, one that is broad enough in scope without being too large for adequate review, should provide the searcher with 20–35 titles. If a searcher retrieves 5–10 and they are exactly what was sought, that result is exceptional and a time-saver. We start with all the aforementioned terms, and if not enough titles are retrieved, we eliminate a term at a time, typically dropping *cytochrome* first, because few older reports include this word in the title or abstract. Expanding the range of years searched is necessary in the case of some older drugs, such as phenytoin, phenobarbital, and many oncology agents. Literature published before 1980 does not directly reflect an understanding of the P450 system, and the searcher may be left making a few leaps and assumptions. In summary, we like to perform a narrow search first. Beginning with a search that is too broad means wading through many titles, usually more than 35. Reading through titles and abstracts that may not be needed takes time.

■ CRITICALLY REVIEWING THE LITERATURE

Case Reports

Individual cases are often the first clue to a potential drug interaction and were particularly so in the days before human liver microsome studies. Although controls are not involved and confounding variables exist, cases have great merit, especially if they occur with enough frequency to lead to further study, as occurred with terfenadine. A strong case report includes information on pre- and post-administration serum levels of drugs, with corresponding clinical effects. Too often, serum levels are missing from case reports. We find it helpful to routinely monitor serum levels of drugs with toxic metabolites or narrow therapeutic windows, especially before administering a new drug with potential interactions, and to obtain another measurement of levels (at the appropriate time) if a drug interaction is suspected. These data greatly strengthen a case report's credibility. Presentation of a finding of a serum level exceeding clinical standards after administration of a second drug, associated with a significant clinical event, is also common in a strong case report. Monahan et al. (1990), Katial et al. (1998), and Armstrong and Schweitzer (1997) have written excellent case reports.

Reports of In Vitro Studies

In the United States, drugs must now be tested for P450-mediated interactions in the laboratory. This testing is done with human liver microsome studies, which permit thorough evaluation of the metabolisms of drugs at the level of the hepatocyte and determine which enzymes will be studied and probed in healthy volunteers and patient volunteers. Human liver samples are centrifuged, and microsomes are then incubated with the cofactors and enzymes needed for reactions to complete, as well as with test drugs or probe drugs. After completion of the reactions, high-performance liquid chromatography is used for detection of drug or metabolite concentrations. Numerous drugs can be tested by these methods, quickly and without need for subjecting volunteers to drug effects. Zhao et al. (1999) conducted an excellent human liver microsome study. More recently, *Escherichia coli* have been used to manufacture recombinant human enzymes, thus fully automating in vitro assays. In this new manner, individual enzymes can be tested with drugs in the laboratory (McGinnity and Riley 2001). Human liver microsome studies and recombinant enzyme studies sometimes provide data that do not translate to clinical populations. This lack of clinical correlation is multifactorial and includes differences in culture concentrations and conditions compared with in vivo conditions (Venkatakrishnan et al. 2001).

Reports of In Vivo Studies

Studies involving human volunteers are the gold standard. Studies involving healthy volunteers are usually small ($n \leq 8$–15), randomized, placebo-controlled studies, sometimes crossover in design. These studies are helpful in testing drug interactions predicted by in vitro studies. The small size of these studies, the frequent use of the single-dose design, and the use of healthy volunteers may limit their generalizability to the general population. Studies involving actual patients, whose ages, diseases, and drug histories vary widely, are some of the strongest studies, particularly if confounding variables are well controlled. Drug concentration, area under the curve, and maximal drug concentration are typically measured in these studies. When these parameters as well as pharmacodynamic effect (e.g., psychomotor effects in studies of hypnotics) are studied, the clinical information gleaned can be very helpful. Villikka et al. (1997) conducted an in vivo study with pharmacodynamic correlation. Hesslinger et al. (1999) studied potential drug interactions in psychiatrically ill patients receiving multiple agents.

Review Articles

Review articles are necessary compilations of primary research reports. Reviews allow the sorting and evaluating of research necessary to understand a topic as a whole. These articles help introduce readers to an area of research and provide another viewpoint. A drawback of most reviews is the loss of specific data or of finer arguments and points within individual reports. Many reviews cover only a few drugs or a portion of the P450 system, so several reviews are necessary to compile a full picture. We recommend that reviews be used as guideposts in making clinical decisions. We postpone making final clinical decisions in critical cases until we have examined some of the more specific reports cited by the reviewers themselves or found in our own literature searches.

Jefferson and Greist (1996) wrote an excellent introduction to the P450 system. Tseng and Foisy (1997) provided tables and text, clearly and with good references, to guide the reader through a complicated area of medicine. Other good reviews include a review by Tredger and Stoll (2002) and a series of reviews for child psychiatrists by Oesterheld and Shader (1998) and Flockhart and Oesterheld (2000). Finch et al. (2002) provided a thorough review of rifampin and its metabolism, especially its induction of most metabolic enzymes. These authors included reviews and discussion of case reports, in vitro and in vivo data, and P-glycoproteins across many drug classes.

Epidemiological Reports

Population studies help guide the need for drug-interaction research. Jankel and Fitterman (1993) and Hamilton et al. (1998) provided the big-picture reasoning for drug-interaction study. Jankel and Fitterman (1993) found that 3% of hospitalizations each year are due to drug-drug interactions. Hamilton and colleagues (1998) confirmed that use of azole antifungals and rifamycins increases the risk of hospitalization because of these drugs' significant P450-mediated drug interactions.

Manufacturer Package Inserts

Manufacturers are important sources of information about their products. *Physicians' Desk Reference* (2002) contains the texts of the package inserts of all drugs marketed in the United States and is also available on-line at PDR.net. Most newer drugs have discrete sections in the manufacturer's insert pertaining to their P450-mediated interactions. We have on many occasions called a manufacturer to obtain postmarketing or not-yet published information about its drugs. Discussions with manufacturers' doctorate-level professionals are generally rewarding and informational.

■ SUMMARY

A thorough review of the literature concerning a particular drug interaction usually involves reading the package insert and then a few review articles, followed by taking a more focused look at in vitro and in vivo data. All these research tools are necessary to develop a full understanding of the data available on any drug interaction. Because there are no perfect sources, a compilation similar to this Concise Guide is what each provider should develop about his or her own frequently prescribed drugs.

■ REFERENCES

Armstrong SC, Cozza KL: Consultation-liaison drug-drug interaction update. Psychosomatics 41:155–156, 2000

Armstrong SC, Schweitzer SM: Delirium associated with paroxetine and benztropine combination (letter). Am J Psychiatry 154:581–582, 1997

Finch CK, Chrisman CR, Baciewicz AM, et al: Rifampin and rifabutin drug interactions: an update. Arch Intern Med 162:985–992, 2002

Flockhart DA, Oesterheld JR: Cytochrome P450-mediated drug interactions. Child Adolesc Psychiatr Clin N Am 9:43–76, 2000

Hamilton RA, Briceland LL, Andritz MH: Frequency of hospitalization after exposure to known drug-drug interactions in a Medicaid population. Pharmacotherapy 18:1112–1120, 1998

Hesslinger B, Normann C, Langosch JM, et al: Effects of carbamazepine and valproate on haloperidol plasma levels and on psychopathologic outcome in schizophrenic patients. J Clin Psychopharmacol 19:310–315, 1999

Jankel CA, Fitterman LK: Epidemiology of drug-drug interactions as a cause of hospital admissions. Drug Saf 9:51–55, 1993

Jefferson JW, Greist JH: Brussels sprouts and psychopharmacology: understanding the cytochrome P450 enzyme system. Psychiatr Clin North Am 3:205–222, 1996

Katial RK, Stelzle RC, Bonner MW, et al: A drug interaction between zafirlukast and theophylline. Arch Intern Med 158:1713–1715, 1998

McGinnity DF, Riley RJ: Predicting drug pharmacokinetics in humans from in vitro metabolism studies. Biochem Soc Trans 29:135–139, 2001

Monahan BP, Ferguson CL, Killeavy ES, et al: Torsades de pointes occurring in association with terfenadine use. JAMA 264:2788–2790, 1990

Oesterheld JR, Shader RI: Cytochromes: a primer for child psychiatrists. J Am Acad Child Adolesc Psychiatry 37:447–450, 1998

Physicians' Desk Reference, 56th Edition. Montvale, NJ, Medical Economics, 2002

Tredger JM, Stoll S: Cytochrome P450—their impact on drug treatment. Hospital Pharmacist 9:167–173, 2002

Tseng AL, Foisy MM: Management of drug interactions in patients with HIV. Ann Pharmacother 31:1040–1058, 1997

Venkatakrishnan K, von Moltke LL, Greenblatt DJ: Human drug metabolism and the cytochromes P450: application and relevance of in vitro models. J Clin Pharmacol 41:1149–1179, 2001

Villikka K, Kivisto KT, Luurila H, et al: Rifampin reduces plasma concentrations and effects of zolpidem. Clin Pharmacol Ther 62:629–634, 1997

Zhao XJ, Koyama E, Ishizaki T: An in vitro study on the metabolism and possible drug interactions of rokitamycin, a macrolide antibiotic, using human liver microsomes. Drug Metab Dispos 27:776–785, 1999

Appendix

TRADE AND GENERIC DRUG NAMES USED IN THIS BOOK

■ DRUGS LISTED BY TRADE NAME

Trade name	Generic name	Trade name	Generic name
Accolate	zafirlukast	Anturane	sulfinpyrazone
Aciphex	rabeprazole	Aptin	alprenolol
Actos	pioglitazone	Aralen	chloroquine
Adalat	nifedipine	Aricept	donepezil
Adriamycin	doxorubicin	Arimidex	anastrozole
Agenerase	amprenavir	Arkin	vesnarinone
Aldactone	spironolactone	Atarax	hydroxyzine
Aldesleukin	interleukin-2	Ativan	lorazepam
Aldomet	methyldopa	Atromid-S	clofibrate
Alfenta	alfentanil	Aurorix	moclobemide
Allegra	fexofenadine	Avandia	rosiglitazone
Aller-Chlor	chlorpheniramine	Avapro	irbesartan
Amaryl	glimepride	Avelox	moxifloxacin
Ambien	zolpidem	Aventyl	nortriptyline
Amdray	valspodar	Avlosulfin	dapsone
Amerge	naratriptan	Axert	amiotriptan
Amoxil	amoxicillin	Axid	nizatidine
Anafranil	clomipramine	Aygestin	norethindrone
Ansaid	flurbiprofen	Baratol	indoramin
Antabuse	disulfiram	Baycol	cerivastatin

■ DRUGS LISTED BY TRADE NAME *(continued)*

Trade name	Generic name	Trade name	Generic name
Belustine	lomustine	Celexa	citalopram
Benadryl	diphenhydramine	CellCept	mycophenolate mofetil
Benecid	probenecid	Celontin	methsuximide
Benylin	dextromethorphan	Cerubidine	daunorubicin
Bextra	valdecoxib	Chibroxin	norfloxacin
Biaxin	clarithromycin	Chlo-Amine	chlorpheniramine
BiCNU	carmustine	Chloromycetin	chloramphenicol
Blocarden	timolol	Chlor-Trimeton	chlorpheniramine
Bolvidon	mianserin	Cipro	ciprofloxacin
Buprenex	buprenorphine	Claritin	loratadine
BuSpar	buspirone	Clinoril	sulindac
Butazolidin	phenylbutazone	Clozaril	clozapine
Calan	verapamil	Cogentin	benztropine
Camptosar	irinotecan	Cognex	tacrine
Cantor	minaprine	Comtan	entacapone
Carbatrol	carbamazepine	Concerta	methylphenidate
Cardene	nicardipine	Cordarone	amiodarone
Cardizem	diltiazem	Coreg	carvedilol
Ceclor	cefaclor	Coumadin	warfarin
Celebrex	celecoxib	Coumarin	coumadin

DRUGS LISTED BY TRADE NAME (continued)

Trade name	Generic name	Trade name	Generic name
Covera	verapamil	Dilacor XR	diltiazem
Cozaar	losartan	Dilantin	phenytoin
Crixivan	indinavir	Dilaudid	hydromorphone
Cytadren	aminoglutethimide	Diltia XT	diltiazem
Cytoxan	cyclophosphamide	Diovan	valsartan
Darvon	propoxyphene	Diprivan	propofol
DaunoXome	daunorubicin	Disalcid	salsalate
Daypro	oxaprozin	Dolobid	diflunasil
Decadron	dexamethasone	Dolophine	methadone
Delsym	dextromethorphan	Dopar	L-dopa
Deltasone	prednisone	Doxil	doxorubicin
Demadex	torsemide	DTIC-Dome	dacarbazine
Demerol	meperidine	Duragesic	fentanyl
Depakene	valproic acid	Dynabac	dirithromycin
Depo-Provera	medroxyprogesterone	DynaCirc	isradipine
Deprenyl	selegiline	Ebastel	ebastine
Desyrel	trazodone	Ecotrin	aspirin
DiaBeta	glyburide	Effexor	venlafaxine
Diflucan	fluconazole	Efudex	fluorouracil
Digibind	digitoxin	Elavil	amitriptyline

■ DRUGS LISTED BY TRADE NAME *(continued)*

Trade name	Generic name	Trade name	Generic name
Eldepryl	selegiline	Feldene	piroxicam
Eldisine	vindesine	Fentanyl Oralet	fentanyl
Ellence	epirubicin	Fepron	fenoprofen
Emfib	gemfibrozil	Flagyl	metronidazole
Empirin	aspirin	Flexeril	cyclobenzaprine
E-mycin	erythromycin	Floxin	ofloxacin
Endep	amitriptyline	Fluoroplex	fluorouracil
Enkaid	encainide	Fluothane	halothane
Epivir	lamivudine	Forane	isoflurane
Equanil	meprobamate	Fortovase	saquinavir
Eskalith	lithium	Frova	frovatriptan
Estinyl	ethinyl estradiol	Fulvicin	griseofulvin
Estrace	estradiol	Gabitril	tiagabine
Ethmozine	moricizine	Geodon	ziprasidone
Ethrane	enflurane	Gliadel	carmustine
Eulexin	flutamide	Glucotrol	glipizide
Evipal	hexobarbital	Grifulvin	griseofulvin
Exelon	rivastigmine	Halcion	triazolam
Fareston	toremifene	Haldol	haloperidol
Felbatol	felbamate	Halfan	halofantrine

■ DRUGS LISTED BY TRADE NAME (continued)

Trade name	Generic name	Trade name	Generic name
Hismanal	astemizole	Lanoxin	digoxin
Hivid	zalcitabine	Lasix	furosemide
Ifex	ifosfamide	Lescol	fluvastatin
Imitrex	sumatriptan	Levaquin	levofloxacin
Imodium	loperamide	Lexapro	S-citalopram
Imovane	zopiclone	Liazal	liarozole
Imuran	azathioprine	Librium	chlordiazepoxide
Inderal	propranolol	Lipitor	atorvastatin
Indocin	indomethacin	Lithobid	lithium
INH	isoniazid	Lomotil	diphenoxylate
Intron A	interferon-α_{2b}	Lopressor	metoprolol
Ismelin	guanethidine	Loxitane	loxapine
Isoptin	verapamil	Ludiomil	maprotiline
Ixoten	trofosfamide	Luvox	fluvoxamine
Kaletra	lopinavir/ritonavir	Malarone	atovaquone/proguanil
Keppra	levetiracetam	Maxalt	rizatriptan
Ketek	telithromycin	Manerix	moclobemide
Klonopin	clonazepam	Marinol	tetrahydrocannabinol
Lamictal	lamotrigine	Maxaquin	lomefloxacin
Lamisil	terbinafine	Mebaral	mephobarbital

■ DRUGS LISTED BY TRADE NAME (continued)

Trade name	Generic name	Trade name	Generic name
Meclomen	meclofenamate	Motrin	ibuprofen
Medrol	methylprednisolone	MSIR	morphine
Medrone	methylprednisolone	Mucomyst	acetylcysteine
Mellaril	thioridazine	Mycobutin	rifabutin
Meprospan	meprobamate	Myleran	busulfan
Meridia	sibutramine	Mysoline	primidone
Methylin	methylphenidate	Nalline	nalorphine
Metoflane	methoxyflurane	Naprosyn	naproxen
Mevacor	lovastatin	Narcan	naloxone
Mexitil	mexiletine	Naropin	ropivacaine
Micronase	glyburide	Navane	thiothixene
Micronor	norethindrone	Navelbine	vinorelbine
Miltown	meprobamate	NegGram	naladixic acid
Minipress	prazosin	Nembutal	pentobarbital
Mirapex	pramipexole	Neoral	cyclosporine
Moban	molindone	Neosar	cyclophosphamide
Mobic	meloxicam	Neurontin	gabapentin
Modalim	ciprofibrate	Nexium	esomeprazole
Mogadon	nitrazepam	Nidrel	nitrendipine
Monistat	miconazole	Nimotop	nimodipine

DRUGS LISTED BY TRADE NAME *(continued)*

Trade name	Generic name	Trade name	Generic name
Nizoral	ketoconazole	Orthoclone OKT3	muromonab-CD3
Nolvadex	tamoxifen	Orudis	ketoprofen
Norcuron	vecuronium	Ovrette	norgestrel
Norebox	reboxetine	Oxsoralen	methoxsalen
Norflex	orphenadrine	OxyContin	oxycodone
Noroxin	norfloxacin	Paludrine	proguanil
Norpramin	desipramine	Pamelor	nortriptyline
Norval	mianserin	Paraflex	chlorzoxazone
Norvasc	amlodipine	Parafon Forte DSC	chlorzoxazone
Norvir	ritonavir	Parlodel	bromocriptine
Novantrone	mitoxantrone	Parnate	tranylcypromine
Novocain	procaine	Pavulon	pancuronium
Nubain	nalbuphine	Paxil	paroxetine
Numorphine	oxymorphine	Peflox	pefloxacin
Oleoresin	capsaicin	Penetrex	enoxacin
Oncovin	vincristine	Pepcid	famotidine
Orap	pimozide	Periactin	cyproheptadine
Orapred	prednisolone	Permax	pergolide
Orinase	tolbutamide	Phenergan	promethazine
Orlaam	levomethadyl	Phenob	phenobarbital

435

■ **DRUGS LISTED BY TRADE NAME** *(continued)*

Trade name	Generic name	Trade name	Generic name
Plan B	levonorgestrel	Prolixin	fluphenazine
Plaquenil	hydroxychloroquine	Prometrium	progesterone
Platinol	cisplatin	Pronestyl	procainamide
Plavix	clopidogrel	Propulsid	cisapride
Plendil	felodipine	ProSom	estazolam
Pletal	cilostazol	Protonix	pantoprazole
Ponstel	mefenamic acid	Provigil	modafinil
Posicor	mibefradil	Prozac	fluoxetine
Pravachol	pravastatin	Purinethol	6-mercaptopurine
Prelone	prednisolone	Quinaglute	quinidine
Prevacid	lansoprazole	Quinidex	quinidine
Preveon	adefovir	Rapamune	sirolimus
Priftin	rifapentine	Raxar	grepafloxacin
Prilosec	omeprazole	Redux	dexfenfluramine
Primaquine	primaquine	Reglan	metoclopramide
Procanbid	procainamide	Relefan	nabumetone
Procardia	nifedipine	Relpax	eletriptan
Profenal	suprofen	Remeron	mirtazapine
Prograf	tacrolimus	Reminyl	galantamine
Proleukin	interleukin-2	Requip	ropinirole

■ DRUGS LISTED BY TRADE NAME *(continued)*

Trade name	Generic name	Trade name	Generic name
Rescriptor	delavirdine	Sandimmune	cyclosporine
Restoril	temazepam	SangCya	cyclosporine
Retrovir	zidovudine	Sarafem	fluoxetine
ReVia	naltrexone	Seconal	secobarbital
Rezulin	troglitazone	Seldane	terfenadine
Rheumatrex	methotrexate	Serax	oxazepam
Ricamycin	rokitamycin	Serentil	mesoridazine
Rifadin	rifampin	Seroquel	quetiapine
Rilutek	riluzole	Serzone	nefazodone
Rimactane	rifampin	Sevorane	sevoflurane
Risperdal	risperidone	Sinemet	carbidopa/levodopa
Ritalin	methylphenidate	Sinequan	doxepin
Rivizor	vorozole	Singulair	montelukast
Rohypnol	flunitrazepam	Slo-bid	theophylline
Romazicon	flumazenil	Slo-phyllin	theophylline
Roxicodone	oxycodone	Sonata	zaleplon
Rubex	doxorubicin	Sporanox	itraconazole
Rythmol	propafenone	Stelazine	trifluoperazine
Sabril	vigabatrin	Sterapred	prednisone
Salacid	salicylic acid	Subutex	norbuprenorphine

■ DRUGS LISTED BY TRADE NAME *(continued)*

Trade name	Generic name	Trade name	Generic name
Sufenta	sufentanil	Theolair	theophylline
Sular	nisoldipine	Thorazine	chlorpromazine
Sulfazole	sulfaphenazole	Tiazac	diltiazem
Surmontil	trimipramine	Ticlid	ticlopidine
Sustiva	efavirenz	Tofranil	imipramine
Symmetrel	amantadine	Tolectin	tolmetin
Synercid	quinupristin/dalfopristin	Tolvin	mianserin
Tagamet	cimetidine	Tonocard	tocainide
Tambocor	flecainide	Topamax	topiramate
Tao	troleandomycin	Toposar	etoposide
Tasmar	tolcapone	Toprol XL	metoprolol
Taxol	paclitaxel	Toradol	ketorolac
Taxotere	docetaxel	Trandate	labetolol
Tedolan	etodolac	Trental	pentoxifylline
Tegretol	carbamazepine	Trilafon	perphenazine
Tequin	gatifloxacin	Trileptal	oxcarbazepine
Teslac	testololactone	Trovan	trovafloxacin
Tespamine	thiotepa	Tylenol	acetaminophen
Theo-24	theophylline	Ultiva	remifentanil
Theo-Dur	theophylline	Ultram	tramadol

■ DRUGS LISTED BY TRADE NAME *(continued)*

Trade name	Generic name	Trade name	Generic name
Uniphyl	theophylline	Wellbutrin	bupropion
Valium	diazepam	Xanax	alprazolam
Vancocin	vancomycin	Xylocaine	lidocaine
Velban	vinblastine	Yocon	yohimbine
VePesid	etoposide	Yohimex	yohimbine
Verelan	verapamil	Zaditen	ketotifen
Versed	midazolam	Zagam	sparfloxacin
Vesanoid	tretinoin	Zanosar	streptozocin
Vesprin	triflupromazine	Zantac	ranitidine
Viagra	sildenafil	Zarontin	ethosuximide
Vicodin	hydrocodone	Zerit	stavudine
Videx	didanosine	Ziagen	abacavir
Vioxx	rofecoxib	Zithromax	azithromycin
Viracept	nelfinavir	Zocor	simvastatin
Viramune	nevirapine	Zofran	ondansetron
Vistaril	hydroxyzine	Zoloft	sertraline
Vistide	cidofovir	Zomig	zolmitriptan
Vivactil	protriptyline	Zonegran	zonisamide
Voltaren	diclofenac	Zyban	bupropion
Vumon	teniposide	Zyprexa	olanzapine
		Zyrtec	cetirizine

■ DRUGS LISTED BY GENERIC, OR NONPROPRIETARY, NAME

Generic name	Trade name	Generic name	Trade name
abacavir	Ziagen	azathioprine	Imuran
acetaminophen	Tylenol	azithromycin	Zithromax
acetylcysteine	Mucomyst	benztropine	Cogentin
adefovir	Preveon	bromocriptine	Parlodel
alfentanil	Alfenta	buprenorphine	Buprenex
alprazolam	Xanax	bupropion	Wellbutrin, Zyban
alprenolol	Aptin	buspirone	BuSpar
amantadine	Symmetrel	busulfan	Myleran
aminoglutethimide	Cytadren	capsaicin	Oleoresin
amiodarone	Cordarone	carbamazepine	Carbatrol, Tegretol
amiotriptan	Axert	carbidopa/levodopa	Sinemet
amitriptyline	Elavil, Endep	carmustine	BiCNU, Gliadel
amlodipine	Norvasc	carvedilol	Coreg
amoxicillin	Amoxil	cefaclor	Ceclor
amprenavir	Agenerase	celecoxib	Celebrex
anastrozole	Arimidex	cerivastatin	Baycol
aspirin	Ecotrin, Empirin	cetirizine	Zyrtec
astemizole	Hismanal	chloramphenicol	Chloromycetin
atorvastatin	Lipitor	chlordiazepoxide	Librium
atovaquone/proguanil	Malarone	chloroquine	Aralen

■ DRUGS LISTED BY GENERIC, OR NONPROPRIETARY, NAME *(continued)*

Generic name	Trade name	Generic name	Trade name
chlorpheniramine	Aller-Chlor, Chlo-Amine, Chlor-Trimeton	coumadin	Coumarin
		cyclobenzaprine	Flexeril
chlorpromazine	Thorazine	cyclophosphamide	Cytoxan, Neosar
chlorzoxazone	Paraflex, Parafon Forte DSC	cyclosporine	Neoral, Sandimmune, SangCya
cidofovir	Vistide	cyproheptadine	Periactin
cilostazol	Pletal	dacarbazine	DTIC-Dome
cimetidine	Tagamet	dapsone	Avlosulfin
ciprofibrate	Modalim	daunorubicin	Cerubidine, DaunoXome
ciprofloxacin	Cipro	delavirdine	Rescriptor
cisapride	Propulsid	desipramine	Norpramin
cisplatin	Platinol	dexamethasone	Decadron
citalopram	Celexa	dexfenfluramine	Redux
S-citalopram	Lexapro	dextromethorphan	Benylin, Delsym
clarithromycin	Biaxin	diazepam	Valium
clofibrate	Atromid-S	diclofenac	Voltaren
clomipramine	Anafranil	didanosine	Videx
clonazepam	Klonopin	diflunasil	Dolobid
clopidogrel	Plavix	digitoxin	Digibind
clozapine	Clozaril	digoxin	Lanoxin

■ DRUGS LISTED BY GENERIC, OR NONPROPRIETARY, NAME *(continued)*

Generic name	Trade name	Generic name	Trade name
diltiazem	Cardizem, Dilacor XR, Diltia XT, Tiazac	esomeprazole	Nexium
		estazolam	ProSom
diphenhydramine	Benadryl	estradiol	Estrace
diphenoxylate	Lomotil	ethinyl estradiol	Estinyl
dirithromycin	Dynabac	ethosuximide	Zarontin
disulfiram	Antabuse	etodolac	Tedolan
docetaxel	Taxotere	etoposide	Toposar, VePesid
donepezil	Aricept	famotidine	Pepcid
L-dopa	Dopar	felbamate	Felbatol
doxepin	Sinequan	felodipine	Plendil
doxorubicin	Adriamycin, Doxil, Rubex	fenoprofen	Fepron
ebastine	Ebastel	fentanyl	Duragesic, Fentanyl Oralet
efavirenz	Sustiva	fexofenadine	Allegra
eletriptan	Relpax	flecainide	Tambocor
encainide	Enkaid	fluconazole	Diflucan
enflurane	Ethrane	flumazenil	Romazicon
enoxacin	Penetrex	flunitrazepam	Rohypnol
entacapone	Comtan	fluorouracil	Efudex, Fluoroplex
epirubicin	Ellence	fluoxetine	Prozac, Sarafem
erythromycin	E-mycin	fluphenazine	Prolixin

■ DRUGS LISTED BY GENERIC, OR NONPROPRIETARY, NAME *(continued)*

Generic name	Trade name	Generic name	Trade name
flurbiprofen	Ansaid	hydrocodone	Vicodin
flutamide	Eulexin	hydromorphone	Dilaudid
fluvastatin	Lescol	hydroxychloroquine	Plaquenil
fluvoxamine	Luvox	hydroxyzine	Atarax, Vistaril
frovatriptan	Frova	ibuprofen	Motrin
furosemide	Lasix	ifosfamide	Ifex
gabapentin	Neurontin	imipramine	Tofranil
galantamine	Reminyl	indinavir	Crixivan
gatifloxacin	Tequin	indomethacin	Indocin
gemfibrozil	Emfib	indoramin	Baratol
glimepiride	Amaryl	interferon-α_{2b}	Intron A
glipizide	Glucotrol	interleukin-2	Aldesleukin, Proleukin
glyburide	DiaBeta, Micronase	irbesartan	Avapro
grepafloxacin	Raxar	irinotecan	Camptosar
griseofulvin	Fulvicin, Grifulvin	isoflurane	Forane
guanethidine	Ismelin	isoniazid	INH
halofantrine	Halfan	isradipine	DynaCirc
haloperidol	Haldol	itraconazole	Sporanox
halothane	Fluothane	ketoconazole	Nizoral
hexobarbital	Evipal	ketoprofen	Orudis

■ DRUGS LISTED BY GENERIC, OR NONPROPRIETARY, NAME *(continued)*

Generic name	Trade name	Generic name	Trade name
ketorolac	Toradol	lovastatin	Mevacor
ketotifen	Zaditen	loxapine	Loxitane
labetolol	Trandate	maprotiline	Ludiomil
lamivudine	Epivir	meclofenamate	Meclomen
lamotrigine	Lamictal	medroxyprogesterone	Depo-Provera
lansoprazole	Prevacid	mefenamic acid	Ponstel
levetiracetam	Keppra	meloxicam	Mobic
levofloxacin	Levaquin	meperidine	Demerol
levomethadyl	Orlaam	mephobarbital	Mebaral
levonorgestrel	Plan B	meprobamate	Equanil, Meprospan, Miltown
liarozole	Liazal	6-mercaptopurine	Purinethol
lidocaine	Xylocaine	mesoridazine	Serentil
lithium	Eskalith, Lithobid	methadone	Dolophine
lomefloxacin	Maxaquin	methotrexate	Rheumatrex
lomustine	Belustine	methoxyflurane	Metoflane
loperamide	Imodium	methoxysalen	Oxsoralen
lopinavir/ritonavir	Kaletra	methsuximide	Celontin
loratadine	Claritin	methyldopa	Aldomet
lorazepam	Ativan	methylphenidate	Concerta, Methylin, Ritalin
losartan	Cozaar	methylprednisolone	Medrol, Medrone

DRUGS LISTED BY GENERIC, OR NONPROPRIETARY, NAME *(continued)*

Generic name	Trade name	Generic name	Trade name
metoclopramide	Reglan	nabumetone	Relefan
metoprolol	Lopressor, Toprol XL	naladixic acid	NegGram
metronidazole	Flagyl	nalbuphine	Nubain
mexiletine	Mexitil	nalorphine	Nalline
mianserin	Bolvidon, Norval, Tolvin	naloxone	Narcan
mibefradil	Posicor	naltrexone	ReVia
miconazole	Monistat	naproxen	Naprosyn
midazolam	Versed	naratriptan	Amerge
minaprine	Cantor	nefazodone	Serzone
mirtazapine	Remeron	nelfinavir	Viracept
mitoxantrone	Novantrone	nevirapine	Viramune
moclobemide	Aurorix, Manerix	nicardipine	Cardene
modafinil	Provigil	nifedipine	Adalat, Procardia
molindone	Moban	nimodipine	Nimotop
montelukast	Singulair	nisoldipine	Sular
moricizine	Ethmozine	nitrazepam	Mogadon
morphine	MSIR	nitrendipine	Nidrel
moxifloxacin	Avelox	nizatidine	Axid
muromonab-CD3	Orthoclone OKT3	norbuprenorphine	Subutex
mycophenolate mofetil	CellCept	norethindrone	Aygestin, Micronor

■ DRUGS LISTED BY GENERIC, OR NONPROPRIETARY, NAME (continued)

Generic name	Trade name	Generic name	Trade name
norfloxacin	Chibroxin, Noroxin	pergolide	Permax
norgestrel	Ovrette	perphenazine	Trilafon
nortriptyline	Aventyl, Pamelor	phenobarbital	Phenob
ofloxacin	Floxin	phenylbutazone	Butazolidin
olanzapine	Zyprexa	phenytoin	Dilantin
omeprazole	Prilosec	pimozide	Orap
ondansetron	Zofran	pioglitazone	Actos
orphenadrine	Norflex	piroxicam	Feldene
oxaprozin	Daypro	pramipexole	Mirapex
oxazepam	Serax	prazosin	Minipress
oxcarbazepine	Trileptal	pravastatin	Pravachol
oxycodone	OxyContin, Roxicodone	prednisolone	Orapred, Prelone
oxymorphine	Numorphine	prednisone	Deltasone, Sterapred
paclitaxel	Taxol	primaquine	Primaquine
pancuronium	Pavulon	primidone	Mysoline
pantoprazole	Protonix	probenecid	Benecid
paroxetine	Paxil	procainamide	Procanbid, Pronestyl
pefloxacin	Peflox	procaine	Novocain
pentobarbital	Nembutal	progesterone	Prometrium
pentoxifylline	Trental	proguanil	Paludrine

■ DRUGS LISTED BY GENERIC, OR NONPROPRIETARY, NAME *(continued)*

Generic name	Trade name	Generic name	Trade name
promethazine	Phenergan	rizatriptan	Maxalt
propafenone	Rythmol	rofecoxib	Vioxx
propofol	Diprivan	rokitamycin	Ricamycin
propoxyphene	Darvon	ropinirole	Requip
propranolol	Inderal	ropivacaine	Naropin
protriptyline	Vivactil	rosiglitazone	Avandia
quetiapine	Seroquel	salicylic acid	Salacid
quinidine	Quinaglute, Quinidex	salsalate	Disalcid
quinupristin/dalfopristin	Synercid	saquinavir	Fortovase
rabeprazole	Aciphex	secobarbital	Seconal
ranitidine	Zantac	selegiline	Deprenyl, Eldepryl
reboxetine	Norebox	sertraline	Zoloft
remifentanil	Ultiva	sevoflurane	Sevorane
rifabutin	Mycobutin	sibutramine	Meridia
rifampin	Rifadin, Rimactane	sildenafil	Viagra
rifapentine	Priftin	simvastatin	Zocor
riluzole	Rilutek	sirolimus	Rapamune
risperidone	Risperdal	sparfloxacin	Zagam
ritonavir	Norvir	spironolactone	Aldactone
rivastigmine	Exelon	stavudine	Zerit

■ DRUGS LISTED BY GENERIC, OR NONPROPRIETARY, NAME (continued)

Generic name	Trade name	Generic name	Trade name
streptozocin	Zanosar	thiotepa	Tespamine
sufentanil	Sufenta	thiothixene	Navane
sulfaphenazole	Sulfazole	tiagabine	Gabitril
sulfinpyrazone	Anturane	ticlopidine	Ticlid
sulindac	Clinoril	timolol	Blocarden
sumatriptan	Imitrex	tocainide	Tonocard
suprofen	Profenal	tolbutamide	Orinase
tacrine	Cognex	tolcapone	Tasmar
tacrolimus	Prograf	tolmetin	Tolectin
tamoxifen	Nolvadex	topiramate	Topamax
telithromycin	Ketek	toremifene	Fareston
temazepam	Restoril	torsemide	Demadex
teniposide	Vumon	tramadol	Ultram
terbinafine	Lamisil	tranylcypromine	Parnate
terfenadine	Seldane	trazodone	Desyrel
testololactone	Teslac	tretinoin	Vesanoid
tetrahydrocannabinol	Marinol	triazolam	Halcion
theophylline	Slo-bid, Slo-phyllin, Theo-24, Theo-Dur, Theolair, Uniphyl	trifluoperazine	Stelazine
		triflupromazine	Vesprin
thioridazine	Mellaril	trimipramine	Surmontil

DRUGS LISTED BY GENERIC, OR NONPROPRIETARY, NAME *(continued)*

Generic name	Trade name	Generic name	Trade name
trofosfamide	Ixoten	vincristine	Oncovin
troglitazone	Rezulin	vindesine	Eldisine
troleandomycin	Tao	vinorelbine	Navelbine
trovafloxacin	Trovan	vorozole	Rivizor
valdecoxib	Bextra	warfarin	Coumadin
valproic acid	Depakene	yohimbine	Yocon, Yohimex
valsartan	Diovan	zafirlukast	Accolate
valspodar	Amdray	zalcitabine	Hivid
vancomycin	Vancocin	zaleplon	Sonata
vecuronium	Norcuron	zidovudine	Retrovir
venlafaxine	Effexor	ziprasidone	Geodon
verapamil	Calan, Covera, Isoptin, Verelan	zolmitriptan	Zomig
vesnarinone	Arkin	zolpidem	Ambien
vigabatrin	Sabril	zonisamide	Zonegran
vinblastine	Velban	zopiclone	Imovane

INDEX

*Page numbers printed in **boldface** type refer to tables or figures.*

452